MOLECULAR STRUCTURE AND FUNCTION OF FOOD CARBOHYDRATE

An industry–university co-operation Symposium organised under the auspices of the National College of Food Technology, University of Reading, on 10*th and* 11*th April,* 1973

THE SYMPOSIUM COMMITTEE

GORDON G. BIRCH, B.Sc., Ph.D., F.R.I.C., M.R.S.H., F.C.S.
Lecturer at National College of Food Technology,
Reading University, Weybridge, Surrey.

LESLIE F. GREEN, B.Sc., A.R.I.C., F.C.S., F.I.F.S.T.
Applied Projects Manager, Beecham Products,
Randalls Road, Leatherhead, Surrey.

H. VIZARD ROBINSON, A.C.I.S.
Secretary at National College of Food Technology,
Reading University, Weybridge, Surrey.

MOLECULAR STRUCTURE AND FUNCTION OF FOOD CARBOHYDRATE

Edited by

G. G. BIRCH and L. F. GREEN

A HALSTED PRESS BOOK

JOHN WILEY & SONS
NEW YORK — TORONTO

PUBLISHED IN THE U.S.A. AND CANADA BY
HALSTED PRESS
A DIVISION OF JOHN WILEY & SONS, INC., NEW YORK

Library of Congress Cataloging in Publication Data

Main entry under title:

Molecular structure and function of food carbohydrate.

"A Halsted Press book."

"An industry–university co-operation symposium organised under the auspices of the National College of Food Technology . . . on 10th and 11th April, 1973."

1. Carbohydrates—Congresses. 2. Food—Congresses. I. Birch, Gordon Gerard, ed. II. Green, Leslie Frank, ed. III. National College of Food Technology.

[DNLM: 1. Carbohydrates—Congresses. QU75 M718 1973]

TX553.C28M64 547'.78 73-16299

ISBN 0-470-07323-3

WITH 30 TABLES AND 82 ILLUSTRATIONS

Printed in Great Britain by Galliard (Printers) Ltd Great Yarmouth

List of Contributors

W. BANKS
Flour Milling and Baking Research Association, Chorleywood, Herts., England.

J. E. G. BARNETT
Department of Physiology and Biochemistry, University of Southampton, Southampton, England.

G. G. BIRCH
National College of Food Technology, University of Reading, Weybridge, Surrey, England.

J. G. BRENNAN
National College of Food Technology, University of Reading, Weybridge, Surrey, England.

J. D. BROOKE
Human Performance Laboratory, Salford University, Salford, Lancs., England.

R. A. M. DELANEY
Moorepark Research Centre, Agricultural Institute, Fermoy, Ireland.

J. K. DONNELLY
Moorepark Research Centre, Agricultural Institute, Fermoy, Ireland.

N. FISHER
Flour Milling and Baking Research Association, Chorleywood, Herts., England.

C. T. GREENWOOD
Flour Milling and Baking Research Association, Chorleywood, Herts., England.

YORAM HOUMINER
Department of Organic Chemistry, The Hebrew University, Jerusalem, Israel.

R. E. HUGHES
Department of Applied Biology, University of Wales Institute of Science and Technology, Cardiff, Wales.

R. KHAN
Philip Lyle Memorial Research Laboratory, Reading, Berkshire, England.

G. LISINSKA
Department of Food Technology and Storage of the Agricultural University in Wroclaw, Poland.

H. B. MCMICHAEL
Middlesex Hospital, London, England.

D. J. MCWEENY
Food Science Division, Ministry of Agriculture, Fisheries and Food, Norwich, Norfolk, England.

G. B. MADSEN
Novo Industrias, Copenhagen, Denmark.

E. R. MORRIS
Unilever Research, Unilever Limited, Colworth House, Sharnbrook, Beds., England.

D. D. MUIR
Flour Milling and Baking Research Association, Chorleywood, Herts., England.

B. E. NORMAN
Novo Industrias, Copenhagen, Denmark.

A. C. O'SULLIVAN
Moorepark Research Centre, Agricultural Institute, Fermoy, Ireland.

G. L. S. PAWAN
Metabolic Division, Department of Medicine, The Middlesex Hospital Medical School, London, England.

R. J. PRIESTLEY
National College of Food Technology, University of Reading, Weybridge, Surrey, England.

R. S. SHALLENBERGER
New York State Agricultural Experiment Station, Cornell University, Geneva, New York 14456, *USA.*

G. SODAH-AYERNOR
National College of Food Technology, University of Reading, Weybridge, Surrey, England.

DOUW G. STEYN
Emeritus Professor of Pharmacology, Medical Faculty, University of Pretoria, Republic of South Africa.

Contents

Opening Remarks

E. J. Rolfe

Principal, National College of Food Technology, University of Reading, Weybridge, Surrey, England

It has been shown in numerous cases when attempting to understand the complex chemical changes which occur in biological systems that it is not sufficient to be aware of the chemical formula for each of the substances involved, but also it is necessary to have information concerning the spatial configuration of the molecules. As a consequence, in a relatively few years molecular biology has become perhaps the most intensively studied area of biochemistry, and is applied to problems as varied as muscular contraction and the oxygenation of haemoglobin. Perutz has mapped the chain of amino acids that constitute haemoglobin. The apparent lack of symmetry in the tertiary folding pattern is striking—the polypeptide chain is coiled and convoluted about itself in an apparent haphazard arrangement. But it is clear that the folding of the molecule is not haphazard, and the correct primary sequence of amino acids is essential to ensure the correct pattern of the functional protein. Apparently trivial alterations or errors in the assembly of proteins can destroy their biochemical function and render them useless to the cell, *e.g.* the substitution of glutamic acid (normally present at position No. 6 in each of the β-chains) by valine in haemoglobin is sufficient to change the shape of the red blood cells into the abnormal form characteristic of sickle-cell anaemia.

Carbohydrates present us with a similar situation to the proteins, in that the former also form a series of complex three-dimensional molecules including polymers of high molecular weight. It is being found that in order to understand the properties of these molecules, not only in terms of chemical reactivity, but particularly physiological aspects (*e.g.* the ability to elicit a sweet taste) and physical properties, it is necessary to have regard to the configuration and structure of the molecules. If the relationship between structural characteristics and behaviour can be elucidated then it becomes possible to attempt modification of the molecules in a systematic fashion so that a new compound is obtained which satisfies more precisely the performance required. Present attempts in this direction are made largely by trial and error, but studies in progress (some of which are reported at this symposium) are moving towards providing information which will permit such developments on a logical and scientific basis.

The major areas of interest to which the relationship between the structure and behaviour of carbohydrates is presently relevant are:

1. nutrition including absorption and metabolism;
2. physiological properties;
3. technological applications to food processing and manufacture.

1. NUTRITION

In the 18th century, sugar was still a luxury and restricted to the rich man's table, but now the average intake of sucrose in Western countries is about 50 kg per annum and consumption in the UK is one of the highest. Glucose syrups are being used widely in manufactured foods and are introducing into our diet previously unfamiliar carbohydrates. No doubt other changes in our consumption of sugars will occur, *e.g.* it has been predicted that within a few years fructose will be of great commercial importance, for current developments in the use of enzymes attached to solid polymer reactors will make it possible to produce the sugar cheaply from wheat starch. The effects of such dramatic changes in our diet need to be and are being studied.

Diseases of teeth and their supporting structures are more widespread than any other disease, and include particularly chronic periodontitis and dental caries. Presently there is not a clear understanding of these two diseases but the dental plaque appears to be a factor common to both.[1] The plaque present in the natural erupted tooth consists of a closely packed mass of micro-organisms in a matrix of high branched dextrans. The bacteria produce the dextrans to deal with the problem of large quantities of fermentable carbohydrate and possibly also acid end products and to bind essential organic and inorganic nutrients which are present only in small quantities. A positive correlation between the degree of dental caries and the amount of sugar taken in solid foods in those who did not clean their teeth has been demonstrated.[2] The cariogenic nature of sucrose seems to be because it is a better precursor of dextran than any of the other dietary carbohydrates, and dextran is an especially good pabulum for the growth and activity of the cariogenic *Streptococcus acidophilus.* Heavy masticatory activity reduces interstitial stagnation sites of plaque adjacent to the tooth where attack occurs, and it appears therefore that the introduction of diets based on foods lacking in fibrous texture and containing greater amounts of fermentable carbohydrate is a principal factor in initiating these two dental diseases.

It has been reported that some sugars are more prone to induce body fat formation.[3] Adult male rats which had been fed for six months on diets containing sucrose, or more especially fructose, had more carcass fat than rats fed diets containing glucose syrup, dextrose or a standard laboratory diet. Baboons fed isocaloric diets achieved more abdominal fat on a high sucrose diet than on a high glucose syrup diet.

But more sinister is the implication of sucrose in ischaemic heart disease.[2] In rats, sucrose has been shown to produce an increase of plasma triglyceride. Males are much more susceptible to heart disease than females, and sucrose diets have been shown to produce higher levels of triglyceride in the fasting serum of men than of premenopausal women.[4,5] Baboons show a sex difference in the response of the serum total phospholipids to a sucrose diet.[6] Baboons were fed for 13 weeks on a diet containing 75% sucrose. In the fasting serum before the diet the level of phospholipids, male: female, was 1:2, but after the diet the level in the male fasting serum increased to the level of that of the female, which remained approximately constant. Evidence is accumulating to suggest that the activity of certain phospholipid fractions may play a part in platelet adhesiveness and possibly ischaemic heart disease. There is as yet no suggestion that the concentration of phospholipid in the serum is in any way a reflection of phospholipid activity. However, because of the possible connection between sucrose intake and ischaemic heart disease coupled with the overwhelming prevalence of the disease in men as opposed to premenopausal women of the same age, it has been suggested that the disease could be due to interrelated hormonal changes induced by sucrose.[2] Continued investigation is needed, particularly as other evidence has been produced which is said to refute the claim that sucrose in the diet is a major cause of coronary heart disease,[7] rather the total caloric intake and changes in body weight are more important than the type of dietary carbohydrate. From a consideration of available evidence it has been concluded that it does not significantly incriminate sugar in the causation of coronary heart disease.[8]

Relatively slight structural modifications can effect dramatically, for example, enzyme activity and active transport across the mucosal membrane of the small intestine and subsequent phosphorylation. Fructose in its transport into cells and reactions as far as triose phosphates is independent of insulin. This is in strong contrast to glucose and explains the usefulness of fructose in treatment of diabetes. However, insulin deficiency by allowing an increase in the activity of gluconeogenic enzymes unfortunately causes greater conversion of fructose to glucose and this imposes a limit on its use in diabetics who are severely insulin-deficient.

2. PHYSIOLOGY

Of the physiological properties of carbohydrates that of inducing the sensation of sweetness is of prime importance. Shallenberger's hypothesis expressed in its simplest form is that the sweet taste response is due to an intermolecular bonding phenomenon between the sweet tasting compound and the taste bud receptor site. Some supporting evidence is available for the idea that bonding with taste bud proteins is an essential stage in eliciting a taste response. It has been reported that the back of the tongue is an area particularly sensitive to bitter tastes. A protein fraction isolated from the epithelial tissue taken from the back of porcine tongues was examined for complex formation with quinine, brucine, naringenin and caffeine at various concentrations.[9] The association constant, which describes the relation between the degree of binding and concentration, was determined for each compound and ranking in order was in good agreement with the relative bitterness of the compounds. The free energy associated with the interaction was also calculated and indicated weak physical interactions operative in the binding mechanism characteristic of the strength of hydrogen bonds rather than covalent interactions. The protein fraction elicited no response with the sugars, but a similar preparation from the tip of porcine tongues responded to sugars but gave no response to bitter compounds. More recently it has been shown that Dastoli's sweet-sensitive protein is found not only in the papillae but also to an equal extent in the surrounding epithelium of the tongue which is devoid of taste buds, and no protein could be detected which occurred only in the papillae extracts.[10] Assuming that there are specific taste-sensitive areas of the tongue, and a protein is the sensor, then it is difficult to understand why it is present in other areas of the tongue in such large quantities.

3. TECHNOLOGY

There are numerous examples of the importance of the configuration of the carbohydrate molecule in food technology, particularly with respect to water retention, increasing the viscosity of liquids and producing gels. New natural polysaccharides have become available, *e.g.* alginates with dramatic water binding properties to form gels have been derived from seaweeds. A range of sweetening agents with graded properties is available as glucose syrups. Starch can be hydrolysed to give a mixture, the composition of which may range from carbohydrates consisting of smaller dextrose polymers to essentially dextrose itself. Gelatinised starch treated with α- or β-amylase yields maltose as the essential intermediate product which is subsequently hydrolysed to dextrose by glucoamylase. Acid hydrolysis of starch is completely random and most of the sugars formed are reducing sugars, but the composition is complicated by secondary reversion reactions. By varying the production process and making use of both methods of hydrolysis the composition of a glucose syrup may be modified to suit it for a particular need, but at the moment there are limits to the control that can be exercised over the composition. The composition is also influenced by the special behaviour of branched chain molecules of amylopectin towards hydrolysis.

Starch has been traditionally used as a thickening agent for sauces, but with the introduction of new food processes and new food products it has been found that the available starch does not possess the required properties. If gravies and sauces prepared with ordinary starch are frozen then very extensive breakdown of the texture occurs on thawing accompanied by extensive syneresis. The use instead of waxy rice starch (consisting essentially of the branched chain molecules of amylopectin) yields products which show no syneresis until after 20 freeze–thaw cycles.[11,12] The stability is due in part to the branched structure inhibiting association of the molecules, but further study is needed to explain this unusual stability of waxy rice starch.

From an understanding of the physical and chemical aspects of thickening and gel formation, and a knowledge of the configuration and structure of the constituent macromolecules, we can build up an appreciation of the texture characteristics of many foods and systematically and logically develop improvements. The food technologist must be aware of such work because of its potential to improve processing methods and the quality and nutritive value of the food.

The modification of the structure of the starch molecule by chemical and other methods as a means of introducing new properties has to a large extent been the result of experimental trial and error. It is to be expected that further progress will depend greatly on the extent of our basic knowledge of the chemistry and structure of the molecules concerned. Examples of such developments include the following.

(*a*) *Cross-linked starches.* Aqueous suspensions of waxy cereal starches gelatinise with heat to produce excessively stringy cohesive pastes which, however, have the advantages of high clarity and water binding, and resistance to retrogradation. Introduction of cross-bonding controls the swelling of the granules and reduces stringiness without interfering with the other desirable characteristics. The cross-linked starches for food use may be prepared by the reaction of ungelatinised starch with, for example, epichlorohydrin[13] or water-soluble metaphosphates.[14]

(*b*) *Starches with improved resistance to retrogradation.* The intermolecular association that causes retrogradation may be reduced by replacing some of the hydroxyl groups with acetyl or propionyl groups, or by introducing ionising groups which cause the molecules to repel one another. The recently developed starch phosphates in which at least part of the phosphate groups are monoesters and therefore not involved in cross-bonding are highly resistant to retrogradation and thawing. Their polyelectrolyte character also confers clarity and high water-binding capacity and prevents gel formation. The viscosity and extent of cold water dispersibility depends upon the degree of substitution, amount of cross-bonding and extent of degradation which have occurred during manufacture.

(*c*) *Staling of bread.* All the changes which occur during staling cannot be explained simply by the retrogradation of starch, but it appears to be the most important single factor. A widely used method to inhibit staling is the addition of a surface-active agent, particularly polyoxyethylene monostearate or glyceryl monostearate. Their ability to form complexes with amylose has been reported, but as staling is thought to involve only the amylopectin fraction of the starch, this complexing with amylose is probably not significant. It has been suggested that these surface-active agents form helical complexes with the outer linear branches of the amylopectin molecules and as a consequence restrict their dilation.[15] This could explain the mechanism of the anti-staling activity because the complexing of the outer branches of amylopectin molecules would inhibit aggregation.

The above examples serve to indicate that the behaviour and properties of carbohydrates cannot be explained simply in terms of chemistry relative to the reactive groups within the molecule, but the overriding factor is the configuration and structure of the molecule. The papers presented at this symposium illustrate the wide diversity of situations where such considerations are vital in elucidating the problem.

REFERENCES

1. Poole, D. F. G. and Newman, H. N. (1971). *Nature* (*Lond.*), **234,** p. 329.
2. Yudkin, J. (1972). *Nature* (*Lond.*), **239,** p. 197.
3. Brook, M. and Noel, P. (1969). *Nature* (*Lond.*), **222,** p. 563.
4. Macdonald, I. (1965). *Amer. J. Clin. Nutrit.,* **16,** p. 458.
5. Klugh, C. A. and Irwin, M. I. (1966). *Fed. Proc.,* **25,** p. 672.
6. Coltart, T. M. (1969). *Nature* (*Lond.*), **222,** p. 575.
7. Keys, A. (1971). *Atherosclerosis,* **14**(2), p. 193.

8. Walker, A. R. P. (1971). *Atherosclerosis*, **14**(2), p. 137.
9. Dastoli, F. R., Lopickes, D. I. and Doig, A. R. (1968). *Nature* (*Lond.*), **218,** p. 884.
10. Kayama, N. and Kurihara, K. (1971). *J. Gen. Physiol.,* **57,** p. 297.
11. Hanson, H. L., Campbell, A. and Lineweaver, H. (1951). *Food Technol.,* **5,** p. 432.
12. Davis J. G., Anderson, J. H. and Hanson, H. L. (1955). *Food Technol.,* **9,** p. 13.
13. Konigsberg. M. (1950). US Patent 2,500,950; *Chem. Abstr.,* **44,** p. 6666.
14. Keer, R. W. and Cleveland, F. C. (1957). US Patent 2,801,242; *Chem. Abstr.,* **51,** p. 18666.
15. Gray, V. M. and Schoch, T. J. (1962). *Stärke,* **14,** p. 239.

1

Configuration, Conformation and the Properties of Food Sugars

G. G. BIRCH

National College of Food Technology, University of Reading, Weybridge, Surrey, England

R. S. SHALLENBERGER

New York State Agricultural Experiment Station, Cornell University, Geneva, New York, USA

ABSTRACT

The thesis is presented that conformation and configuration underlie all the properties of the food sugars and even apparently minor structural alterations in sugar molecules cause profound chemical and physical differences in the ways that they may react in foodstuffs. These intrinsic differences in stereochemistry within the food sugars also affect their sensory differences and the nutritional and metabolic characteristics with which they may be attributed. Selected examples of both rare and common food sugars are discussed with reference to their stereochemical features.

INTRODUCTION

The configuration of any hydroxyl group in a sugar structure governs the amount of non-bonded interaction which it experiences with its neighbours. If this exceeds a certain limiting value the entire sugar ring may alter its shape (invert) producing a different ring form or change in conformation. Hence configuration and conformation are interdependent and for any individual sugar (which by definition is configurationally exactly characterised) there exists one favoured conformation in which its properties may most conveniently be described.

It is the thesis of this introductory paper that configuration and conformation underlie all the properties of the food sugars, and indeed offer the only reliable means for understanding the technological or nutritional potential of carbohydrate in the diet. Configuration and conformation first of all affect the very distribution of sugars in nature and hence the availability of those to which we have become metabolically most accustomed. Next they govern the chemical and physical properties of dietary carbohydrates and hence determine the analytical techniques by which we monitor and control their level in foodstuffs. Thirdly, configuration and conformation affect the sensory, nutritional and metabolic values of foods and govern the fine differences between their induced metabolic responses which are only now being examined in depth and detail.

In this paper the stereochemical basis for many properties of common and rare food sugars will be described with particular emphasis on those areas in which we have had some especial interest.

CONFIGURATION

Configuration may be regarded as the disposition of substituents in an asymmetric carbon atom. This introduces an element of handedness or 'chirality' to the asymmetric carbon atom which is considered in each case in relation to the reference compound D-glyceraldehyde. Hence the hydroxyl groups of the sugars are seen as projecting either above or below the plane of the ring when viewed in the conventional manner of Haworth rings (*i.e.* the plane of the ring at right angles to the plane of the paper). More correctly we should speak of the equatorial character of the hydroxyl groups (for those about in the plane of the ring) and the axial character (for those at right angles to the plane of the ring). Configuration defines which anomeric forms of a sugar (α or β) are possible. Configuration may be altered only by severence of covalent bonds.

CONFORMATION

Conformation may be defined as those changes in ring shape which are possible when rotating substituents about a bond linking two carbon atoms. The two common ring sizes of the sugars are the six-membered pyranose ring and the five-membered furanose ring. The former may exist in two possible 'chair' conformations and six possible 'boat' conformations as well as innumerable skew conformations, whereas the latter may exist as puckered 'twist' or 'envelope' conformations (Fig. 1). Thus the number of stereospecific entities

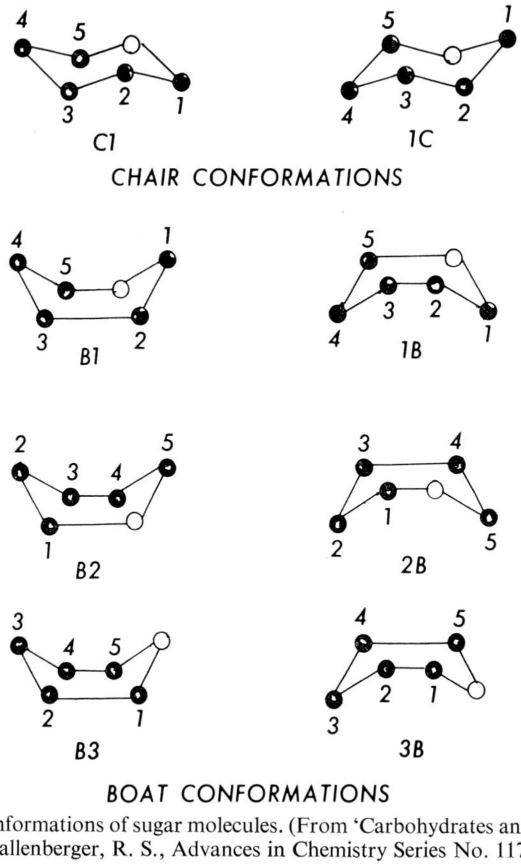

FIG. 1. Conformations of sugar molecules. (From 'Carbohydrates and Solution', Shallenberger, R. S., Advances in Chemistry Series No. 117.)

which are possible for one particular sugar is enormous and hence attempts to find the stereochemical basis of many biological effects may be practically impossible.

The two possible chair forms for a pyranose ring should be specified in terms of the chirality of the system to which the chair forms belong, *e.g.* $C1_D$, $1C_D$ or $C1_L$ or $1C_L$. For many sugars one particular conformation (usually a chair form) is favoured for energetic reasons so that g.l.c. analysis or p.m.r. spectroscopy may reveal 95% or more of the molecules existing in that form.

MULTIPLE GROUP STEREO-GEOMETRY

There is a third element of stereochemistry important to the properties of sugars in foods which we call 'multiple group stereo-geometry'. In β-D-glucopyranose (in its favoured C1 chair structure) the primary feature of its conformation is that all OH groups are equatorially disposed and all ring protons are axially disposed. This relation to ring shape is a second feature of conformation. As the result of ring conformation and carbon atom substituent configuration, the

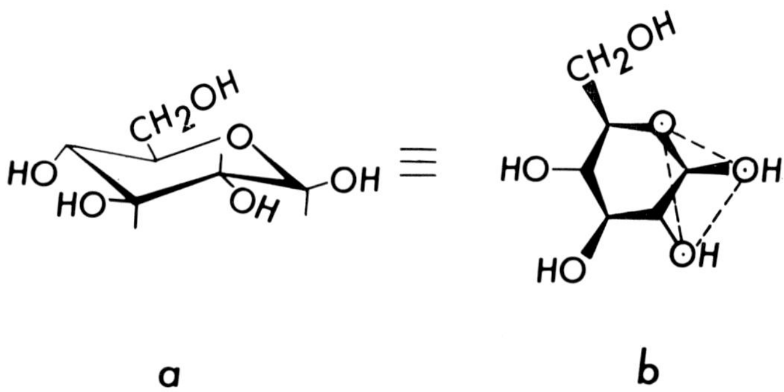

FIG. 2. Multiple group stereo-geometry.

geometric relation of atoms or groups in the molecule to each other constitute a third element of chirality, or third feature of conformation. Thus, the geometric relation of the ring oxygen atom and the hydroxyl oxygen atoms at carbon atoms one and two describes a chiral oblique planar triangle as shown in Fig. 2, which is not superimposable on its mirror image. Such group-geometry relations may have important bearing on the taste of the sugars.

CONFIGURATIONAL EFFECTS IN THE PROPERTIES OF FOOD SUGARS

The best known example of configuration affecting the properties of food sugars lies in the function of the anomeric centre. The two possible anomeric forms of one of the sugar rings are called the α and β forms depending on whether the hydroxyl groups at the anomeric centre project downwards or upwards respectively in the usual Haworth representation of the ring (Fig. 3). Although a sugar will crystallise with all its molecules in one or other of the forms shown in Fig. 3, any of these forms will revert to an equilibrium mixture of all possible types as shown in Fig. 3 once the sugar is dissolved in water. This change is accompanied by an alteration in optical rotation and hence is referred to as 'mutarotation'. In all

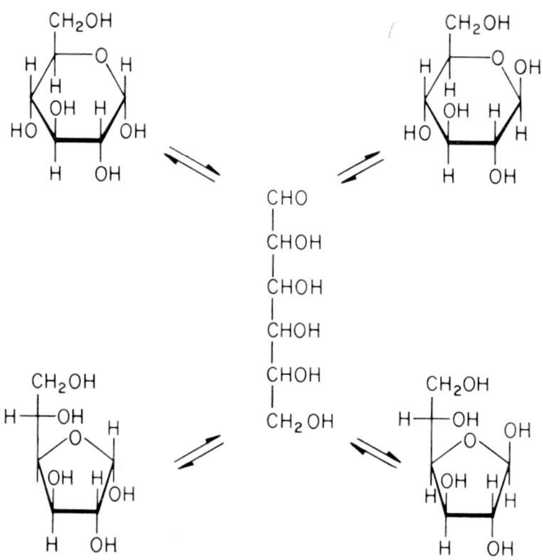

FIG. 3. Mutarotation of sugars into complex tautomeric mixtures.

the analyses which are employed in the quality control of foods in today's industry this reaction is liable to play a significant part, governing the magnitude of the polarimetric measurements which may be undertaken, specific reactions with analytical enzymes and rates of crystallinity and solubility. The technological and textural properties of foods may depend on the size, solubility and distribution of crystalline forms of a particular sugar. In sweetened condensed milk for example it is an even distribution of α-lactose monohydrate crystals which confers the desired texture. Incorrect temperature and processing conditions could lead to the β-modification and a slimy product of low consumer acceptability.

The sugars have several centres of atomic (configurational) chirality which leads to a family of diastereoisomers. D-Glucose and D-galactose differ in the spatial disposition of carbon atom substituents on the fourth carbon atom in such a manner that glucose has the *dextro* configuration and galactose has the *laevo* configuration. In their favoured (C1) conformation, this leads to an equatorial disposition for the glucose OH group and an axial disposition for the galactose OH group. Since an axial OH group is an element of conformational instability, presumably leading to

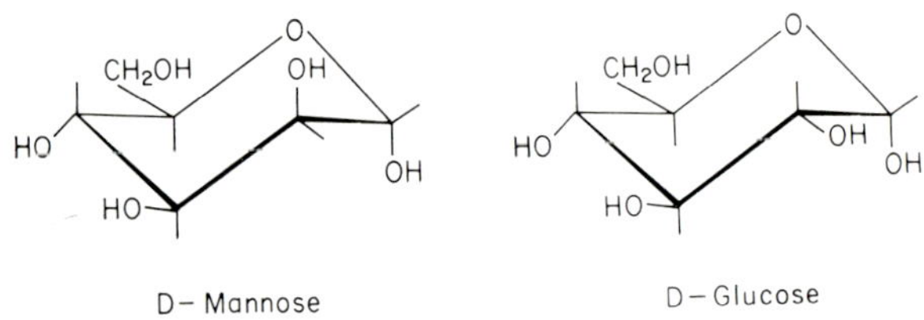

FIG. 4. Configurational difference between D-mannose and D-glucose.

easier formation of the aldehydo form of the sugar in solution, galactose is more prone to enter into the so-called non-enzymic browning reaction in foods.

Digestibility and nutritional response among the sugars depend on single configurational criteria and can thus result in profound differences between rare and common food sugars.[1] D-Mannose is found to be poorly absorbed, like many other rare food sugars, and differs from the abundant D-glucose only in the disposition of the

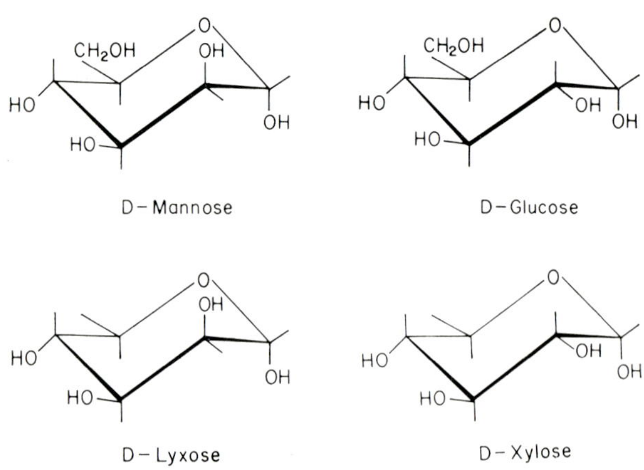

FIG. 5. Configurational analogies in glucose, mannose, xylose and lyxose.

second hydroxyl group (Fig. 4). D-Mannose bears the same configurational relationship to D-lyxose as does D-glucose to D-xylose, *i.e.* the absence of a primary alcohol group in the pentose in each case (Fig. 5). The last two mentioned sugars are absorbed and, at least to some extent in the case of xylose, metabolised. Thus it is interesting that mannose is poorly utilised and rather 'inert' whereas lyxose has been reported as highly toxic to rats.[2] However, if mannose is conveyed into the bloodstream by a transfusion method it appears to be quite toxic to humans[3,4] in modest quantities. This emphasises the need for a chemical understanding of nutritional and indeed therapeutic uses of the sugars before their indiscriminate use, either for dietary experiments or as food additives.

CONFORMATIONAL PROPERTIES OF THE FOOD SUGARS

Like configuration, conformation can affect the technological and biological properties of food sugars and it may well be that a particular configurational form is most suited to a conformational change which can be induced by a food processing operation. For example, the anhydro derivative laevoglucosan (Fig. 6) is formed by the action of heat and acid on D-glucose and could account for the

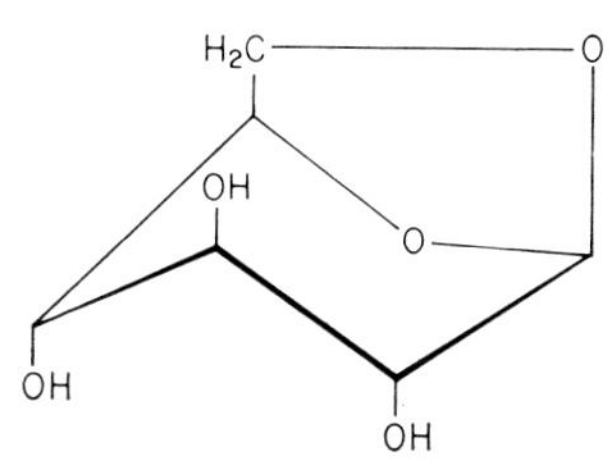

FIG. 6. Conformational structure of laevoglucosan.

disappearance of glucose from foods. Furthermore, its presence at low levels can be detected by gas chromatography[5] and, in glucose syrups, this constitutes a method for assessing the degree of acid treatment which the syrups have undergone and hence their method of manufacture.

Since conformation represents the real form in which a molecule is able to exert a particular biological effect, it enables us to recognise molecular analogies which, in turn, lead to analogous biological effects. For this reason D-galactose is an analogue of L-arabinose (Fig. 7), both sugars being absorbed into the bloodstream and both being cataractogenic. The former is able to induce cataract in rats whereas the latter is able only to enhance a cataract already set up.[6]

Of intrinsic relationship to the stereochemical structure of the sugars is their taste. This is best understood in terms of a stereospecific AH,B system of reciprocating hydrogen bonds,[7-10] and if sweetness is indeed a truly fundamental sensation we are well on the way to understanding the basic stereochemical requirements for an ideal saporous molecule within the sugar series. D-Fructose is still the sweetest sugar known and previously one of us[7] has assigned the 1,2-glycol arrangement as the AH,B system of the molecule.

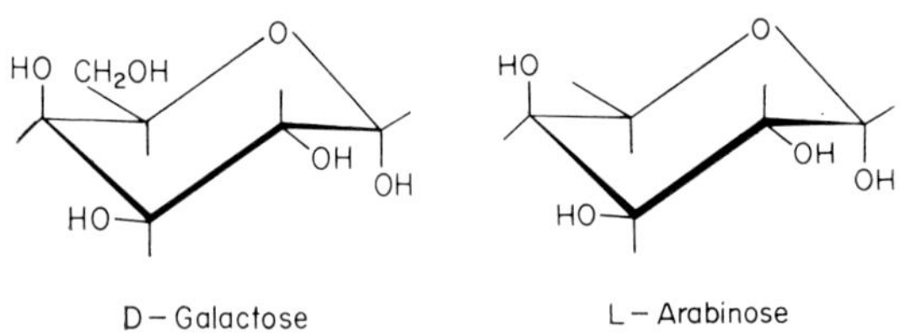

FIG. 7. Configurational analogy between D-galactose and L-arabinose.

Although it may be argued that the elimination of hydroxyl groups at positions 2, 3 and 4 is needed to substantiate the claim, a recent discovery[11] that D-arabinose and 2-deoxy-D-fructose (*i.e.* 1-deoxy-D-mannose) are each less sweet (Fig. 8) than D-fructose leaves little doubt about the original assignment.

Analogies such as these help us to grasp which functions of the sugar ring are specifically involved in binding to the taste bud protein both in mono- and oligo-saccharides. In the latter it is likely that only one sugar residue binds to the taste bud protein,[12] the other being excluded presumably for steric reasons. This effect is so marked that molecules above the molecular weight of trisaccharide probably have no sweetness at all.

In exploring the sweet taste of other compounds, such as the nitroaniline series, Kier[13] deduced that a third 'dispersion' site is needed to explain the varying sweetness of a closely related series of compounds. In addition to an AH,B unit, a dispersion component at a distance of about 3·5 Å from one of the electronegative atoms of the AH,B unit and about 5·5 Å from the other electronegative atom is needed. This constitutes the third element of stereochemistry referred to as 'multiple group stereo-geometry' and mentioned earlier in this treatise. It has recently been invoked by one of us[14] to account for the varying odorous notes and note intensities of volatile enantiomers.

In a sense, it would appear that the sugar enantiomers have the same sweetness in most cases because they do not generally possess a

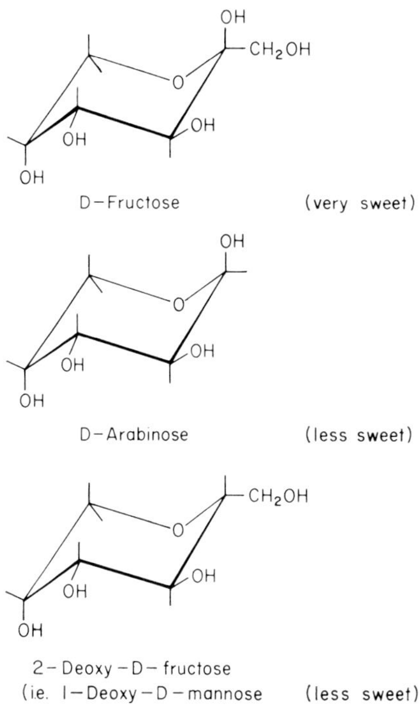

FIG. 8. Location of the saporific AH,B system in D-fructose.

third 'dispersion' or hydrophobic site. D- and L-Fructose are an exception, and the high sweetness of D-fructose, originally attributed to the lipophilicity of the ring methane carbon atom,[15] may be due to the fact that the methane carbon atom is the third site required for increased sweetness intensity. In that case, since the tripartite site imparts a multiple group element of chirality, one fructose enantiomer may indeed be sweeter than the other.

CONCLUSION

An interplay of configurational and conformational effects probably accounts for all the properties which have been observed in the food sugars and although all the conformational possibilities which occur in foodstuffs are by no means yet understood, research in certain areas is well described in terms of these possibilities. Perhaps the determination of configurational and conformational changes in foods by sophisticated analytical techniques such as gas chromatography, n.m.r. spectrometry and mass spectrometry will provide the type of control over food carbohydrate quality which must be our objective.

REFERENCES

1. Birch, G. G. (1969). *Fd. Wrld.,* **4,** p. 5.
2. Heggeness, F. W. (1960). *Amer. J. Physiol.,* **198,** p. 625.
3. Birch, G. G. (1971). *Lancet,* **7739**(2), p. 1419.
4. Wood, F. C. and Cahill, G. F. (1963). *J. Clin. Invest.,* **42,** p. 1300.
5. Kheiri, M. S. A. and Birch, G. G. (1969). *Cereal Chem.,* **46**(4), p. 400.
6. Patterson, J. W. (1955). *Arch. Biochem. Biophys.,* **58,** p. 24.
7. Shallenberger, R. S. (1963). *J. Fd. Sci.,* **28,** p. 584.
8. Shallenberger, R. S. (1964). *Agric. Sci. Rev.,* **2,** p. 11.
9. Shallenberger, R. S. (1964). *New Scient.,* **407**(3), p. 569.
10. Shallenberger, R. S., Acree, T. E. and Guild, W. E. (1965). *J. Fd. Sci.,* **30,** p. 560.
11. Birch, G. G. and Lindley, M. G. (1973). Unpublished results.
12. Birch, G. G., Cowell, N. D. and Eyton, D. (1970). *J. Fd. Technol.,* **5,** p. 277.
13. Kier, L. B. (1972). *J. Pharm. Sci.,* **61,** p. 1394.
14. Shallenberger, R. S. (1973). *Proc. 5th International Congr. Pharmacology,* S. Karger, Basel, in the press.
15. Shallenberger, R. S. and Acree, T. E. (1971). In *Handbook of Sensory Physiology,* IV, *Chemical Senses,* Part 2, Taste, Ed. L. M. Beidler, Springer-Verlag, Berlin, p. 221.

DISCUSSION

Chairman: You have given us an extremely lucid description of your hypothesis. I was most interested to see how you had advanced the initial concepts to cover a wide range of points. I would like to open the discussion by asking you if you could account for degrees of sweetness on the basis of your theory—for instance, why is sucrose as sweet as it is? I believe it is the third sweetest sugar. Is there any simple reason for that?

Shallenberger: One requirement for sweetness I did not mention was the idea of lipophilicity. Apparently for a compound to taste sweet it must have some element of what we call the greasy factor which was suggested by Dr Lemieux. One of the reasons that β-D-fructose is so sweet is the greasy methane carbon atom that none of the other ordinary sugars have. Sucrose has the AH,B unit as described by Gordon Birch. Professor Kier has recently explained this third element required for sweetness, this lipophilicity. In sucrose the AH of the AH,B system is exactly 5·5 Å from this third site, and this, I think, is also the reason why fructose tastes so sweet. I have not yet sat down with my model and I don't know which form to pull the ring into to calculate distances, but I think he is correct and that is why sucrose is as sweet as it is.

Radley: You have been dealing with one set of reactions which produce sweetness. I am completely ignorant as to the structure or function—not function, but number of functions—which any taste bud exercises. This is something like eyes with rods and cones responsive to various factors. Taste it, and the sweetness reacts for sweetness!

Shallenberger: No. This is one problem. In a sweet α-glycol arrangement the distance between the centres of the two oxygen atoms is about 3 Å. If you get something reacting with AH,B of the receptor and AH,B of the sweetener reacting at the same time, that is sweetness. You don't have to stretch your imagination too far to get sourness. All you have to do is have a hydrogen atom reacting with B alone to cause sour taste, and it doesn't take too much imagination to get saltiness—all you need is a chlorine atom in association with sodium. And you can reduce the AH,B distance from 3 Å to 1·5 Å, and that is one of the requirements for bitterness. I am saying that one taste bud receptor can respond to our four arbitrary classifications of taste—that is the simplistic chemist's way.

Rolfe: Can you account by your theory how it is that halides of low molecular weight taste salty, *e.g.* NaCl, LiBr, but become increasingly bitter as molecular weight is increased, *e.g.* RbCl and KI?

Shallenberger: We can define sensations to each other by reference to standard compounds. How do you define sweetness? I can give you sucrose and say 'That tastes sweet, do you recognise it?' and give you sodium chloride and say 'That tastes salty'. Unfortunately, in any deviation from sodium chloride you are involved in another taste sense, where it is due to the interaction or double interaction if you are introducing an element of varying taste, and any deviation from sodium chloride begins to get bitter. The sensations you get from sodium chloride or potassium chloride have a bitter taste. Some of the sugars taste bitter, *e.g.* β-D-mannose. We worked with people who had no sweet taste whatever and I wanted to know how saturated solutions of glucose would taste to these people, and we varied the sweetness of the sugars by creating a molecular hydrogen bond which should create a bitter taste. I haven't answered your question. I am thinking about it.

McMichael: Does the hydrophobic part of the sweetness configuration correspond with part of the sweetness receptor site or does it suggest transfer across the lipid cell membrane?

Shallenberger: Probably both. I am beginning to think in terms of both. The major operation is AH,B. The third point is the lipophilicity.

McMichael: Is there evidence that the taste moiety, the taste process, involves energy release?

Shallenberger: Let's argue that one out over a bottle of beer. I don't know. I really don't know. I think it is energy input rather than energy release. I know that everybody has to think in terms of any reaction like water flowing downhill. I think the sweet taste response is energy input.

2

The Role of Carbohydrate in Non-Enyzmic Browning

D. J. McWeeny

Food Science Division, Ministry of Agriculture, Fisheries and Food, Norwich, England

ABSTRACT

The use of the term 'non-enzymic browning' as the general description customarily applied to a group of quite diverse chemical reactions will be discussed. Some of these reactions have been studied in detail and the so-called Maillard reaction between reducing sugars and amino acids is now generally accepted as involving the successive formation of mono-glycosylamines, di-glycosylamines, deoxy-osuloses and unsaturated osuloses in the early stages of reaction; the later stages are still poorly understood and the nature of the pigment has not been established. It seems likely that the pigment, although often of high molecular weight, is not a true polymer and has a composition which varies according to the extent and conditions of reaction as well as being dependent upon the particular reactants involved.

Maillard-type reactions will be compared with other carbohydrate-based browning reactions and with browning reactions which do not involve the participation of carbohydrates; the comparison will cover the nature of the intermediates, the effects of retarders and the characteristics of the pigment. These show some similarities but the confusion likely to arise when information about one type of browning is incautiously related to another type of browning will be illustrated.

Apart from chemical effects, soluble carbohydrates may also have a physical effect upon the reaction through their effect on the water activity of the reaction system, which in some situations can have a marked effect on reaction rates.

There are a number of excellent reviews of the chemistry of non-enzymic browning as it relates to foods[1-3] and the role of carbohydrates is discussed in these at some length. It does not seem appropriate to attempt a detailed review in a short paper like this and the aim will be rather different, *i.e.* to identify certain features of non-enzymic browning which for one reason or another tend to get little mention in the scientific literature and then to use these points to illustrate how the role of carbohydrates is similar to (and differs from) the role of alternative reactants.

GENERAL FEATURES

First it seems important to get an appreciation (if not a precise definition) of what is meant by non-enzymic browning and this is not particularly easy. One of the factors which has contributed to confusion on this is psychological in that we, as chemists, are accustomed to giving specific reactions a name and to associating this name with specific precursors and products; we have probably all been brought into contact with organic chemistry for the first time in association with things like the Wurtz synthesis and the Friedel–Crafts reaction. So when we hear about 'the non-enzymic browning reaction' we are conditioned to thinking of it as a specific reaction of particular reactants leading through a series of predictable intermediates to an identifiable product. This is quite remote from the truth and it only causes confusion to think in this way. In fact, non-enzymic browning is a general description of quite diverse reactions, the common feature of which is that they involve carbonylic intermediates and lead to the formation of products whose distinguishing feature is an intense absorption in the UV with some residual absorption above 400 nm which decreases at longer wavelengths.

Within this general description, the initial reactants may be as chemically different as a reducing sugar and an oxidised fat; either of these may be reacting with, for instance, an amino acid, a protein or a phospholipid; the early intermediates include some simple carbonyls, unsaturated carbonyls, di- and polycarbonyls, acyclic and cyclic carbonyls; later intermediates include linear and cyclic condensation products with amino compounds; the coloured products may be relatively small molecules which are soluble in water—or on the other hand they may be oil soluble—they may be very large molecules which are virtually insoluble. Against that background it seems difficult to suggest that there is a basic common reaction involved! Yet there seems to be a psychological need to find a common pattern and in the past there has been an emphasis on the common features of these reactions—for instance on the similarities in coloured products or on the fact that sulphites are always effective to some degree in limiting the development of these brown pigments. In fact, it is probably more accurate to regard this last observation as a reflection of the versatility of sulphites as chemically active compounds rather than as an indication of some underlying and essential common feature of the mechanism by which brown pigments are produced.

This is not to say that there are no common features but rather that one should establish with some care the precise nature of the features of one type of browning reaction which do have a parallel in another type of browning, and having done so determine whether or not these are quantitatively significant similarities; what may be a key step in one reaction may exist, but be quantitatively irrelevant, in another. A simple illustration of this might be the role of 5-hydroxymethyl furfuraldehyde which appears to be an important intermediate in the high-temperature caramelisation of sugar. It is also found in slightly acid reaction mixtures of reducing sugars with amino acids (Maillard reactions) at moderate temperatures, but can easily be demonstrated as being quantitatively unimportant as an intermediate in this latter situation.[4]

Since the so-called Maillard reaction (which is not really a specific series of events as is usual in the case of a 'named' chemical reaction) has been studied more thoroughly than other types of browning reactions, it is appropriate to describe the salient features of the Maillard reaction and to compare these with other types of browning, emphasising the role of carbohydrates as the comparison proceeds.

In the specific case of glucose and glycine, there now seems to be fairly general acceptance of a series of reactions as indicated in Fig. 1. This illustrates the ways in which various types of carbonylic intermediates can be formed. The extent to which each type of intermediate is formed may be influenced by temperature, pH and concentration —it will also be influenced by substituting other carbohydrates for glucose, *e.g.* the stereochemistry of the hydroxyl group at C-4 can affect the geometrical isomerism of an olefinic bond formed at the 3,4 position, and consequently the ease with which cyclisation occurs (either before or after condensation with an amino group); the stereochemistry at C-5 may also have a role to play in some cyclisation reactions.

If, instead of aldoses, one considers ketoses and their reactions, it is immediately obvious that relatively little work has been done with these, although it is known from the work of Heyns *et al.* that

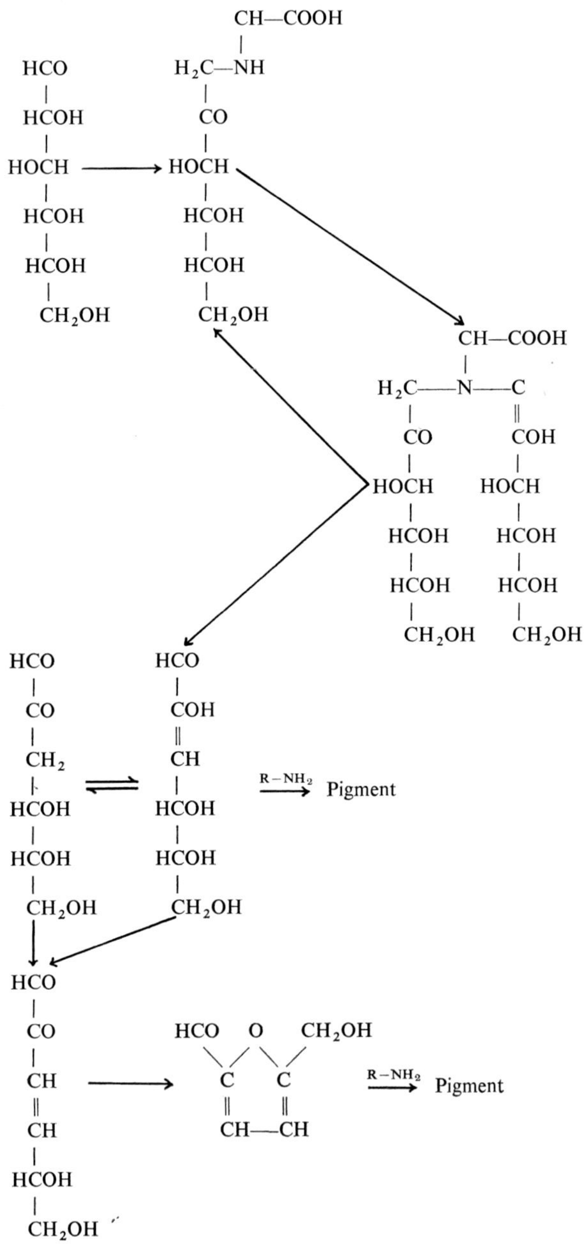

FIG. 1. Schematic diagram of early stages in the Maillard reaction.

in the case of fructose, the 2-amino-2-deoxyglucoses are formed from amino acids[5]—these are analogous to the 1-amino-1-deoxyfructoses from glucose. Further stages in the reaction have not been studied in much detail; however, it is clear that the browning reactions of fructose are quite different, *e.g.* the loss of amino acid or of free amino groups of casein is very low with fructose as compared to glucose.

To take another example, if one considers other carbohydrates (for instance ascorbic acid) then there is even less information available. Reynolds[3] summarises the position, indicating a number of di-carbonylic intermediates, but there is no reference to nitrogenous intermediates produced from reaction of these with amino acids.

There is information about the relative rates at which colour is developed with various sugars; xylose and arabinose tend to produce colour very rapidly,[6–8] as does dehydroascorbic acid.[9] Similarly, xylose and arabinose bind the free amino groups of protein (and reduce its biological value) much more rapidly than glucose, which in turn does so more rapidly than lactose and maltose,[8] but this will not be dealt with in detail here. For the present it is intended to consider the influence of carbohydrate on the nature of the pigment and its properties as well as the intensity of colour.

In terms of the colour intensity produced, as related to particular carbohydrate precursors, orders of relative reactivity are sometimes quoted[6,7,10]—it is important to realise that not only do these relative rates apply only to the particular conditions (concentration, pH and temperature) employed, they also relate only to the time interval studied, *e.g.* initially fructose and glycine usually produce more colour than glucose and glycine but the position can be reversed if the reaction is allowed to continue. Again, non-reducing disaccharides will be very slow to brown at first, but if hydrolysis releases a reactive reducing monosaccharide, it may subsequently brown very quickly.

The question of what the coloured compounds are is unresolved; certainly they vary even from the same reactants. In terms of the relative incorporation of the carbon residues of sugars and amino acids it can vary from 6:1 to 1:1 according to the relative amounts of the reactants (8:1 and 1:10 respectively)[11,12] and there is no evidence of a repeating unit. If the carbohydrate is changed and ascorbic acid is substituted for glucose, the properties of the pigment change. For instance, the extinction coefficient becomes markedly pH-sensitive,[9] a fact which seems to have escaped notice when the effect of pH on reaction rates has been studied; colour measurement must be made at a standard pH in measurements of reaction rate in terms of production of a pH-sensitive pigment. This may not have been necessary for studies of the production of the glucose–glycine pigment and illustrates the importance of determining carefully where similarities *do* exist between different browning systems—and where they *do not*.

Carbohydrates also have an effect on the physical properties of the pigment, *i.e.* its solubility. The water solubility of many pigments from non-enzymic browning reactions appears to reflect the solubility properties of the carbohydrate reactant; if, on the other hand, one replaces the carbohydrate by a lipid-soluble unsaturated aldehyde (such as might be found in an oxidising fat), then the reaction produces a lipid-soluble pigment.[13]

As mentioned above, the pigment varies even with the same reactants, according to the conditions used. Indeed, even if the concentrations, etc. are standardised, it varies according to the reaction time, *i.e.* a severely browned glucose/glycine mixture cannot be diluted to give the same colour as the mixture had at an earlier stage of colour development; the shades are distinctly different even if the absorbance at some arbitrary wavelength in the 400–500 nm region is the same.[14] This may imply, for instance, that as browning develops the original chromophoric grouping has been chemically modified in a way which increases the absorbance in the visible region; if the incorporation of an additional olefinic group in the conjugated system gives a bathochromic shift, which markedly affects the absorption at, say, 450 nm, then the absorbance may double whilst the actual weight of pigmented material increases only very slightly. There should be grave reservations about the validity of judging the rate of a reaction by measuring something which is not in fact the same entity at different times during the reaction—though there is no evidence in the literature that this has been appreciated and one can find elegant mathematical treatments of the kinetics of browning reactions which ignore this fundamentally important possibility.

SULPHITE EFFECTS

It is well known that sulphites cause a decrease in colour development from non-enzymic browning reactions. What is perhaps not so widely appreciated is that ways in which sulphites achieve this may vary widely. To take a very simple experiment, we may compare the effects on glucose/glycine and ascorbic acid/glycine systems.[13] Figure 2 shows that in the first case sulphite has an inhibiting effect, in the latter it is only a retarder. Furthermore, the effect of adding sulphite once colour has developed in an unsulphited control is different. Although in both cases the colour is partially bleached, in the first case the colour achieved from adding sulphite at the beginning of the reaction is markedly less than that achieved by

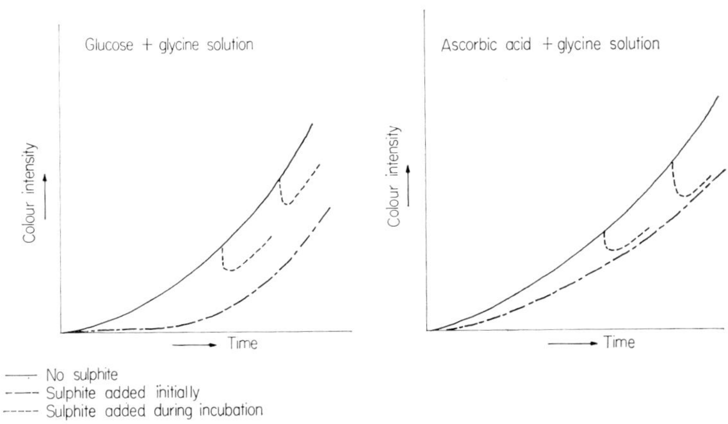

FIG. 2. Effect of sulphite on colour development at 50°C.

adding it later; in the second case the final colours are fairly comparable. If one was to carry out the same experiment with an unsaturated aldehyde (of the type which might be found in an oxidising fat) in place of the carbohydrate, then the observation would be broadly similar to that with glucose.

The reasons for these differences in sulphite action in different browning reactions are not well understood but there have been some advances in our appreciation of the various ways in which sulphite can exert an effect and these help towards a qualitative appreciation of the reasons for the differences. Figure 3 depicts some of these sulphite effects. Disregarding the first one which is usually a weak effect due to the large excess of sugar over bisulphite and the unfavourable equilibrium condition, all the classes of compounds with which sulphite is now thought to react are likely to be found, to some extent, in all non-enzymic browning reactions. What are important, in understanding the differences in sulphite effects, are the relative abundances of the various classes of compounds. At least in the early stages of reaction one might expect to find dicarbonylic intermediates more abundantly in ascorbic acid-based reactions than in those based on an oxidising fat; the position may be reversed in terms of $\alpha\beta$-unsaturated aldehydes. Consequently, the dominant mechanisms by which sulphite exerts its anti-browning effect may

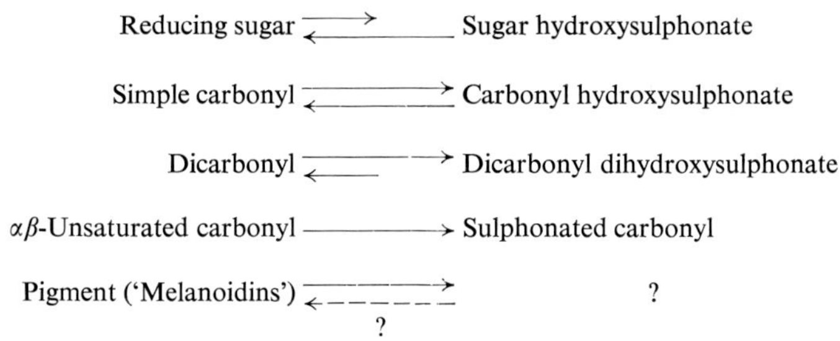

FIG. 3. Sulphite effects on non-enzymic browning.

be different in the two cases. For instance, the reaction with dicarbonyls is a reversible equilibrium[15] and one would therefore expect a retardation, as is observed with ascorbic acid; on the other hand, the reaction with unsaturated aldehydes is an irreversible addition and one might expect an inhibition phase, as is found with reducing sugars.

PHYSICAL EFFECTS

Having given some examples illustrating the general features of the role of carbohydrates in the chemistry of non-enzymic browning, one should not forget one of their physical effects, *viz.* the effect of soluble carbohydrates on water activity. It is, of course, well known that sugars lower the a_w of systems to which they are added; the preservative action of sugar in, for instance, jams relies on the lowering of a_w to the point at which microbiological growth is no longer possible.

There are several references[16–19] in Reynolds' reviews to studies on non-enzymic browning in various dehydrated fruits and vegetables where the effects of moisture content or equilibrium relative humidity (and hence water activity) on browning rates have been studied; there are more recent studies on model systems by Labuza

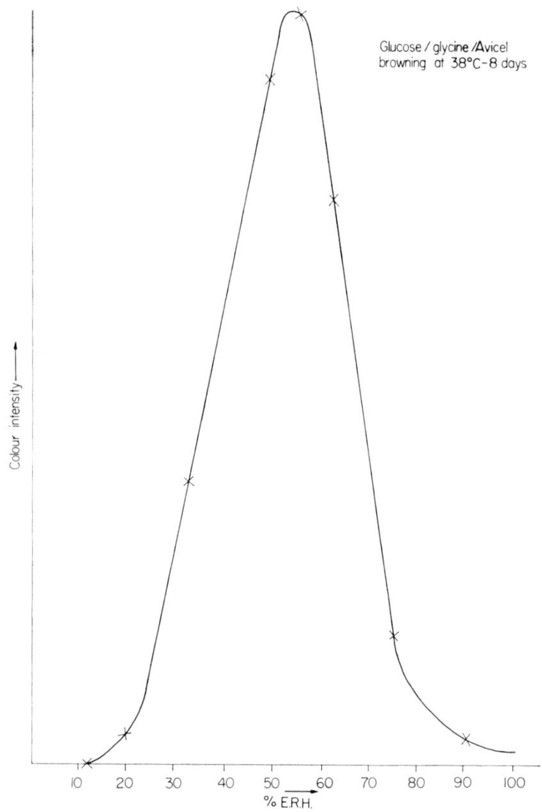

FIG. 4. Effect of ERH on browning.

et al.[20] The effect can be seen very clearly in some model experiments on glucose and glycine dispersed on an Avicel (cellulose) support under various ERH conditions at 37°C.[21] Figure 4 shows the very sharp dependence of browning rates on ERH and it is interesting to add that as browning progresses the ERH at which browning is fastest changes as the reaction proceeds; we have not studied the reaction with other substrates but it might be useful to compare this picture with the one obtained with ascorbic acid or an unsaturated aldehyde in place of glucose. There is no particular reason to assume the ERH for optimal reaction rate will be the same with these reactants as it is with glucose.

Whilst there are only a limited number of examples of the use of soluble carbohydrates to lower a_w to the 0·5 to 0·65 region, the trend towards the so-called intermediate moisture foods (already an important pet food item in North America) may bring to light more cases where addition of sugars and other carbohydrates in order to reduce a_w (and hence preserve the food) may predispose products to unexpectedly high rates of non-enzymic browning.

CONCLUSION

In discussing the various types of browning reaction in relation to foods it is important to realise that a variety of substrates can be involved; the course of the reaction, the properties of the products and the effectiveness of retarders will vary according to the type of substrate which dominates the reaction.

In the past it has been found that the rate of browning in foods can often be related to the reducing sugar content—it tends to be assumed that (with a few known exceptions) it is always so. The comparisons which have been made may provide the basis for verifying this assumption in new or existing food products. Since non-enzymic browning has its beneficial effects in foods (notably in some of its flavour effects which, regrettably, it has not been possible to consider in this paper) as well as its undesirable ones, it is important to appreciate the different roles which carbohydrates and the other reactants can play so as perhaps to take advantage of them. In the past, the browning reactions have come to be regarded by the food processor as a problem; until recently the beneficial aspects, in terms of flavour production, had received relatively little attention. This imbalance is not now so great and it may be that our increasing understanding of the chemistry of the browning reactions will be employed more in the controlled production of flavours and less in further attempts to control colour. The role of specific carbohydrates in this is likely to be both important and subtle—some of the peculiarities of the browning reactions mentioned in this paper may indicate why this should be so.

ACKNOWLEDGEMENT

I wish to thank my colleagues, particularly Dr M. E. Knowles and Dr B. Wedzicha, for their agreement to the use in this paper of previously unpublished observations from our various joint investigations.

REFERENCES

1. Danehy, J. P. and Pigman, W. W. (1951). *Adv. Fd. Res.,* **3,** p. 241.
2. Reynolds, T. M. (1963). *Adv. Fd. Res.,* **12,** p. 1.
3. Reynolds, T. M. (1965). *Adv. Fd. Res.,* **14,** p. 167.
4. Burton, H. S., McWeeny, D. J. and Biltcliffe, D. O. (1963). *J. Sci. Fd. Agric.,* **14,** p. 291.
5. Heyns, K., Breuer, H. and Paulsen, J. (1957). *Chem. Ber.,* **90,** p. 1374.
6. Maillard, L. C. (1912). *Compt. Rend.,* **154,** p. 66.
7. Spark, A. A. (1969). *J. Sci. Fd. Agric.,* **20,** p. 308.
8. Lewis, V. M. and Lea, C. H. (1950). *Biochim et Biophys Acta,* **4,** p. 532.
9. Wedzicha, B. and McWeeny, D. J. (1972). To be published.
10. Burton, H. S. and McWeeny, D. J. (1963). *Nature,* **197,** p. 266.
11. Reynolds, T. M. (1962). Unpublished results (quoted in Ref. 2, p. 40).
12. Wolfrom, M. L., Schlicht, R. C., Langer, A. W. and Rooney, C. S. (1953). *J. Amer. Chem. Soc.,* **75,** p. 1013.
13. McWeeny, D. J., Burton, H. S. and Biltcliffe, D. O. (1963). Unpublished data.
14. McWeeny, D. J. and Spark, A. A. (1968). Unpublished data.
15. Knowles, M. E. (1971). *Chem. Ind.,* p. 910.
16. Wolfrom, M. L. and Rooney, C. S. (1953). *J. Amer. Chem. Soc.,* **75,** p. 5435.
17. Stadtman, E. R., Barker, H. A., Mrak, E. M. and Mackinney, G. (1946). *Ind. Eng. Chem.,* **38,** p. 99.
18. Legault, R. R., Hendel, C. E., Talburt, W. F. and Pool, M. F. (1951). *Fd. Technol.,* **5,** p. 417.
19. Draudt, H. N. and I-Yih Huang (1966). *J. Agric. Food Chem.,* **14,** p. 170.
20. Labuza, T. P., Tannenbaum, S. R. and Karel, M. (1970). *Fd. Technol.,* **24,** p. 543.
21. McWeeny, D. J. (1971). Unpublished data.

DISCUSSION

Chairman: Thank you very much indeed, Dr McWeeny. I do congratulate you for having even attempted to speak on such a very broad and complex subject as non-enzymic browning of carbohydrates. It is one of those subjects on which I think we could have done with having a round table discussion alone, because it is a topic of interest not only to sugar manufacturers in every field but to refiners and users and to glucose and fructose producers also, and of course throughout the food industry. Non-enzymic browning is a field on which we could usefully spend time—I feel somehow we will have to get together and arrange our own round table on this.

Radley: Do these reactions take place in completely de-oxygenated conditions?

McWeeny: So far as I am aware, yes. There is no real requirement for oxygen. It goes a great deal faster in the presence of oxygen but with the exclusion of oxygen you get colour development. You obviously have a specific reason for asking that question and we will pursue it together later.

Shallenberger: It is interesting to note that in model system studies of the browning reaction, glycine is invariably used. The formaldehyde produced must inhibit the very reaction being studied. It amazes me. Have none of these people ever heard of the formal titration?

McWeeny: Well, maybe we should pursue that one too.

3

Sucrochemistry*

R. KHAN

Philip Lyle Memorial Research Laboratory, Reading, England

ABSTRACT

In view of the possible industrial and biological applications of the halogen derivatives of sucrose, new synthetic routes to various chlorodeoxy derivatives have been investigated. The nucleophilic substitution reaction of the sulphonate or chlorosulphate derivatives of sucrose, using chloride as nucleophile, has been reported to give chlorodeoxy derivatives. The direct synthesis of mono-, di- and trichlorodeoxy derivatives by reaction of sucrose and its appropriately protected derivatives with methanesulphonyl chloride in N,N-*dimethyl formamide is described.*

1′,2,3,3′,4,4′-*Hexa*-O-*benzoyl sucrose on treatment with methanesulphonyl chloride in* N,N-*dimethyl formamide gave the* 6,6′-*dichloro*-6,6′-*dideoxy derivative. Similar treatment of* 2,3,3′,4,4′-*penta*-O-*benzoyl sucrose with methanesulphonyl chloride in* N,N-*dimethyl formamide afforded a mixture of* 6,6′-*dichloro*-6,6′-*dideoxy sucrose pentabenzoate and* 1′,6,6′-*trichloro*-1′,6,6′-*trideoxy sucrose pentabenzoate. When sucrose was treated with methanesulphonyl chloride in* N,N-*dimethyl formamide it gave the expected mixture of di- and trichlorodeoxy derivatives from which* 6,6′-*dichloro*-6,6′-*dideoxy sucrose and* 1′,6,6′-*trichloro*-1′,6,6′-*trideoxy sucrose were isolated, indicating that this reaction can result in the specific substitution of primary hydroxyl groups, under the appropriate conditions.*

INTRODUCTION

Our interest in the study of the basic chemistry of sucrose is in exploring novel and potentially profitable non-food outlets for

* Read by Dr K. J. Parker.

sugar. The application of reactions, such as the nucleophilic substitution of sulphonates and chlorosulphates, esterification, elimination, halogenation and oxidation, have led to a large number of rigorously characterised derivatives of sucrose. The potential value of these derivatives, for example, as biologically active materials, polymerisation intermediates, pesticides, food additives and surface active agents, awaits development.

Sucrose is systematically named β-D-fructofuranosyl-α-D-glucopyranoside (1). It has three primary hydroxyls at C-1′, C-6 and C-6′ and five secondary hydroxyl groups at C-2, C-3, C-4, C-3′ and C-4′. The expected difference in the reactivity of these two sets of hydroxyls has been well established. The primary hydroxyls at C-6 and C-6′ have been shown to react preferentially in the diesterification reaction of sucrose.[1,2] Study of the nucleophilic substitution reactions of the sucrose sulphonates and chlorosulphates has revealed the reactivity to be in the order of C-6 > C-6′ > C-4 > C-1′.[3-5]

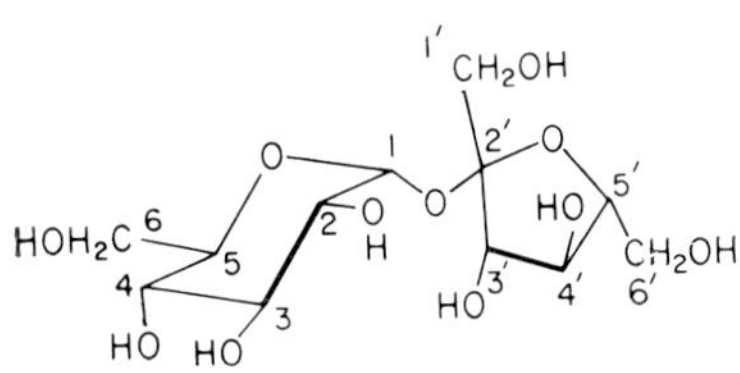

(1)

ANHYDRO DERIVATIVES OF SUCROSE

Trimolar tosylation of sucrose has been reported by Lemieux and Barrette to afford a mixture of products from which 1′,6,6′-tri-*O*-tosylsucrose (2) was claimed to have been isolated in 29% yield.[6] Evidence for the structure (2) was based on its conversion into 1′,2:3,6:3′,6′-trianhydrosucrose (3).[7] However, when 1′,6,6′-tri-*O*-tosylsucrose, prepared by an unambiguous route, was treated under similar conditions with sodium methoxide in methanol, it gave a different trianhydride, namely 1′,4′:3,6:3′6′-trianhydrosucrose (4).[8,9] On the basis of the investigation carried out in this laboratory, the conclusion was drawn that the tritosylate (2) could not have been a precursor of the trianhydride (3) and must have arisen from some other tri-*O*-tosylsucrose such as 2,6,6′-tri-*O*-tosylsucrose.[9]

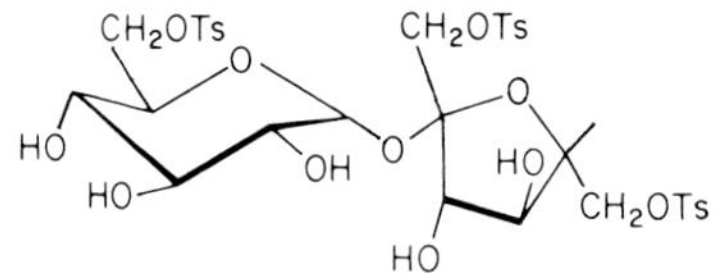

(2)

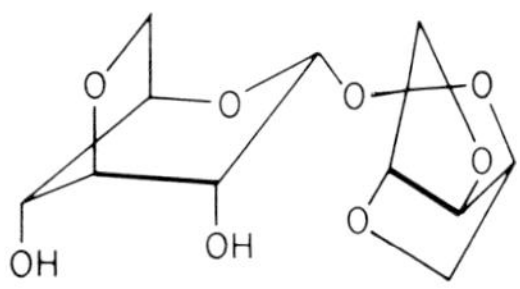

(4)

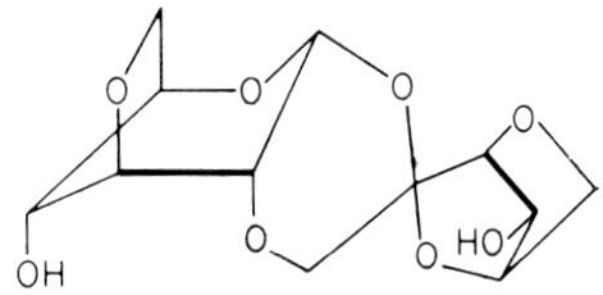

(3)

Treatment of 1′,4,6′-tri-*O*-tosylsucrose pentaacetate with sodium methoxide in methanol has been reported to give 3,6-anhydro-α-D-galactopyranosyl-1′,4′:3′,6′-dianhydro-β-D-fructofuranoside (5).[10] Similarly, 3,6:3′,6′-dianhydrosucrose (6),[3] 1′,4′-3′,6′-dianhydrosucrose (7)[11] and 3′,6′-anhydrosucrose (8)[12] were obtained from 6,6′-di-*O*-tosyl-, 1′,6′-di-*O*-tosyl- and 6′-*O*-tosylsucrose respectively.

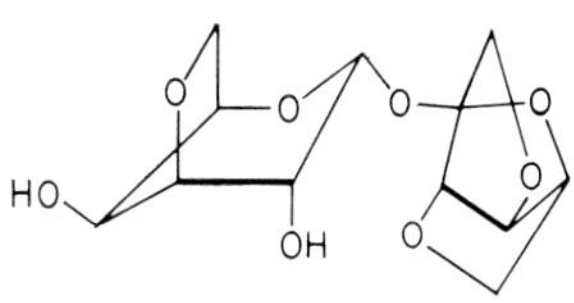

(5)

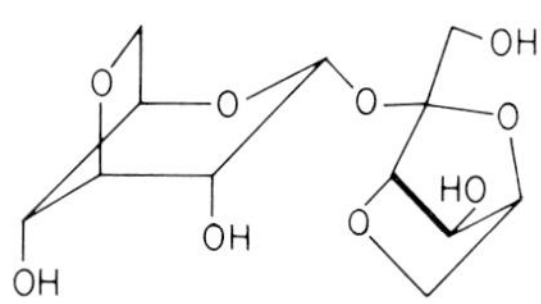

(6)

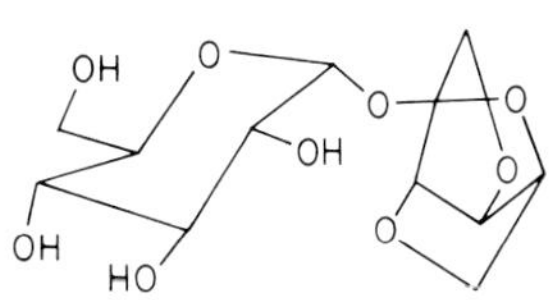

(7)

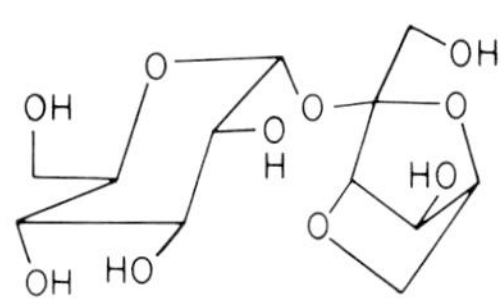

(8)

NUCLEOPHILIC SUBSTITUTION REACTIONS OF SUCROSE SULPHONATES

6,6′-Di-*O*-tosylsucrose hexabenzoate (9) and the corresponding hexaacetate (10) underwent bimolecular nucleophilic substitution when treated with anions such as halides, azide, benzoate, thiocyanate, etc., in aprotic solvents.[3] The disulphonate (9) on refluxing with sodium iodide in butanone gave crystalline 6,6′-diiodo-6,6′-dideoxysucrose hexabenzoate (11). Subsequent hydrogenation of the diiodide (11) gave 6,6′-dideoxysucrose hexabenzoate (12).[3] The p.m.r. spectrum revealed two doublets at τ8·53 and 8·8, and thus confirmed the location of the methyl groups at C-5 and C-5′.

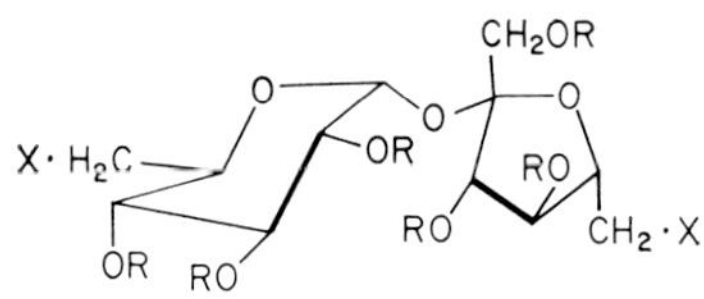

(9) R = Bz, X = OTs (13) R = H, X = N_3

(10) R = Ac, X = OTs (14) R = H, X = NH_2

(11) R = Bz, X = I

(12) R = Bz, X = H

Interest in amino derivatives of sucrose was stimulated by the frequent occurrence of amino sugars as components of antibiotics[13] and bacterial polysaccharides.[14] Synthesis of 6,6′-diazido-6,6′-dideoxysucrose (13)[4,15] a precursor of the 6,6′-diamino-6,6′-dideoxysucrose (14) has been described. Catalytic hydrogenation of the 6,6′-diazide (13) gave the corresponding 6,6′-diamine (14).[15]

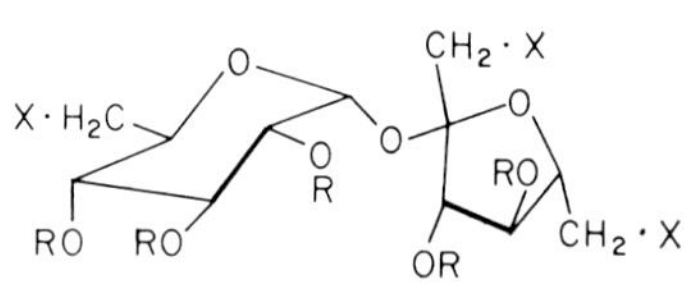

(15) R = Bz, X = OTs (18) R = H, X = NH_2

(16) R = Bz, X = N_3

(17) R = H, X = N_3

1′,6,6′-Tri-*O*-tosylsucrose pentabenzoate (15) underwent nucleophilic substitution with azide in hexamethylphosphoric triamide to afford 1′,6,6′-triazido-1′,6,6′-trideoxysucrose pentabenzoate (16).

Catalytic de-esterification of (16) gave 1′,6,6′-triazido-1′,6,6′-trideoxysucrose (17) which was subsequently hydrogenated to give 1′,6,6′-triamino-1′,6,6′-trideoxysucrose (18).[16]

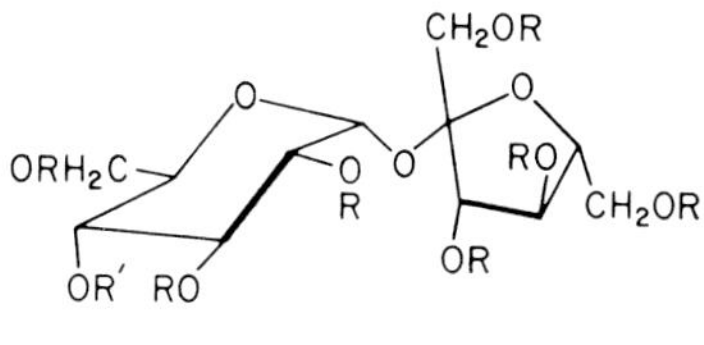

(19) R = Ac, R′ = Ms

(20) R = Ac, R′ = Ts

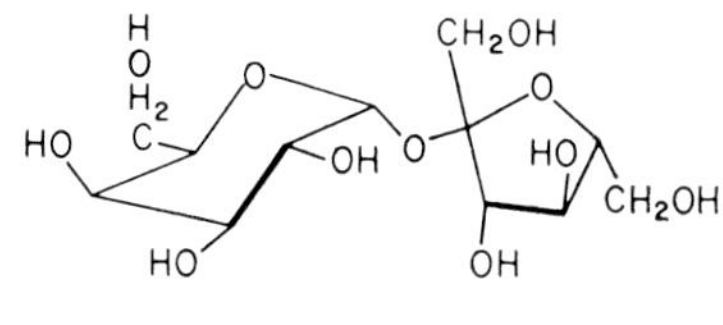

(21)

S_N2 displacement reaction of 4-*O*-sulphonate derivatives of sucrose (19) and (20) with sodium benzoate in hexamethylphosphoric triamide gave a product with inversion of configuration at C-4, which on catalytic de-esterification afforded crystalline α-D-galactopyranosyl-β-D-fructofuranoside (21) in 62% yield.[17] It was of interest to note that the change of the hydroxyl group configuration at C-4 in sucrose caused almost complete loss of sweetness.

EXOCYCLIC VINYL ETHER DERIVATIVES OF SUCROSE

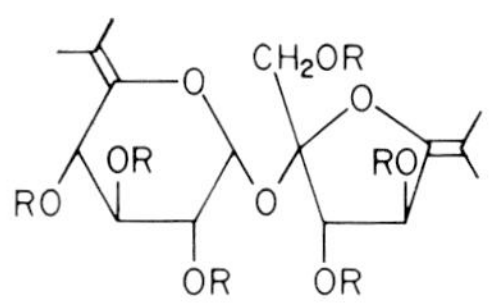

(22) R = Bz

(23) R = Ms

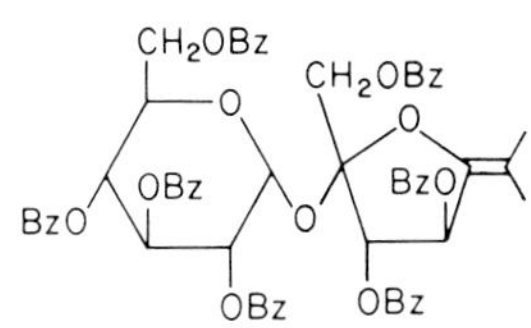

(24)

The potential importance of exocyclic, vinyl ether derivatives of sucrose as polymer and biological intermediates has stimulated considerable interest. Reactions of the 6,6′-diiodide (11) and 6,6′-diiodo-6,6′-dideoxysucrose hexamesylate with silver fluoride in pyridine gave the crystalline 5,5′-diene esters (22) and (23), respectively.[3] Similar treatment of 6′-iodo-6′-deoxysucrose heptabenzoate with silver fluoride in pyridine afforded, after chromatographic fractionation, 6-deoxy-5′-enosucrose heptabenzoate (24).[18]

REACTION WITH SULPHURYL CHLORIDE

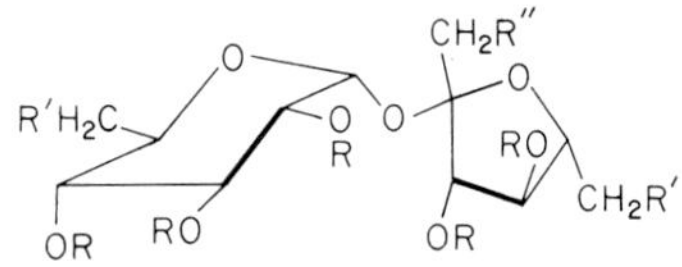

(25) R = Bz, R″ = OBz, R′ = OH

(26) R = Bz, R′ = R″ = OH

(27) R = Bz, R″ = OBz, R′ = OSO_2Cl

(28) R = Bz, R′ = R″ = OSO_2Cl

(29) R = H, R″ = OH, R′ = Cl

Reaction of sulphuryl chloride with sucrose has been reported by Jones *et al.*[19] to give a mixture of products from which 4,6,1′-trichloro-4,6,1′-trideoxysucrose-2,3:3′,6′-disulphate and 4,6,6′-trichloro-4,6,6′-trideoxysucrose tetrakis (chlorosulphate) were isolated.[20] The structure of these compounds still needs to be confirmed. On the other hand, the controlled reaction of sulphuryl chloride with sucrose hexabenzoate (25)[21] and sucrose pentabenzoate (26)[9] has been reported to give hexa-*O*-benzoylsucrose-6,6′-bis(chlorosulphate) (27) and penta-*O*-benzoylsucrose-1′,6,6′-tris(chlorosulphate) (28), respectively.[22] Hough *et al.* have reinvestigated the reaction of sucrose with sulphuryl chloride and have obtained amongst other chlorodeoxy derivatives of sucrose, 6,6′-dichloro-6,6′-dideoxysucrose in 29% yield.[23,24]

REACTION WITH METHANESULPHONYL CHLORIDE–*N,N*-DIMETHYL FORMAMIDE COMPLEX[25]

The value of 6,6′-dichloro-6,6′-dideoxysucrose (29)[3] as an intermediate in the synthesis of other derivatives such as deoxy-, bromo-, anhydro-, azido- and amino-deoxysucrose is well recognised. In this context, reaction of sucrose with methanesulphonyl chloride in

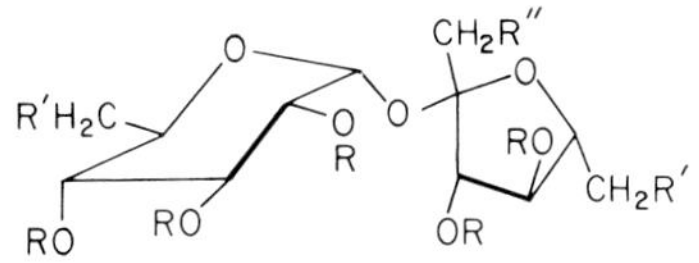

(30) R = AC, R″ = OAC, R′ = Cl

(31) R = AC, R′ = R″ = Cl

(32) R = Bz, R″ = OBz, R′ = Cl

(33) R = Bz, R″ = OH, R′ = Cl

(34) R = Bz, R″ = R″ = Cl

N,*N*-dimethyl formamide was investigated and 6,6′-dichloro-6,6′-dideoxysucrose (29) was obtained in 85% yield.[26] The high yield and ease in working up constitutes a great improvement over other methods. When the same reaction is carried out at higher temperature, it gives a mixture of products from which 6,6′-dichloro-6,6′-dideoxysucrose hexaacetate (30), 1′-6,6′-trichloro-1,6,6′-trideoxysucrose pentaacetate (31) and a second, so far uncharacterised, trichlorotrideoxysucrose pentaacetate were obtained in the yields of 40%, 25% and 10%, respectively.[26] The latter compound according to m.s. data showed two chlorine atoms in the pyranosyl and one chlorine in the ketofuranosyl residue.

Similar reaction of methanesulphonyl chloride–*N*,*N*-dimethyl formamide complex $(Me_2N^+ = CHOMs)Cl^-$ with sucrose hexabenzoate (25) and sucrose pentabenzoate (26) afforded 6,6′-dichloro-6,6′-dideoxysucrose hexabenzoate (32) and 6,6′-dichlorodideoxysucrose pentabenzoate (33), respectively.[27] 1′,6,6′-Trichloro-1,6,6′-trideoxysucrose pentabenzoate (34) from (26) was obtained in 30% yield when the reaction was conducted at higher temperature.[27]

PHYSICAL METHODS

The structures of most of the sucrose derivatives have been confirmed by 100 MHz p.m.r. spectroscopy. Electron-impact ionisation mass spectrometry is extensively used in the structural studies of sucrose derivatives.[36] The initial fragmentation of acetates, benzoates and trimethylsilyl derivatives of sucrose reveal hexapyranosyl (35) and

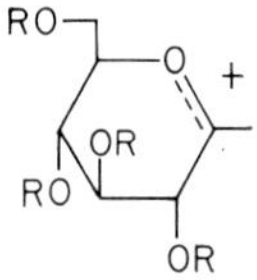

(35)

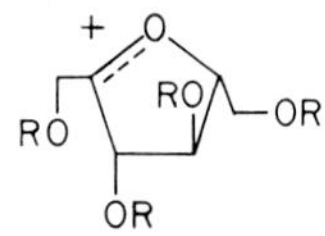

(36)

fructofuranosyl (36) cations, followed by a sequence of fragmentation reactions of the glycosyl residue.[23,24,26,28] This technique permits the rapid and precise identification of sucrose derivatives, prior to the final configurational analysis by p.m.r. spectroscopy.

ACNOWLEDGEMENTS

I am grateful to Professor A. J. Vlitos, Chief Executive, Tate & Lyle Group Research and Development, for his interest and encouragement; to the International Sugar Research Foundation, Inc. (Bethesda, USA) under whose aegis part of this work was undertaken, and to Dr K. J. Parker and Dr K. S. Mufti for helpful discussions.

REFERENCES

1. Reinefeld, E. and Klandinos, S. (1968). *Zucker,* **21,** p. 330.
2. Lemieux, R. U. and McInnes, S. (1962). *Can. J. Chem.,* **40,** p. 2394.
3. Bolton, C. H., Hough, L. and Khan, R. (1972). *Carbohyd. Res.,* **21,** p. 133.
4. Hough, L. and Mufti, K. S. (1972). *Carbohyd. Res.,* **25,** p. 497.
5. Hough, L. and Mufti, K. S. *Carbohyd. Res.,* in press.
6. Lemieux, R. U. and Barrette, J. P. (1959). *Can. J. Chem.,* **37,** p. 1964.
7. Lemieux, R. U. and Barrette, J. P. (1959). *Can. J. Chem.,* **38,** p. 656.
8. Isaacs, N. W., Kennard, C. H. L., O'Donnell, G. W. and Richards, G. N. (1970). *Chem. Commun.,* p. 360.
9. Khan, R. (1972). *Carbohyd. Res.,* **22,** p. 441.
10. Lemieux, R. U. and Barrette, J. P. (1958). *J. Amer. Chem. Soc.,* **80,** p. 2243.
11. Buchanan, J. G. and Cummerson, D. A. (1972). *Carbohyd. Res.,* **21,** p. 293.
12. Buchanan, J. G., Cummerson, D. A. and Turner, D. M. (1972). *Carbohyd. Res.,* **21,** p. 283.

13. Dutcher, J. D. (1963). *Advan. Carbohyd. Chem.*, **18,** p. 259.
14. Sharon, N. (1965). In *The Amino Sugars,* Vol. 1a, Eds. E. A. Balazs and R. W. Jeanloz, Academic Press, New York, p. 1.
15. Khan, R. (unpublished results).
16. Khan, R., Mufti, K. S. and Jenner, M. R. (in press).
17. Khan, R. (1972). *Carbohyd. Res.,* **25,** p. 232.
18. Khan, R. and Jenner, M. R. (unpublished data).
19. Bragg, P. D., Jones, J. K. N. and Turner, J. C. (1959). *Can. J. Chem.,* **37,** p. 1412.
20. Kollonitsch, V. (1970). *Sucrose Chemicals,* C. H. Kline & Co., p. 85.
21. Hough, L., Mufti, K. S. and Khan, R. (1972). *Carbohyd. Res.,* **21,** p. 144.
22. Khan, R. (1972). *Carbohyd. Res.,* **25,** p. 504.
23. Ballard, J. M., Hough, L. and Richardson, A. C. (1972). *Chem. Commun.,* p. 1097.
24. Ballard, J. M., Hough, L., Richardson, A. C. and (in part) Fairclough, P. H. *Carbohyd. Res.,* Part XII (in press).
25. Evans, M. E., Long, L. Jnr and Parrish, F. W. (1968). *J. Org. Chem.,* **33,** p. 1074.
26. Khan, R. and Mufti, K. S. *Carbohyd. Res.* (in press).
27. Khan, R., Mufti, K. S. and Jenner, M. R. (unpublished data).
28. Binkley, W. W., Dougherty, A. C., Horton, D. and Wander, J. D. (1971). *Carbohyd. Res.,* **17,** p. 127.
29. Mckeown, G. G., Serenius, R. S. E. and Hayward, L. D. (1957). *Can. J. Chem.,* **35,** p. 28.
30. Hough, L. and Mufti, K. S. *Carbohyd. Res.,* Part IX (in press).
31. Suami, T., Kato, N., Kawamura, M. and Nishimura, T. (1971). *Carbohyd. Res.,* **19,** p. 407.
32. Ballard, J. M., Hough, L. and Richardson, A. C. (1972). *Carbohyd. Res.,* **22,** p. 441.
33. Bredereck, H., Tinner, H., Wagner, A., Faber, G., Greiner, W. and Huber W. (1958). *Chem. Ber.,* **19,** p. 2824.
34. Jezo, I. (1971). *Chem. Zvesti,* **25,** p. 364.
35. Otake, T. (1970). *Bull. Chem. Soc. Japan,* **43,** p. 3199.
36. Khan, R. (unpublished data).
37. Khan, R., Birch, G. G. and Lindley, M. (unpublished data).
38. Linstead, R. P., Rutenberg, A., Dauben, W. G., and Evans, W. L. (1940). *J. Amer. Chem. Soc.,* **62,** p. 3260.
39. Ness, R. K. and Fletcher, H. G. Jnr. (1952). *J. Amer. Chem. Soc.,* **74,** p. 5344.
40. Hockett, R. C. and Zief, M. (1950). *J. Amer. Chem. Soc.,* **72,** p. 1839.

A list of some characterised derivatives of sucrose

	Melting point	$[\alpha]_D$	Ref.
6,6′-Di-*O*-tosylsucrose	112–114°	+60° (c 1·2, Pyridine)	7, 3
6,6′-Di-*O*-tosylsucrose hexaacetate	64–67°	+55° (c 2·4, CH_2Cl_2)	3
6,6′-Di-*O*-tosylsucrose hexabenzoate	93–96°	+26·3° (c 1·1, CH_2Cl_2)	3
6,6′-Di-*O*-tosylsucrose hexamesylate	97–100°	+32° (c 2·0, $CHCl_3$)	3
6,6′-Diiodo-6,6′-dideoxysucrose hexaacetate			3
6,6′-Diiodo-6,6′-dideoxysucrose hexabenzoate	178–179°	−1·6° (c 1·5, $CHCl_3$)	3
6,6′-Diiodo-6,6′-dideoxysucrose hexamesylate	218–219°	+41·8° (c 2·0, acetone)	3
6,6′-Dideoxysucrose hexabenzoate	118–120°	+19·6° (c 1·42, $CHCl_3$)	3
6,6′-Dideoxysucrose hexamesylate	191–192°	+44·4° (c 2·45, acetone)	3
6,6′-Diazido-6,6′-dideoxysucrose	163–164°	+78·8° (c 0·98, H_2O)	4,15
6,6′-Diazido-6,6′-dideoxysucrose hexaacetate	Syrup	+5·8° (c 5·4, $CHCl_3$)	4
6,6′-Diazido-6,6′-dideoxysucrose hexabenzoate	75–78°	+42·5° (c 1·6, CH_2Cl_2)	3
6,6′-Diazido-6,6′-dideoxysucrose hexamesylate	189–190°	+41·4° (c 1·2, Pyridine)	3

6,6′-Dichloro-6,6′-dideoxysucrose	85–88°	+60° (c 0·5, H_2O)	4
6-6′-Dichloro-6,6′-dideoxysucrose hexaacetate	117–118°	+55° (c 0·55, $CHCl_3$)	4
6-6′-Dichloro-6,6′-dideoxysucrose hexabenzoate	165–167°	+5·8° (c 1, $CHCl_3$)	3, 22
6,6′-Dichloro-6,6′-dideoxy-1′-chlorosulphate sucrose pentabenzoate	136–137°	+11·5° (c 1.12, $CHCl_3$)	22
6,6′-Dichloro-6,6′-dideoxysucrose hexamesylate	139–140°	+52·5° (c 1·0, acetone)	30
6,6′-Dibromo-6,6′-dideoxysucrose hexabenzoate	176–178°	+0·3° (c 0·33, $CHCl_3$)	30
6,6′-Dibromo-6,6′-dideoxysucrose hexamesylate	171–173°	+39·5° (c 0·89, acetone)	30
6,6′-Dithiocyanato-6,6′-dideoxysucrose hexaacetate	169–171°	+71° (c 1·0, $CHCl_3$)	3
6,6′-Dithiocyanato-6,6′-dideoxysucrose hexabenzoate	92–95°	+31·9° (c 1·4, CH_2Cl_2)	3
6,6′-Dithiocyanato-6,6′-dideoxysucrose hexamesylate	177–180°	+68·5° (c 1·2, acetone)	3
6,6′-Diamino-6,6′-dideoxysucrose	105–110°	+51·6° (c 1·53, H_2O)	15
6,6′-Diacetamido-6,6′-dideoxysucrose	85–88°	+44·5° (c 0·86, CH_3OH)	15
6,6′-Diacetamido-6,6′-dideoxysucrose hexaacetate	86–89°	+70·5° (c 1.14, $CHCl_3$)	15
6,6′-Dideoxy-5,5′-dienesucrose hexabenzoate	145–147°	−5° (c 1·0, $CHCl_3$)	3

A list of some characterised derivatives of sucrose—contd.

	Melting point	$[\alpha]_D$	Ref.
6,6′-Dideoxy-5,5′-dienesucrose hexamesylate	110–111°	+13·7° (c 1·9, acetone)	3
6,6′-Bis(chlorosulphate)sucrose hexabenzoate	Syrup	+13.1° (c 1·43, $CHCl_3$)	22
6,6′-Di-*O*-tritylsucrose	134–136°	+43° (c 0·2, $CHCl_3$)	21
6,6′-Di-*O*-tritylsucrose hexaacetate	104–105°	+64·6° (c 0·2, $CHCl_3$)	21
6,6′-Di-*O*-tritylsucrose hexabenzoate	107–110°	+3° (c 0·2, $CHCl_3$)	21
1′,6′-Di-*O*-tritylsucrose hexaacetate	95–98°	+65·3 (c 0·53, $CHCl_3$)	11
1′,2,3,3′,4,4′-Hexa-*O*-benzoylsucrose	Syrup	+23° (c 0·61, $CHCl_3$)	21
1′,6,6′-Tri-*O*-tritylsucrose	128–130°	+62·2° (c 0·87, $CHCl_3$)	21
1′,6,6′-Tri-*O*-tritylsucrose pentaacetate	235–236°	+68·9° (c 2·45, $CHCl_3$)	
1′,6,6′-Tri-*O*-tritylsucrose pentabenzoate	129–131°	+14·9° (c 0·91, $CHCl_3$)	21
2,3,4,3′,4′-Penta-*O*-acetylsucrose	133–134°	+52·5° (c 0·4, $CHCl_3$)	31, 33
2,3,6,3′,4′-Penta-*O*-acetylsucrose	155–156°	+22° (c 3·1, $CHCl_3$)	29

2,3,4,3′,4′-Penta-*O*-benzoylsucrose	Syrup	+2·1° (c 0·62, $CHCl_3$)	9
1′,6,6′-Tri-*O*-tosylsucrose	Syrup	+41° (c 2·12, $CHCl_3$)	9, 31
1′,6,6′-Tri-*O*-tosylsucrose pentaacetate	135·5–136·5°	+68° (c 0·44, $CHCl_3$)	31
1′,6,6′-Tri-*O*-tosylsucrose pentabenzoate	87–90°	+19° (c 1·91, $CHCl_3$)	9
1′,6,6′-Tri-*O*-mesylsucrose pentabenzoate	99–101°	+27° (c 1·32, $CHCl_3$)	9
6,6′-Diiodo-6,6′-dideoxy-1′-*O*-tosylsucrose pentaacetate	69–71°	+32° (c 0·72, $CHCl_3$)	31
6,6′-Dideoxy-1′-*O*-tosylsucrose pentaacetate	Syrup	+60·3° (c 0·32, $CHCl_3$)	31
1′6,6′-Triazido-1′,6,6′-trideoxysucrose	Syrup	+64° (c 0·58, acetone)	16
1′,6,6′-Triazido-1′,6,6′-trideoxysucrose pentabenzoate	58–60°	+30·6° (c 1·06, $CHCl_3$)	16
1′,6,6′-Triazido-1′,6,6′-trideoxysucrose pentaacetate	Syrup	+101·2° (c 0·57, $CHCl_3$)	16
1′,6,6′-Triazido-1′,6,6′-trideoxysucrose pentamesylate	72–74°	+54·7° (c 0·72, $CHCl_3$)	16
1′,6,6′-Triamino-1′,6,6′-trideoxysucrose	121–125°	+68·5° (c 0·85, H_2O)	16
1′,6,6′-Triacetamido-1′,6,6′-trideoxysucrose	107–110°	+36·4° (c 1, CH_3OH)	16
1′,6,6′-Triacetamido-1′,6,6′-trideoxysucrose pentaacetate	99–101°	+37·3° (c 0·98, $CHCl_3$)	16

A list of some characterised derivatives of sucrose—contd.

	Melting point	$[\alpha]_D$	Ref.
1′,6,6′-Tris(chlorosulphate)sucrose pentabenzoate	133–134°	+19·8° (c 1·31, $CHCl_3$)	22
1′,6,6′-Trichloro-1′,6,6′-trideoxysucrose	Syrup	+52·5° (c 0·66, acetone)	22
1′,6,6′-Trichloro-1′,6,6′-trideoxysucrose pentaacetate	Syrup	+78·3° (c 1·03, $CHCl_3$)	26
1′,6,6′-Trichloro-1′,6,6′-trideoxysucrose pentabenzoate	90–92°	+3·9° (c 0·49, $CHCl_3$)	22
1′,4,6′-Tri-*O*-methylsucrose	Syrup	+67·6° (c 1·74, H_2O)	29
1′,4,6′-Tri-*O*-methylsucrose pentaacetate	Syrup	+57·7° (c 3·72)	29
1′,4,6′-Tri-*O*-tosylsucrose pentaacetate	85–91°	—	10
1′,4,6′-Tri-*O*-mesylsucrose pentaacetate	56–58°	+36·1° (c 0·51, acetone)	5
3′,4′-Di-*O*-acetyl-1′,6′-di-*O*-benzoyl-*β*-D-fructofuranosyl-2,3,6-tri-*O*-acetyl-4-*O*-benzoyl-*α*-D-galactopyranoside	Syrup	+14·9° (c 1·33, $CHCl_3$)	5
3′,4′-Di-*O*-acetyl-6′-*O*-benzoyl-1′-*O*-mesyl-*β*-D-fructofuranosyl-2,3,6-tri-*O*-acetyl-4-*O*-benzoyl-*α*-D-galactopyranoside	Syrup	+15·6° (c 1·7, $CHCl_3$)	5
1′-*O*-Mesyl-*β*-D-fructofuranosyl-*α*-D-galactopyranoside	158–161°	+70·1° (c 0·27, H_2O)	5
1′,4,6′-Triazido-1′,4,6′-trideoxy galactosucrose pentaacetate	57–59°	+40·1° (c 1·0, $CHCl_3$)	5
4,6′-Diazido-4,6′-dideoxy-1′-*O*-mesylgalactosucrose pentaacetate	135–138°	−7·1° (c 0·7, acetone)	5

1′,4,6′-Triazido-1′,4,6′-trideoxy galactosucrose pentamesylate	63–65°	+73·3° (c 0·23, acetone)	5
6,4,6′-Tribromo-6,4,6′-trideoxygalactosucrose pentamesylate	140–141°	+54·8° (c 0·75, acetone)	30
4-Azido-4,6,6′-trideoxygalactosucrose pentamesylate	79–83°	+39·6° (c 1·55, acetone)	30
1′,4,6,6′-Tetrazido-1′,4,6,6′-tetradeoxygalactosucrose tetramesylate	171–173°	+45·7° (c 0·28, acetone)	30
3′,6′-Anhydrosucrose	146°	+104° (c 1·2, CH_3OH)	12
1′,4′:3′,6′-Dianhydrosucrose	184–185°	—	11
3,6:3′,6′-Dianhydrosucrose	Syrup	—	3
3,6:3′,6′-Dianhydrosucrose tetraacetate	69–72°	+32·5° (c 1·0, $CHCl_3$)	3
1′,4′:3,6:3′,6′-Trianhydrosucrose	194–196°	+95° (c 2·4, H_2O)	8, 9
1′,4′:3,6:3′,6′-Trianhydrosucrose diacetate	183–185°	+116° (c 0·75, $CHCl_3$)	9
1′,2:3,6:3′,6′-Trianhydrosucrose	163–164·5°	+117°	6, 10
1′,2:3,6:3′,6′-Trianhydrosucrose diacetate	181·5–182·5°	+128·6° (c 1·8, $CHCl_3$)	10
1′,2:3,6:3′,6′-Trianhydrosucrose ditosylate	164·5–166°	—	6
4,4′-Di-*O*-methyl-1′,2:3,6:3′,6′-trianhydrosucrose	179–181°	+140° (c 1·9, $CHCl_3$)	6
3,6-Anhydro-α-D-galactosyl-1′,4′:3′,6′-dianhydro-β-D-fructofuranoside	191–192·5°	+137·5° (c 1·6. H_2O)	10
3,6-Anhydro-α-D-galactosyl-1′,4′:3′,6′-dianhydro-β-D-fructofuranoside diacetate	137·5–138·5°	+94·3° (c 2, $CHCl_3$)	10
Di-*O*-methyl-3,6-anhydro-α-D-galactosyl-1′,4′:3′,6′-anhydro-β-D-fructofuranoside	105–106°	+48·6° (c 1·45, $CHCl_3$)	10

A list of some characterised derivatives of sucrose—contd.

	Melting point	$[\alpha]_D$	Ref.
2,3,4,6,1′,3′,4′-Hepta-*O*-acetylsucrose	158–160°	+52·5° (c 0·4, $CHCl_3$)	12, 32
6′-Chloro-6′-deoxysucrose heptaacetate	116–117°	+56·3° (c 0·4, $CHCl_3$)	24
6′-*O*-Methylsucrose heptaacetate	Syrup	—	37
6-Chloro-6-deoxysucrose	Syrup	+55° (c 1·0, H_2O)	4
6′-*O*-Benzoyl-6-chloro-6-deoxysucrose hexaacetate	Syrup	+61·9° (c 0·1, $CHCl_3$)	4
6-Chloro-6-deoxysucrose heptamesylate	99–101°	+50° (c 0·15, acetone)	4
6-Azido-6-deoxysucrose heptabenzoate	80–83°	+28·5° (c 0·07, acetone)	4
6-Azido-6-deoxysucrose heptaacetate	78–81°	+62·8° (c 1·0, $CHCl_3$)	34
6-Amino-6-deoxysucrose heptaacetate	90–92°	+54° (c 1·0, CH_3OH)	34
6-*O*-Tritylsucrose	99–101°	+51·7° (c 4, DMF)	35
6′-*O*-Tritylsucrose	221–223°	+40·1° (c 0·86, $CHCl_3$)	11, 35
6′-*O*-Tritylsucrose heptaacetate	118°	+58·5° (c 0·96, $CHCl_3$)	11
6′-Phosphatesucrose	Syrup	—	11
6′-Chloro-6′-deoxysucrose heptamesylate	214–218°	+47·3° (c 0·5, acetone)	24

1′,2,3,3′,4′,6′-Hexa-*O*-acetyl-6′-*O*-tritylsucrose	Syrup	+19·9° (c 3·47, $CHCl_3$)	17
4-*O*-Mesyl-6′-*O*-tritylsucrose hexaacetate	85–87°	+29·4° (c 2·19, $CHCl_3$)	17
4-*O*-Tosyl-6′-*O*-tritylsucrose hexaacetate	82–84°	+31·3° (c 1·98, $CHCl_3$)	17
1′,2,3,3′,4′,6-Hexa-*O*-acetyl-4-*O*-mesylsucrose	Syrup	+22·1° (c 1·46, $CHCl_3$)	17
1′,2,3,3′,4′,6-Hexa-*O*-acetyl-4-*O*-tosylsucrose	Syrup	20·6° (c 2·34, $CHCl_3$)	17
4-*O*-Mesylsucrose heptaacetate	94–95°	+25·2° (c 1·26, $CHCl_3$)	17
4-*O*-Tosylsucrose heptaacetate	Syrup	24·5° (c 2·48, $CHCl_3$)	17
α-D-Galactopyranosyl β-D-fructofuranoside	177–179°	+82·3° (c 0·63, H_2O)	17, 5
2,3,4,6-Tetra-*O*-acetyl-α-D-galactopyranosyl-1′,3′,4′,6′-tetra-*O*-acetyl-β-D-fructofuranoside	Syrup	+52·6° (c 0·47, $CHCl_3$)	17
Galactosucrose octabenzoate	79–81°	+52·6° (c 0·72, $CHCl_3$)	17
4,6-Dichloro-4,6-dideoxy-α-D-galactopyranosyl-3′,4′-anhydro-1′,6′-dichloro-1′,6′-dideoxy-β-D-ribohexulofuranoside-2,3-sulphate	146–148°	+68·5° (c 0·5, $CHCl_3$)	24
4,6-Dichloro-1′,3′,4′,6′-tetradeoxy-β-D-glycerohex-3′-enofuranoside-2,3-sulphate	111–112°	+79° (c 0·4, $CHCl_3$)	24
4,6-Dichloro-4,6-dideoxy-α-D-galactopyranosyl-1′,4′,6′-trichloro-1′,4′,6′-trideoxy-β-D-hexulofuranoside-2,3-sulphate	107–111°	—	24
Octa-*O*-acetylsucrose	69°	+59·6°	38
Octa-*O*-benzoylsucrose	81–84°	+37° (c 1·16, $CHCl_3$)	39
Octa-*O*-mesylsucrose	205–206°	+47° (c 1·85, acetone)	40, 3
Octa-*O*-tosylsucrose	82–86°	+41·78°	40

4

New Speciality Glucose Syrups*

G. B. MADSEN and B. E. NORMAN

Novo Industrias, Copenhagen, Denmark

ABSTRACT

The use of enzymes for the industrial hydrolysis of starch has introduced a range of glucose syrups with widely varying carbohydrate composition on the world market.

These syrups are characterised according to DE and carbohydrate spectrum. The traditional categories (high maltose, high DE and low DE syrups) are no longer sufficient. Isomerised syrups have been introduced. The term 'high DE syrups' was originally used for 60–70 *DE syrups but is now also used for* 90–98 *DE syrups for fermentation or hydrogenation.*

A number of experiments have been carried out on the production of 60–70 *DE as well as* 90–98 *DE syrups to demonstrate the influence of the liquefied starch substrate and the enzyme dosage on the final carbohydrate spectrum.*

The production of high maltose syrups by fungal alpha-amylase is described.

INTRODUCTION

The number of starch hydrolysing enzymes freely available to the starch industry is surprisingly low. In spite of this, there is a wide variety of starch hydrolysates being sold on the world market.

The enzymes can roughly be divided into four groups: bacterial alpha-amylases, glucoamylases, fungal alpha-amylases, and beta-amylases. A fifth group of enzymes, glucose isomerases, is being marketed, but cannot as of this moment be designated 'freely available'.

This paper will primarily be dealing with glucose syrups (*i.e.* starch hydrolysates sold as syrups) with dextrose equivalents above 40.

* Read by Miss G. B. Madsen.

So far the majority of glucose syrups have been produced using acid liquefaction, either alone or followed by an enzymatic treatment. However, the tendency is slowly shifting towards purely enzymatic processes.[1-3]

By varying reaction conditions, using different combinations of the above mentioned enzymes and in some cases using acid liquefaction in connection with the enzymes, a series of speciality glucose syrups has been developed. These syrups are characterised according to dextrose equivalents (DE's) and carbohydrate spectrum.

The traditional categories were: high maltose, high DE and low DE syrups. However, these categories are no longer sufficient. Syrups with DE's of 90–98 are being produced and sold in a liquid form, but must in practice be kept at temperatures above 35°C to avoid crystallisation. In order to avoid misunderstandings the high DE category syrups should therefore be separated into two categories, syrups with DE's from 60 to 70, and syrups with DE's from 90 to 98.

The 60 to 70 DE syrups are the ones that were originally called high DE syrups. Their carbohydrate spectrum is such that crystallisation will not occur at ambient temperature at total solids contents up to 80–83%

The 90–98 DE syrups will crystallise immediately under the same conditions, and these syrups are therefore primarily being produced for fermentation industries located in the neighbourhood of the syrups plant. The 90–98 DE syrups are also suitable for hydrogenation, but preferably only those with DE's above 96.

Finally, a completely new category of syrups must be added, the isomerised syrups.

STARCH HYDROLYSING ENZYMES

Before going into detail about the influence of enzyme dosages, liquefaction methods and other factors on the composition of the final syrups, we would like to give a short description of the mode of action of the different starch hydrolysing enzymes.

Bacterial Alpha-amylase

Bacterial amylases prepared from *Bacillus subtilis* will hydrolyse alpha-1,4 links in amylose and amylopectin at random. These enzymes have an optimum working pH of 6–7 and are relatively stable at high temperatures (85°C) in the presence of starch. They are therefore very suitable for starch liquefaction as this temperature lies above the gelatinisation temperature of most starches.

Fungal Alpha-amylase

Fungal alpha-amylases prepared from *Aspergillus oryzae* will also hydrolyse alpha-1,4 links in amylose and amylopectin. These enzymes are less heat-stable than bacterial amylases and are rapidly inactivated at temperatures above 55°C. They are therefore totally unsuitable for starch liquefaction.

However, fungal alpha-amylases will hydrolyse starch to a much greater extent than bacterial amylases, and large amounts of maltose and maltotriose are formed during the reaction. This makes them particularly useful for the preparation of syrups where large quantities of maltose are required.

Glucoamylase

Glucoamylase enzymes hydrolyse starch and α-1,4-glucans by releasing single glucose units from the non-reducing end of the molecule in a step-wise manner. Alpha-1,6 links are also hydrolysed, although at a much slower rate, and so it is possible to degrade liquefied starch completely to glucose. The optimum working temperature for glucoamylase from *Aspergillus niger* is 60°C at a pH of 4·5.

Beta-amylase

Beta-amylases are widely distributed in cereals such as barley, rye and wheat, in soya beans and sweet potatoes. The most common source of beta-amylase for commercial use is malt extract.

Beta-amylase will hydrolyse amylose, amylopectin and other α-1,4-glucans by releasing maltose units from the non-reducing end of the molecule. The maltose released is in the β-anomeric form, hence the name beta-amylase.

Alpha-1,6-glucosidase activity is absent from beta-amylase and so the branch points in amylopectin are not hydrolysed. The enzyme is not able to bypass these points and unless the amylopectin has been partially degraded with acid or alpha-amylase a so-called beta limit dextrin remains.

SYRUPS

60–70 DE Syrups

The most important requirement of these syrups is that they should have the highest possible DE and still be stable to crystallisation at temperatures above 4°C at 80–83% total solids.

A rule of thumb is that there will be a risk of crystallisation when the glucose concentration lies above 43%, calculated on a d.s. basis. This, of course, is not a very accurate figure. Other factors like the maltose concentration and the oligosaccharide composition should be taken into account. Nevertheless, we are using this 43% rule for the evaluation of the 60–70 DE syrups we have produced in our laboratory.

We have made four series of experiments in which the amounts of fungal alpha-amylase (Fungamyl 1600) and glucoamylase (Amyloglucosidase NOVO (AMG) 150) were varied. In all experiments the temperature was held at 55°C and the pH at 5·0. After 42 hr of saccharification, the syrups were analysed for DE, glucose, maltose and maltotriose content.

We used three different substrates, a 38 DE acid hydrolysed syrup, a 20 DE acid hydrolysed syrup and a 20 DE enzyme hydrolysed syrup.

The first series of experiments was carried out using 75 g of Fungamyl 1600 and varying the AMG dosage between 0 and 250 ml per ton of starch dry weight. The substrate was 38 DE acid hydrolysed syrup. The second series of experiments was carried out using the same substrate but double the amount of Fungamyl 1600, *i.e.* 150 g per ton of starch. From these data the influence of enzyme dosage can be seen.

Figure 1 shows the change in final DE and carbohydrate spectrum with increasing dosage of AMG 150 with a fixed Fungamyl dosage of 75 g per ton of starch. Figure 2 shows the corresponding results when using 150 g of Fungamyl per ton of starch.

If the limit of 43% glucose is taken into consideration, the highest acceptable DE using the high Fungamyl dosage will be approximately 68·5. Approximately the same DE was found with half the amount of Fungamyl. However, there is a difference in the carbohydrate composition of the two syrups. With the low Fungamyl dosage the maltose content is approximately 33% whereas the high dosage results in a syrup with 35% maltose. This means that the risk of

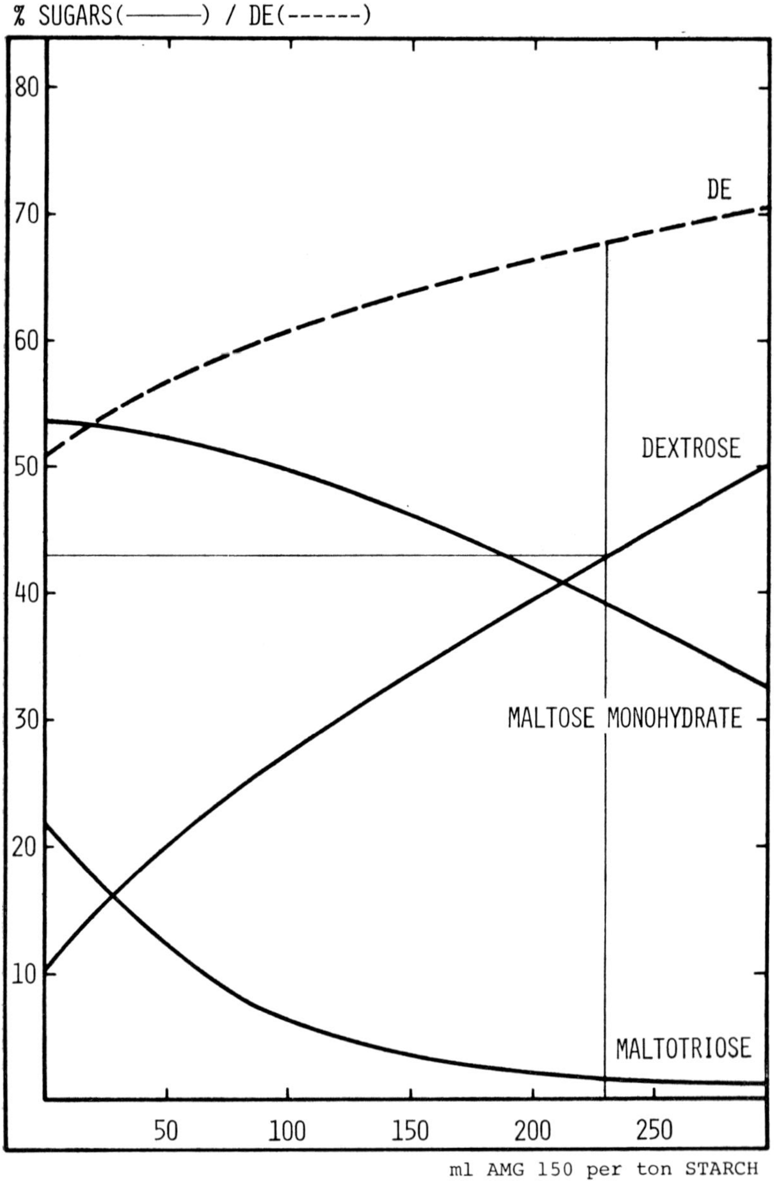

FIG.1. The effect of AMG concentration on syrup composition. Substrate: 38 DE acid converted corn starch—45% w/w. Temperature: 55°C. pH: 5·0. Reaction time: 42 hr. Enzyme dosage: 75 g Fungamyl 1600 per ton of starch.

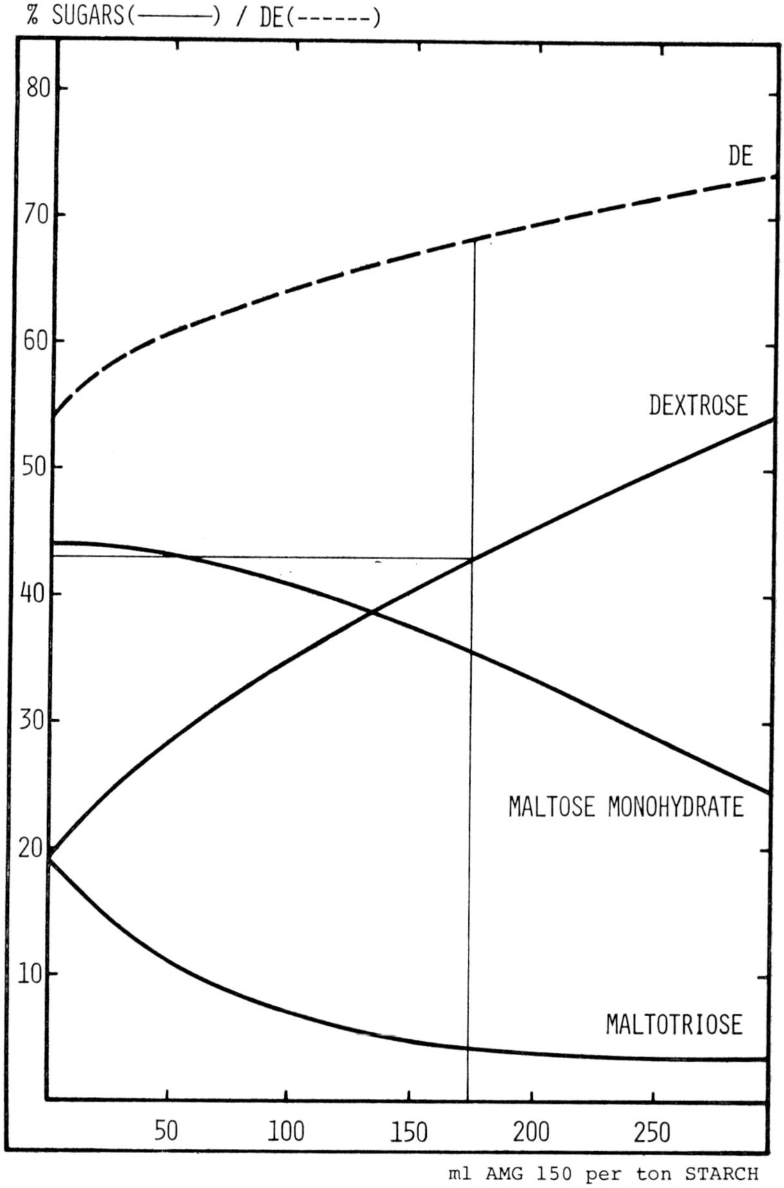

FIG. 2. The effect of AMG concentration on syrup composition. Substrate: 38 DE acid hydrolysed corn starch—45% w/w. Temperature: 55°C. pH: 5·0. Reaction time: 42 hr. Enzyme dosage: 150 g Fungamyl 1600 per ton of starch.

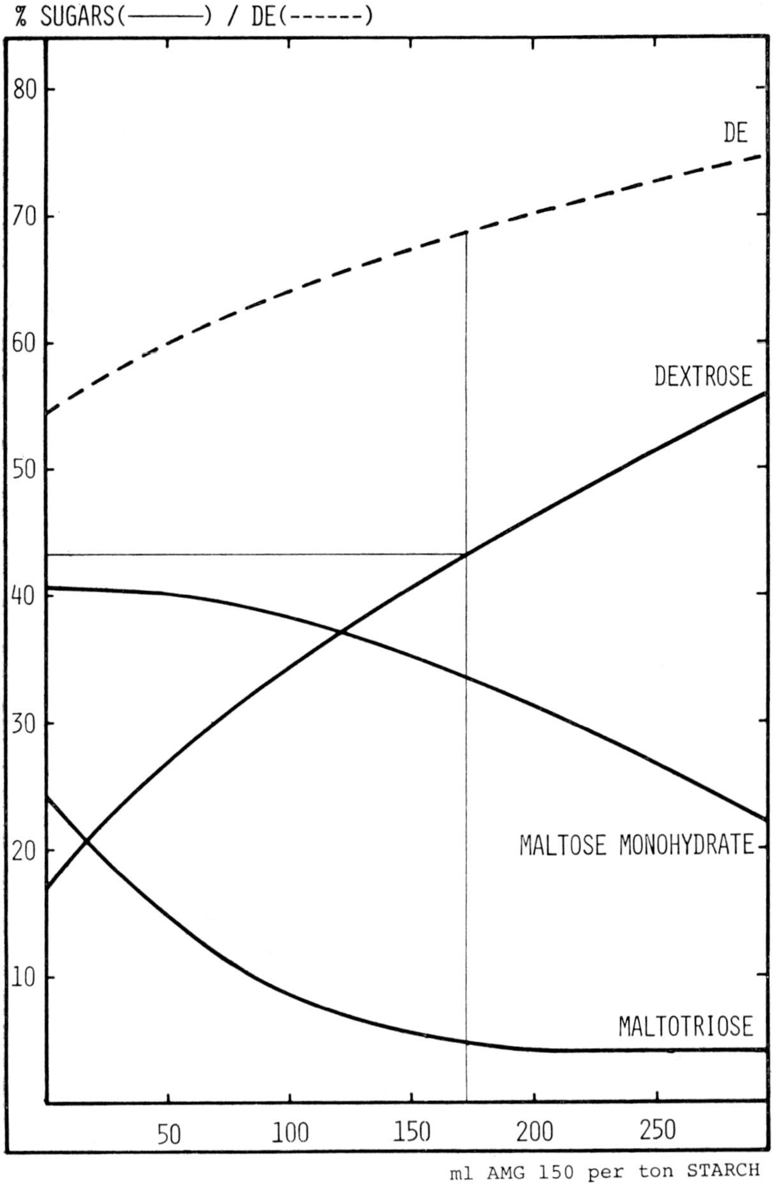

FIG. 3. The effect of AMG concentration on syrup composition. Substrate: 20 DE acid hydrolysed corn starch—45% w/w. Temperature : 55°C. pH: 5·0. Reaction time: 42 hr. Enzyme dosage: 150 g Fungamyl 1600 per ton of starch.

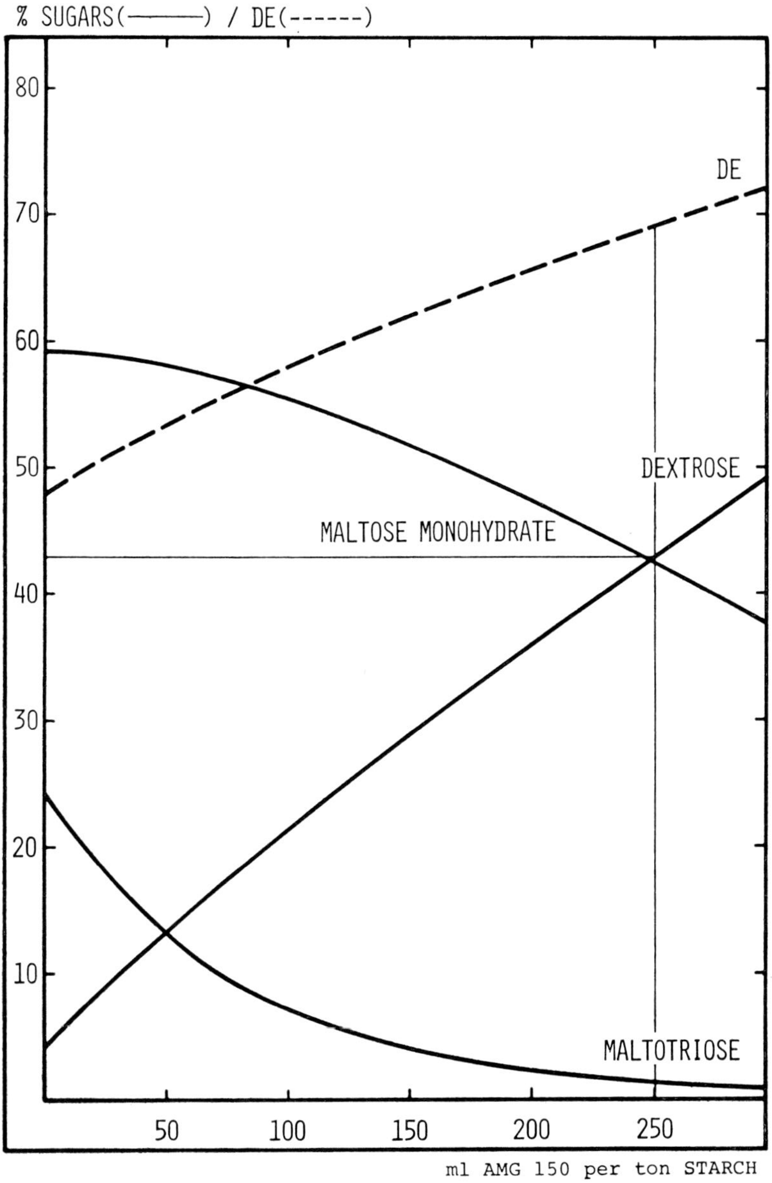

FIG. 4. The effect of AMG concentration on syrup composition. Substrate: 20 DE enzyme hydrolysed corn starch—45% w/w. Temperature: 55°C. pH: 5·0. Reaction time: 42 hr. Enzyme dosage: 150 g Fungamyl 1600 per ton of starch.

crystallisation is reduced with increasing dosage of fungal alpha-amylase.

In continuation of the second series of experiments, the influence of the substrate was examined. 20 DE acid liquefied syrup and 20 DE enzyme liquefied syrup were saccharified using 150 g Fungamyl per ton of starch and a varying AMG dosage.

Figure 3 shows the composition of the syrups made from the acid hydrolysed substrate. The syrup containing 43 % glucose has a DE of approximately 68, a maltose content of 39 % and a triose content of approximately 1·5 %.

Figure 4 shows the composition of the syrups made from enzyme hydrolysed substrate using the same amount of saccharifying enzymes. The syrup containing 43 % glucose has a DE of approximately 69, a maltose content of 42·5 % and a triose content of approximately 1 %. These experiments clearly demonstrate that a much higher maltose content is obtained when using enzymatic liquefaction.

The compositions of the syrups containing 43 % glucose prepared from the three different substrates are listed in Table 1.

TABLE 1

Composition of syrups containing 43 % glucose

Substrate	Acid DE 38	Acid DE 20	Enzyme DE 20
Final DE	68·5	68	69
AMG 150 dosage (ml/ton)	180	230	250
Glucose %	43	43	43
Maltose %	35	39	42·5
Triose %	4	1·5	1
Total fermentable sugars	82	83·5	86·5

The fermentability of the syrup prepared from the enzyme liquefied substrate is considerably higher than that of any of the ones prepared from acid liquefied starch. The glucose/maltose ratio is very favourable in the fully enzymatically produced syrup and the risk of crystallisation is thereby reduced to a minimum. Furthermore, the enzyme syrup is slightly sweeter than the others because of the higher content of maltose.

The 60–70 DE syrups are sold to many different industries. They are also sold to industries for whom the fermentability is the most important factor. To these industries a fermentability of 86·5% is still not quite satisfactory, and the alternative (crystalline dextrose or total sugar) is considerably more expensive. Because of this, the 90–98 DE syrups were developed.

90–98 DE Syrups

As mentioned before, these syrups are not stable to crystallisation so they must be transported in heated and/or insulated tankers and stored at temperatures above 35°C. The dry substance content of the syrups must also be kept fairly low (60–65%), and this means that prolonged storage and transport over long distances should be avoided.

In general the highest possible DE is desirable, because the fermentability of these syrups follows the DE value. The syrups may be produced by either an acid/enzyme process (*i.e.* acid liquefaction and enzymatic saccharification) or a dual enzyme process, but the highest final DE's are obtained when using the dual enzyme process.

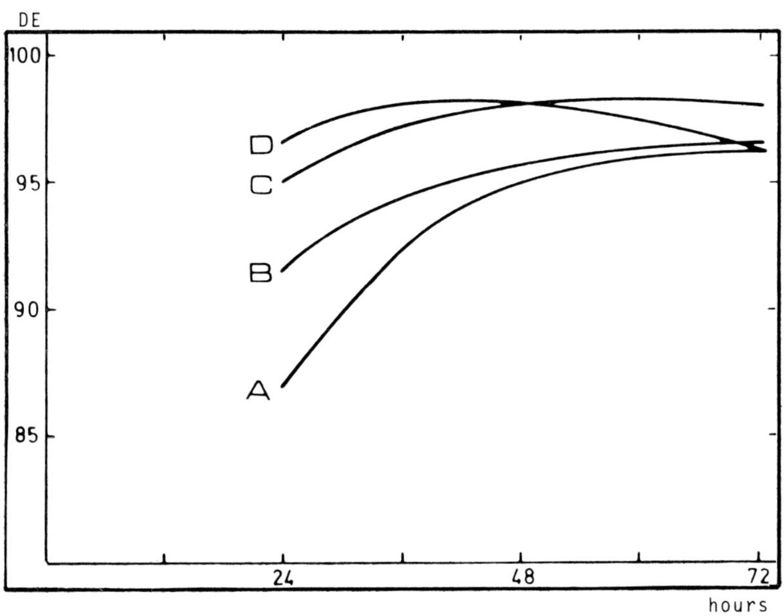

FIG. 5. Effect of enzyme concentration on reaction rate. Substrate concentration: 33%. Temperature: 60°C. pH: 4·5. Enzyme levels: A = 1·5, B = 2·0; C = 3·0; D = 3·5 litres Amyloglucosidase NOVO 75 per ton of starch.

The liquefied substrate is saccharified using a glucoamylase. In our experiments we used Amyloglucosidase NOVO 75 at a temperature of 60°C and a pH of 4·5. All substrates were enzyme liquefied to a DE of approximately 20.

Figure 5 illustrates the effect of enzyme concentration on reaction rate. If the reaction is allowed to continue after the highest DE has been reached, the DE will begin to fall. This effect, which is more noticeable at high enzyme concentrations, is due to the resynthesis of higher sugars from glucose. This reaction is catalysed by all glucoamylase preparations and is not due to the presence of enzyme impurities.

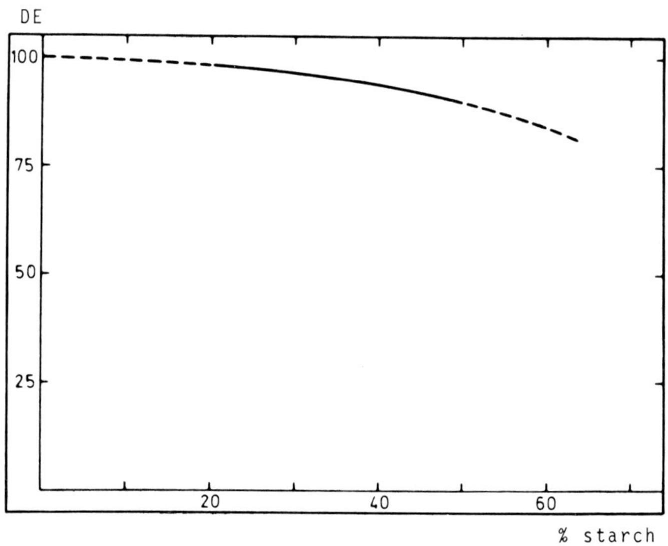

FIG. 6. Dependence of final DE on substrate concentration. Substrate: enzyme liquefied maize starch. Temperature: 60°C. pH: 4·5. Enzyme level: 2·5 litres Amyloglucosidase NOVO 75 per ton of starch.

The two most important sugars formed by this reversion or back polymerisation are maltose and iso-maltose. This means that the reaction must be terminated as soon as the required DE is reached. The general practice is to inactivate the enzyme by heat.

As previously[4] reported, the final DE of the product is also dependent on the substrate concentration. These findings have been confirmed in our laboratories. Figure 6 shows how the DE falls with increasing substrate concentration, and this effect is again due to the resynthesis of higher sugars from glucose. We have found that the concentration of the maltose formed by repolymerisation is determined by the substrate concentration, the higher the dry substance content, the higher the maltose concentration. The amount of isomaltose, however, is more dependent on factors like enzyme concentration and reaction time.

High Maltose Syrups

Both 60–70 DE and 90–98 DE syrups contain fairly large amounts of glucose, and the hygroscopicity of these syrups is therefore relatively high. When a low hygroscopicity is important (*e.g.* for the production of hard-boiled sweets), a completely different type of syrup, the high maltose syrup, is preferred. These syrups are characterised by a very low content of glucose and a high content of maltose.

In the past the bulk of the high maltose syrups have been made using beta-amylases of cereal origin. These enzymes are well suited because of their mode of action. Furthermore, most commercial fungal alpha-amylases contain relatively high amounts of maltase activity. So although relatively high levels of maltose could be reached, the glucose content in the syrup would generally be too high.

However, cereal beta-amylases have their shortcomings. They are strongly inhibited by Cu-ions, and the final maltose concentration is very dependent on the liquefaction. As the beta-amylase is unable to bypass 1,6 linkages, the amylopectin must be broken down to relatively small dextrins during liquefaction in order to avoid a high concentration of beta limit dextrins in the final syrup.

With this in mind, we carried out some experiments with a fungal alpha-amylase, Fungamyl 1600, that has a very low maltase activity. The saccharification was carried out at 50°C and a pH of 5. Three different enzyme dosages, 100 g, 200 g and 400 g per ton of starch, were tested. The substrate was enzyme liquefied corn-starch with a DE of approximately 20.

Figure 7 shows the change in DE, glucose, maltose and triose content with time using the lowest dosage of enzyme. As may be seen, the increase in dextrose is very small. The maltotriose content reaches a maximum after approximately 8 hr and then drops slowly.

Figure 8 shows the change in maltose and glucose concentration with time for the three different dosages of Fungamyl. These curves

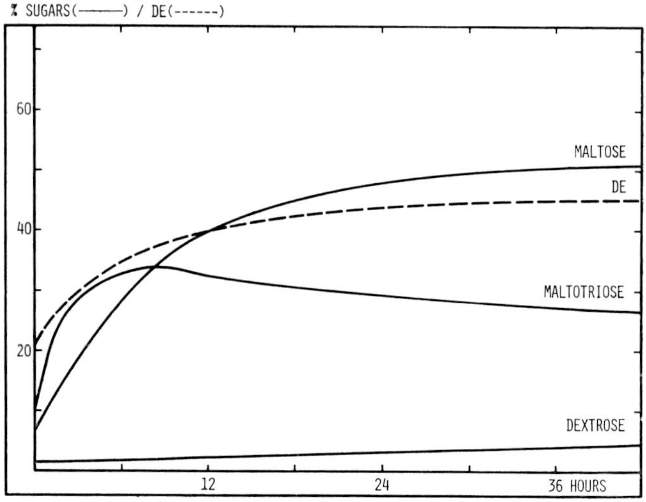

FIG. 7. Change in carbohydrate composition during saccharification. Substrate: 20 DE enzyme liquefied corn starch—40% w/w. Temperature: 50°C. pH: 5·0. Enzyme dosage: 100 g Fungamyl 1600 per ton of starch.

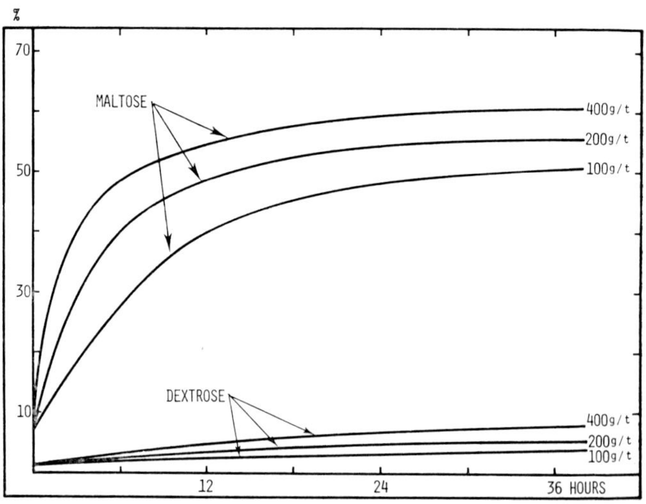

FIG. 8. The effect of Fungamyl dosage on syrup composition. Substrate: 20 DE enzyme liquefied corn starch—40% w/w. Temperature: 50°C. pH: 5·0. Enzyme dosage: 100, 200 and 400 g Fungamyl 1600 per ton of starch.

show that the enzyme is quite stable under the reaction conditions. When using double the amount of enzyme, the reaction time required to reach a certain percentage of maltose is reduced to half. Only with reaction times above 24 hr is a slight decrease in activity noticeable. To reach 45% maltose (anhydrous) using 400, 200 and 100 g Fungamyl per ton of starch the reaction time is 4½, 9 and 18 hr, respectively. To reach 50% maltose, however, the corresponding reaction times will be 7¼, 14½ and 33 hr, respectively. In other words, the lowest dosage needs a reaction time a little longer than expected. With the highest dosage of enzyme, a syrup containing 60% maltose and 7% glucose may be produced in less than 30 hr.

Most of the speciality syrups we have just described are being produced in fairly large quantities today. However, we have tried in each group to go a little beyond what is offered as the standard quality, for example by using enzyme liquefied starch as substrate for 60–70 DE syrups.

The development of microbial enzymes for the hydrolysis of starch has enabled the syrup manufacturers to offer a wide range of syrups to meet their customers' requirements. This development is going to continue and as the number of commercially available enzymes increases, so will the range of speciality syrups.

REFERENCES

1. Barfoed, H. (1967). *Die Stärke,* **19,** p. 2.
2. Madsen, G. B. (1970). *Kongressbericht*, 5, Welt-Getreide-und Brotkongress, **4,** p. 113.
3. Madsen, G. B. (1972). *Vortrag am Internationalen Symposium, Chemie und Technologie der Stärke,* Krakow, 26–27 September.
4. Underkofler, L. A., Denautt, L. J. and Hou, E. F. (1965). *Die Stärke,* **17,** p. 179.

DISCUSSION

Chairman: It is very encouraging to know you have the question of production of glucose syrups under your control and I am sure this will stimulate a lot of interest among people here. It is a very important industry. Even though we have overrun time I think in all fairness I should give Miss Madsen a chance of answering one or two questions at any rate.

Spence: In her early slides Miss Madsen showed maltose concentration on a curve but it was indicated as maltose monohydrate. Does she really mean that?

Madsen: Yes, it has not been calculated back. We are using maltose monohydrate as standard because that is the way we can buy it.

Spence: Commercially available syrups have 33% maltose. Would these be considerably higher?

Madsen: They would be about 34½%.

Spence: What is the fate of maltotriose in high maltose syrup production, since it can only degrade to maltose plus dextrose, and insufficient dextrose is generated to account for this?

Madsen: When taking into account that for each 3% maltotriose disappearing only 1% glucose has to be formed, the decrease in maltotriose shown on the graph is accounted for by the increase in the glucose content.

Tegge: In Fig. 6 you showed a dependence of end DE value on starch concentration. Is this phenomenon dependent on the formation of reversion products as it is in the acid conversion of starch?

Madsen: No, I believe that this is a matter of reaching equilibrium between maltose and glucose: with increasing substrate concentration the equilibrium is pushed to the maltose side.

Hood: Is glucoamylase the only starch hydrolysing enzyme which catalyses the reversion reaction?

Madsen: No, because you don't push the enzymes as far as bacterial amylase. You can get DE's up to above 50 at least but when they are being used in industry they are only letting them go to 15/20 DE, so you only see this when the enzymes go all the way to the end of the reaction.

Hood: Since glucoamylase catalyses reversion reactions, do you think that it is a single enzyme or a multiple enzyme system?

Madsen: Glucoamylase can be separated in two ways but we haven't been able to see any difference in the behaviour of its fractions. It is a multiple enzyme but its components might not be different in the way they react.

Spence: It isn't a transferase enzyme?

Madsen: No, because if we incubate it with maltose we don't get any formation of panose at all.

5

Fructose

G. L. S. PAWAN

Metabolic Division, Department of Medicine,
The Middlesex Hospital Medical School,
London, England

ABSTRACT

A brief account of the chemistry of fructose and its metabolism in man, with particular reference to liver and adipose tissue function, will be presented. The possible usefulness of this sugar in food products and drinks, in certain physiological and pharmacological conditions, and in some pathological disorders will be discussed.

INTRODUCTION

The laevo-rotatory ketose, D-fructose (β-D-fructopyranose, D-laevulose or 'fruit sugar'), occurs naturally in plants and animals. In man it is a normal constituent of blood (0·5–5·0 mg/100 ml), seminal fluid,[1] foetal blood[2–5] and amniotic fluid.[6,7] It is found in some vegetables, *e.g.* the potato and onion, and is widely distributed in fruits where it may be present in the free form, or combined as disaccharides and polysaccharides, and where its concentration will vary with species, ripeness and state of preservation. In honey, fructose constitutes about half the total sugars present; in sucrose, combined with glucose it is present as a five-membered cyclic furanose unit; and in inulin, the fructosan polysaccharide found in the roots and tubers of artichokes, chicory, dandelions, dahlias and other compositae, it is present as some 40 fructose units in combination, which on hydrolysis yields the sugar. In most normal diets fructose contributes about 15 to 50% of the total carbohydrate intake.

It has been known since the early days of organic chemistry that D-fructose can be formed from its isomer, D-glucose (the most abundant of the various polymerised forms of carbohydrate) by a minor change in structure. Until recently, however, this simple transformation has presented difficulties to the chemist because of the simultaneous production of small quantities of many other compounds (such as D-mannose, saccharinic and aldonic acids) by the chemical processes involved. In the last decade, a selection of microbial enzymes has been isolated which can transform D-glucose to D-fructose without the production of these by-products.[8-12] Recently, improved enzymic and chemical processes have made fructose more abundant and cheaper. Pure fructose, as obtained commercially, is a white or cream coloured crystalline powder which is odourless and hygroscopic. It is the sweetest of all the naturally occurring carbohydrates. Fructose is about 1·2–1·8 times as sweet as sucrose and more than twice as sweet as glucose.[13,14] These subjective values of sweetness will, of course, vary with temperature and other factors.

When pure crystalline fructose (β-D-fructopyranose) is dissolved in water it undergoes mutarotation as a result of rapid pyranose–furanose interconversion, yielding a complex equilibrium mixture of isomers, such as β-D-fructopyranose, α-D-fructopyranose, β-D-fructofuranose and α-D-fructofuranose. The relative proportions of these different substances produced from fructose in solution can vary greatly with temperature, pH and other factors. In metabolic studies, therefore, when comparing the effects of D-fructose with the fructose component of sucrose, it should be remembered that when sucrose is dissolved in aqueous solution its fructose moiety, unlike the case with D-fructose itself, is present in only one form—the five-membered furanose with a fixed β-anomeric configuration.[15] Furthermore, on heating or acidifying a concentrated aqueous solution of D-fructose, the sugar undergoes dehydration[16] with the production of a series of crystalline, non-reducing, dimeric dianhydrides which are not fermentable by yeast. It is therefore preferable, in metabolic studies, to sterilise fructose solutions by bacterial filtration rather than by autoclaving.

ABSORPTION OF FRUCTOSE IN MAN

Until fairly recently, it was thought that fructose absorption from the gut occurred by a slow passive diffusion process, and that a large proportion of the fructose was converted in the wall of the intestine into glucose. It is now believed that fructose absorption from the lumen of the intestine, though not as fast as that of glucose, is rapid, linearly related to its concentration and is not inhibited by the presence of glucose.[17,18] There is increasing evidence that an active transport mechanism is involved in fructose absorption from the intestine,[19] and in man the major part of the absorbed fructose passes unchanged via the portal vein for further metabolism in the liver.[20] Conversion of fructose into glucose by the intestinal mucosa, which has been advanced as an argument against the use of fructose as a substitute for glucose in certain conditions, does not appear to be important.[21] At most, about 10–20% of the absorbed fructose is so converted.[20,22] Furthermore, unlike glucose, orally administered fructose does not significantly stimulate release of enteroglucagon and pancreatic insulin.[23,24]

Most normal subjects tolerate 100 g oral fructose loads, but in the author's experience single oral doses of more than 50 g may occasionally produce slight gastro-intestinal distress, epigastric pain and diarrhoea. If larger doses of fructose are to be used, it is advisable to give these as hourly spaced feedings. We have given fructose to normal persons in quantities up to 500 g/day in this manner without untoward symptoms.

INTESTINAL METABOLISM

The fructose-containing disaccharide, sucrose, is hydrolysed in the 'brush border' of the intestinal mucosa by sucrase. This enyzme can be induced by high sucrose, high fructose, and, to a lesser extent, high glucose diets.[25,26] This adaptive increase in sucrase activity by fructose feeding has been used to stimulate sucrase activity in children with sucrose intolerance due to sucrase-isomaltase deficiency. After a few days on a high fructose diet, improvement in tolerance to dietary sucrose has been observed.[27]

In normal individuals after a fructose feed, 80–90% of this sugar on entry into the intestinal epithelial cells passes on unchanged in the blood to the liver. The remaining 10–20% is transformed by the enzyme fructokinase (a specific keto-hexokinase) into fructose-1-phosphate. A small quantity of the fructose may be converted into fructose-6-phosphate by hexokinase in the intestinal mucosa.

In the presence of both fructose and glucose, *e.g.* after sucrose feeding, fructose is metabolised mainly by fructokinase, since glucose competes with fructose for the enzyme, hexokinase. Fructose-1-phosphate is then split by the enzyme fructose-1-phosphate aldolase into the trioses, di-hydroxyacetone phosphate and glyceraldehyde, which are subsequently metabolised by pathways described under the section on the liver (Fig. 1). The activities of the intestinal mucosal enzymes for fructose metabolism are affected by diet,

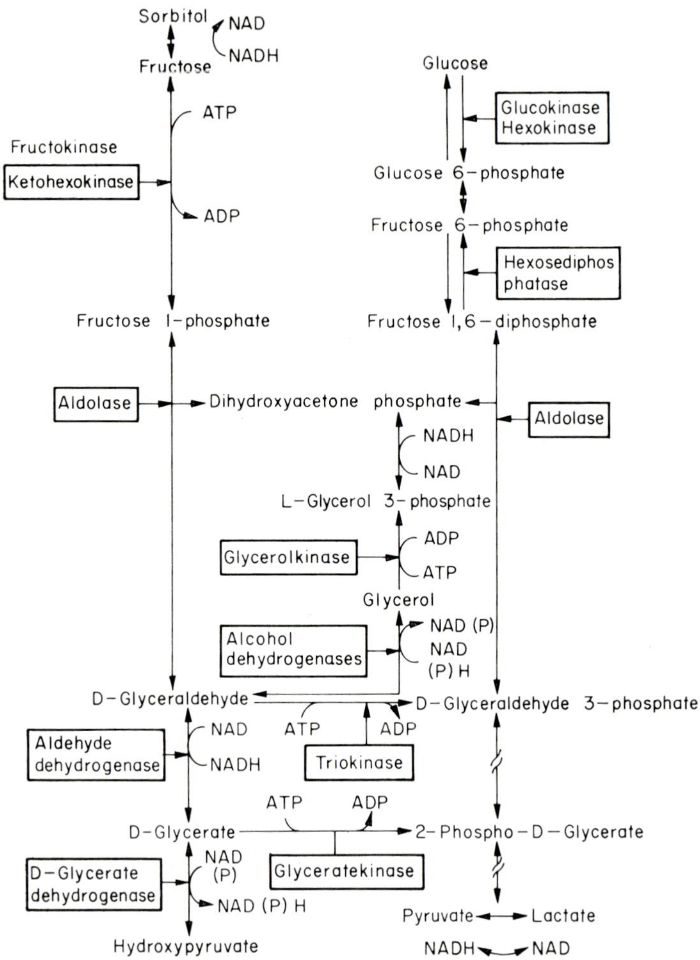

FIG. 1. The metabolism of fructose in liver.

certain vitamins and drugs. Thus, a high fructose or sucrose diet increases activity of fructokinase and fructose-1-phosphate aldolase,[28,29] and folic acid administration, alone or with fructose, increases these two enzymes as well as the gluconeogenic enzyme, fructose-1-6-diphosphatase, and other glycolytic enzymes.[30,31] This ability of folic acid has been used to increase fructose-1-phosphate aldolase in a child with hereditary fructose intolerance and improve her clinical condition.[32] Intestinal fructokinase and fructose-1-phosphate aldolase activity is also increased by phenobarbital[33] and decreased by dexamethasone.[34,35]

LIVER METABOLISM

In the liver of normal subjects and of diabetics with severe insulin deficiency, fructose is rapidly taken up and metabolised to the triose level (Fig. 1). The half-life of intravenously administered fructose, owing to rapid liver utilisation, is approximately 50% of that of glucose.[36] This rapid utilisation of fructose is associated with corresponding increases in blood levels of pyruvate, lactate, α-ketoglutarate and citrate[37] and a fall in serum phosphate.[38]

In the liver (and possibly kidney) the first reaction pathway for fructose is its conversion by the specific ketohexokinase—fructokinase—to fructose-1-phosphate. The fructokinase activity, unlike that of the hexokinase—glucokinase—is insulin independent. The fructose-1-phosphate is then split by liver aldolase B into equal parts of dihydroxyacetone phosphate and glyceraldehyde (Fig. 1). The dihydroxyacetone phosphate is mixed into the triose pool and metabolised further either to pyruvate or to glucose and glycogen, depending on the metabolic state of the subject as to requirements for glycolysis or gluconeogenesis. In liver, glycogen formation from fructose is several times more efficient than from glucose[39] and this process is less impaired in diabetes, liver disease and after surgical operations than is glycogen formation from glucose.[40–42]

In the liver, glyceraldehyde may be metabolised in at least three different ways (Fig. 1): (1) phosphorylation by a triokinase to glyceraldehyde phosphate which may be further metabolised to glucose or pyruvate; (2) reduction by alcohol dehydrogenase to glycerol which is then either further oxidised in the mitochondria, or activated by glycerolkinase to α-glycerol phosphate, and combined with free fatty acids for triglyceride synthesis in the cytoplasm of the cells; or (3) oxidised by aldehyde dehydrogenase and metabolised as shown in Fig. 1. The resulting fate of the trioses formed after a fructose load is influenced by the prevailing metabolic condition of the subject. Thus, when gluconeogenesis is proceeding at a high rate, *e.g.* in fasting, on high fat diets, during recovery after severe exercise and cold exposure, or in severe diabetes mellitus, the triose phosphates generated from fructose are converted mainly to glucose and glycogen. But on high (glucose) carbohydrate diets, and in the presence of raised insulin levels, the trioses are oxidised to pyruvate, lactate and other Krebs cycle intermediates. The increase in lactate formation, manifested by elevated blood lactic acid levels, may give rise to metabolic acidosis. This is of particular importance in subjects with acid-base disturbance when receiving rapid intravenous infusions of large amounts of fructose.[43–45]

It has also been suggested that a large dose of fructose administered intravenously (more than 1 g/kg/hr) may lower ATP and ADP levels in the liver[46] as a result of the rapid phosphorylation of fructose to fructose-1-phosphate.[47–49] The altered ATP and inorganic phosphate levels thus produced may adversely affect purine metabolism and lead to increased serum and urine uric acid levels[50–52] and in susceptible individuals precipitate gouty attacks. Continuous intravenous infusions of smaller amounts of fructose (less than 0·5–0·7 g/kg/hr) do not appear to have much effect on serum urate levels in adult persons.[52–54] Consumption of fructose in food is therefore unlikely to have any significant effect on serum uric acid levels.

MUSCLE TISSUE METABOLISM OF FRUCTOSE

The metabolic utilisation of fructose by skeletal muscle is different from that of liver tissue.[55] Like glucose it is phosphorylated by hexokinase and undergoes subsequent reactions as fructose-6-phosphate. High concentrations of glucose may inhibit fructose metabolism in this tissue, but there is good evidence in man that even at low concentrations fructose is directly utilised by muscle tissue and may be converted to glycogen.[56–59] The effect of fructose on muscle glycogen depends on existing glycogen content. In resting muscle with a normal glycogen content, glucose and fructose produce similar glycogen increments, but in muscle previously depleted of glycogen by heavy exercise, glycogen synthesis from glucose is greater than from fructose. Under working conditions, however, fructose is readily and rapidly utilised by muscle tissue in man.[60] I have been investigating the effects of various dietary carbohydrate supplements in athletes (swimmers and runners) and preliminary results indicate that in certain conditions fructose may be of value in improving performance.

Cardiac muscle appears to metabolise fructose readily, and intravenous administration of this sugar may have some advantage in improving coronary vasodilation and increasing cardiac output.[61,62]

ADIPOSE TISSUE METABOLISM OF FRUCTOSE

Under normal conditions, adipose tissue takes up fructose by means of a carrier system different from that of glucose, and which is stimulated by insulin only in the absence of glucose. The fructose taken up is metabolised at a relatively rapid rate by the adipose tissue. Glycerophosphate is produced, re-esterification of fatty acids occurs, and triglyceride levels are increased in this tissue. Alteration in blood levels of some lipids, particularly triglycerides, have been reported in men and post-menopausal women receiving large amounts of fructose, and suggestions have been made of possible atherogenicity of fructose[63–6] but this has been disputed.[67,68]

METABOLIC DISEASES (INBORN ERRORS) OF FRUCTOSE METABOLISM

Two rare inborn errors caused by a deficiency of enzymes of fructose metabolism have been described—essential fructosuria and hereditary fructose intolerance.[69–72] In essential fructosuria, the enzyme, fructokinase, is deficient or absent, but aldolase activity is normal.[70,73] In these subjects, fructose feeding causes a marked rise in blood fructose with resulting increased urine loss of the unchanged sugar.

In hereditary fructose intolerance, the fructose-1-phosphate aldolase (aldolase B) is abnormal, deficient or absent.[55,74,75] The condition appears to be inherited as an autosomal recessive (or dominant?) trait. In normal persons this aldolase is present in liver, kidney cortex and intestinal mucosa, and provides most of the fructose-1-phosphate splitting and fructose-1,6-diphosphate splitting activity of these organs. In subjects with the disorder the metabolic disturbance caused by fructose ingestion in the absence of adequate fructose-1-phosphate aldolase activity is an accumulation of fructose-1-phosphate derived from the phosphorylation of fructose by fructokinase. The build-up of fructose-1-phosphate appears to exert an inhibitory action on fructokinase, resulting in abnormally high blood levels of fructose and loss of the sugar in the urine. Since in this condition the fructose-1-phosphate is neither metabolised nor converted to glucose and, in addition, inhibits glucose release from the liver, hypoglycaemia ensues. Subjects with this condition must therefore avoid fructose-containing foods and sucrose. Failure to do this results in attacks of low blood sugar, weight loss, liver enlargement, jaundice, vomiting, anorexia and dysfunction of the liver and kidney.[76] The enzyme defect is not demonstrable in the blood cells, but on receiving a fructose load these subjects exhibit a prolonged fall in blood glucose.[77] This has been used as a test to aid diagnosis of the condition.

FRUCTOSE IN NUTRITION

Effect on Alcohol (Ethanol) Metabolism

Administration of various sugars, particularly fructose, has been reported to increase the rate of metabolism of ethanol and to facilitate 'sobering up' of intoxicated persons. Lieber[78] reviewed the available evidence and concluded that the published results of any effect of sugars on ethanol metabolism were equivocal. In my own laboratory we have studied the effects of different sugars (glucose, fructose, galactose and sucrose) on the rate of metabolism of standard amounts of alcohol under controlled conditions in human subjects, and concluded that fructose, in doses of 30 g or more orally, was the only sugar to exert a significant influence on accelerating the rate of ethanol metabolism (Fig. 2).[79-83] Further experiments (Pawan, to be published) indicate that fructose is also of value in preventing and alleviating symptoms of alcoholic 'hangover'. Fructose has also been used intravenously to increase the rate of ethanol metabolism in severely intoxicated persons[84,85] and to treat patients with delirium tremens.[86] Fructose is of considerable value given with ethanol and amino acids in intravenous feeding.

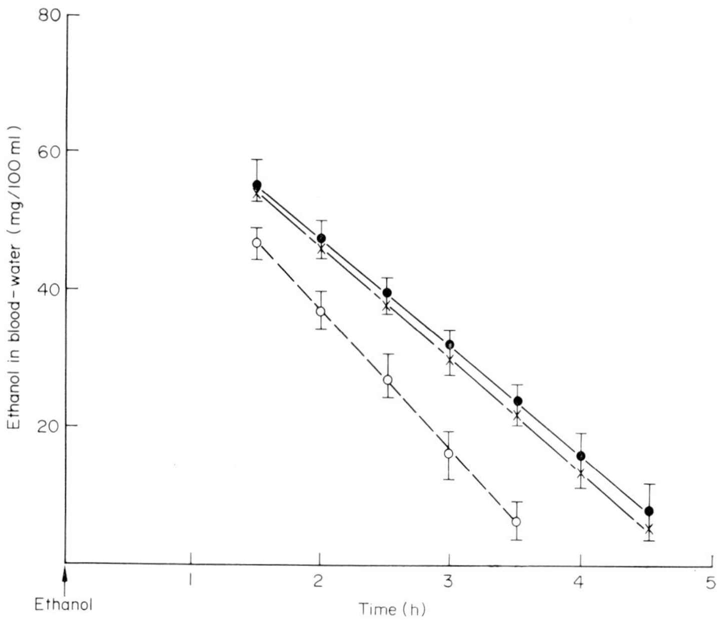

FIG. 2. Plasma alcohol concentrations (●——●) of 12 men given 0·5 g ethanol/kg body weight on three occasions, and the effect of 30 g glucose (×—×) and of 30 g fructose (○ — — —○) taken with this dose of alcohol in the same subjects. The vertical bars represent the standard errors of the mean.

Dental Caries

Some evidence has been advanced indicating that fructose might be less cariogenic and produce less dental plaque formation than sucrose.[87] Further investigation in this area is urgently needed.

Iron Metabolism

Fructose has been shown to increase intestinal absorption of iron to a considerable extent in man[88] as a result of the formation of an iron–fructose chelate complex which is better absorbed than inorganic iron. This effect of fructose on iron absorption is not seen with glucose. The effect of fructose on iron metabolism and iron deficiency anaemia may be a potentially useful area of research.

High Altitude

At high altitude (low atmospheric) conditions, fructose is taken up and utilised much more readily by extra-hepatic tissues like muscle, and possibly brain, than at sea level conditions, and produces smaller increases of lactate and pyruvate in the blood.[89]

Pathological Conditions

Fructose has been used for many years in several countries, *e.g.* Germany and Austria, as a sweetening agent and substantial constituent of the diet in adult diabetics without deterioration in control of the disease.[90] It has several suggested advantages over glucose in various physiological and pathological conditions in man.[22,41,62,91–93] Compared with glucose it is more slowly absorbed from the gut and is utilisable without insulin. Fructose is sweeter on a weight basis than sucrose,[94] hence smaller quantities (fewer calories) are needed for sweetening purposes in diets used for weight reduction in obesity. It is more rapidly utilised than glucose and produces lower total blood sugar levels and smaller urinary losses. It appears to be metabolised normally in post-operative and uraemic patients with glucose intolerance. Fructose can be given intravenously in high concentrations and is less irritating than glucose on the peripheral veins. It is a potent agent for building up liver glycogen stores, exerts an appreciable 'protein sparing' action, improves the utilisation of intravenously administered amino acids and ethanol, and may be of value given intravenously after acute myocardial infarction.[95,96]

FRUCTOSE IN FOOD SCIENCE AND TECHNOLOGY

Apart from its use in diabetic low-calorie foods and drinks, fructose is being increasingly studied in respect of its potential value in the food and drink industry, *e.g.* in confectionery, formulation of brewing sugars, bread making, and various athletic, geriatric and convalescent food preparations. Fructose is much more soluble in water and in alcohol than either sucrose or glucose, and in bulk-handling transport of liquids, syrups containing fructose are less liable to crystallise out than those containing glucose. When heated, fructose decomposes more easily than glucose in the baking process (melanoidine formation) yielding a major product, hydroxymethyl-furfural, which readily condenses with amino groups in proteins, peptides and amino acids to give an attractive brown coloration and improved flavour in baked bread. Fructose has useful humectant properties due to its hygroscopic nature, and this is of value in prolonging storage life in the tobacco, leather and baking industries, and for preventing internal crystallisation and desiccation in confectionery. It may be useful in aroma retention and flavour transfer of natural flavours in foods, for antioxidant properties, for prevention of 'sandiness' in ice icream and for maintaining a smooth texture in cream icings. In certain commercial fruit juices, *e.g.* blackcurrant juice, the use of fructose instead of sucrose or glucose for sweetening purposes would provide fewer calories, better flavour preservation and avoid the bitter 'after taste' of an artificial sweetening agent like saccharin.

Commercially available fructose preparations are sold on the open market in many countries. Chocolate, bread products, cakes, jam, yoghourt, pudding powder, sweets, milk drinks, chocolate creams, tinned fruit, fruit juices, champagne, fruit vermouth and sweet brandy are some products successfully marketed. In the UK the next few years should see an increase in other fructose-containing products.

REFERENCES

1. Mann, T. (1949). *Advances in Enzymology,* **9,** p. 329.
2. Orr, A. P. (1924). *Biochem. J.,* **18,** p. 171.
3. Eymer, P. (1951). *Aerztl. Forschg. Worishofen.,* **5,** 1, p. 442.
4. Huggett, A. St.G. (1950). *Arch. Dis. Child.,* **25,** p. 101.
5. Hagerman, D. D. and Villee, C. A. (1952). *J. clin. Invest.,* **31,** p. 911.
6. Itizyo, M. (1934). *Jap. J. Med. Sci. II. Biochemistry,* **2,** p. 359.
7. Marazzini, F. (1957). *Riv. Ostet.,* **39,** p. 1025.
8. Marshall, R. O. and Kooi, E. R. (1957). *Science,* **125,** p. 648.
9. Tsumura, N. and Sato, T. (1960). *Agr. Biol. Chem.,* **24,** p. 326.
10. Tsumura, N. and Sato, T. (1961). *Agr. Biol. Chem.,* **25,** pp. 616, 620.
11. Tsumura, N. and Sato, T. (1965). *Agr. Biol. Chem.,* **29,** pp. 1123, 1129.
12. Yamanaka, K. (1963). *Agr. Biol. Chem.,* **27,** p. 265.
13. Shallenberger, R. S., Acree, T. E. and Guild, W. E. (1965). *J. Food Sci.,* **30,** p. 560.
14. Allen, R. J. L. and Brook, M. (1967). *Amer. J. clin. Nutrit.,* **20,** p. 163.
15. Barker, S. A. (1970). In *International Symposium on Clinical and Metabolic Aspects of Laevulose*, Calmic Limited, Crewe, pp. 1–7.

16. Hilton, H. W. (1963). In *Methods in Carbohydrate Chemistry,* Vol. 11, Academic Press, London, p. 199.
17. Holdsworth, C. D. and Dawson, A. M. (1964). *Clinical Science,* **27,** p. 371.
18. Gray, G. M. and Ingelfinger, F. J. (1966). *J. clin. Invest.,* **45,** p. 388.
19. Gracey, M., Burke, V. and Oshin, A. (1970). *Lancet,* **2,** p. 827.
20. Cook, G. C. (1969). *Clinical Science,* **37,** p. 675.
21. Dawson, A. M. (1968). *Scientific Basis of Medicine. Annual Reviews,* The Athlone Press, London, pp. 186–205.
22. Miller, M., Craig, J. W., Drucker, W. R. and Woodward, H. Jr (1956). *Yale J. Biol. Med.,* **29,** p. 335.
23. Marks, V. (1970). In *International Symposium on Clinical and Metabolic Aspects of Laevulose,* Calmic Limited, Crewe, pp. 37–41.
24. Marks, V. and Samols, E. (1970). In *Advances in Metabolic Disorders,* Vol. 4, Academic Press, London, pp. 1–38.
25. Rosensweig, N. S. and Herman, R. H. (1968). *J. clin. Invest.,* **47,** p. 2253.
26. Rosensweig, N. S. and Herman, R. H. (1970). *Amer. J. Clin. Nutrit.,* **23,** p. 1373.
27. Greene, H. L., Stifel, F. B. and Herman, R. H. (1971). *Lancet,* **1,** p. 651.
28. Rosensweig, N. S., Stifel, F. B., Herman, R. H. and Zakim, D. (1968). *Biochim. Biophys. Acta,* **170,** p. 228.
29. Rosensweig, N. S., Stifel, F. B., Zakim, D. and Herman, R. H. (1969). *Gastroenterology,* **57,** p. 143.
30. Rosensweig, N. S., Herman, R. H., Stifel, F. B. and Herman, Y. F. (1969). *J. clin. Invest.,* **48,** p. 2038.
31. Rosensweig, N. S., Stifel, F. B., Herman, Y. F. and Herman, R. H. (1969). *Amer. J. Clin. Nutrit.,* **22,** p. 667.
32. Greene, H. L., Stifel, F. B. and Herman, R. H. (1972). Western Soc. Pediat. Res., Carmel, California, pp. 4–6.
33. Rosensweig, N. S., Stifel, F. B. and Herman, R. H. (1969). *Clinical Res.,* **17,** p. 596.
34. Rosensweig, N. S., Herman, R. H. and Stifel, F. B. (1970). *Fed. Proc.,* **29,** p. 256.
35. Rosensweig, N. S., Herman, R. H. and Stifel, F. B. (1970). *Amer. J. Clin. Nutrit.,* **23,** p. 670.
36. Smith, L. H., Ettinger, R. H. and Seligson, D. (1953). *J. clin. Invest.,* **32,** p. 273.
37. Craig, J. W., Miller, M., Mackenzie, M. S. and Woodward, H. Jr (1957). *J. clin. Invest.,* **37,** p. 118.
38. Pletscher, A., Fahlaender, H. and Staub, H. (1951). *Helv. Physiol. Pharmakol. Acta,* **9,** p. 46.
39. Cori, C. F. (1926). *J. biol. Chem.,* **70,** p. 577.
40. Ashare, R., Moore, R. and Ellison, E. H. (1955). *Arch. Surgery,* **70,** p. 428
41. Bergstrom, J. and Hultman, E. (1967). *Acta med. Scand.,* **182,** p. 93.

42. Nilsson, L. H. and Hultman, E. (1970). In *IV World Congress of Gastroenterology,* Copenhagen, pp. 12–18.
43. Bergstrom, J., Hultman, E. and Roch-Norlund, A. E. (1968). *Acta med. Scand.,* **184,** p. 359.
44. Anderson, G., Brohult, J. and Sterner, G. (1968). *Acta Paediat. Scand.,* **58,** p. 301.
45. Kekomaki, M., Raivio, K. O. and Maenpaa, P. H. (1970). *Acta Anaesth. Scand.,* Supplement 37, p. 114.
46. Bode, C., Schumacher, H., Goebell, H., Zelder, O. and Pelzer, H. (1971). *Hormones Metab. Res.,* **3,** p. 289.
47. Maenpaa, P. H., Raivio, K. O. and Kekomaki, M. (1968). *Science,* **161,** p. 1253.
48. Burch, H. B., Max, P. Jr, Chyu, K. and Lowry, O. H. (1969). *Biochem. Biophys. Res. Comm.,* **34,** p. 619.
49. Woods, H. F., Eggleston, L. V. and Krebs, H. A. (1970). *Biochem. J.,* **119,** p. 501.
50. Perheentupa, J. and Raivio, K. (1967). *Lancet,* **2,** p. 528.
51. Stirpe, F., Della Corte, E., Bonetti, E., Abbondanza, A., Abbati, A. and De Stefano, F. (1970). *Lancet,* **2,** p. 1310.
52. Heuckenkamp, P. U. and Zollner, N. (1971). *Lancet,* **1,** p. 808.
53. Curreri, P. W. and Pruitt, B. A. (1970). *Lancet,* **1,** p. 839.
54. Sahebjami, H. and Scalettar, R. (1971). *Lancet,* **1,** p. 366.
55. Hers, H. G. and Joassin, G. (1961). *Enzymol. Biol. Clin.,* **1,** p. 4.
56. Butterfield, W. J. H., Sargent, B. H. and Whichelow, M. J. (1964). *Lancet,* **1,** p. 574.
57. Weinstein, J. J. and Roe, J. H. (1952). *J. Lab. Clin. Med.,* **40,** p. 39.
58. Weichselbaum, T. E., Margraf, H. W. and Elman, R. (1953). *Metabolism,* **2,** p. 434.
59. Hultman, E. (1967). *Scand. J. clin. Lab. Invest.,* **19,** Supplement 94.
60. Pearson, C. M. and Rimer, D. G. (1959). *Proc. Soc. Exper. Biol. Med.,* **100,** p. 671.
61. Danforth, W. H., Hogancamp, C. E., Ballard, F. B. and Bing, R. J. (1959). *Amer. J. Med. Sci.,* **238,** pp. 137, 477.
62. Elliot, W. C., Cohen, L. S., Klein, M. D., Lane, F. J. and Gorlin, R. (1967). *J. Appl. Physiol.,* **23,** p. 865.
63. Macdonald, I. and Braithwaite, D. M. (1964). *Clinical Science,* **27,** p. 23.
64. Macdonald, I. (1966). *Amer. J. clin. Nutrit.,* **18,** p. 369.
65. Antar, M. A. and Ohlson, M. A. (1965). *J. Nutrition,* **85,** p. 329.
66. Nikkila, E. A. and Pelkonen, R. (1966). *Proc. Soc. Exper. Biol. Med.,* **123,** p. 91.
67. Antonis, A., Iles, C. and Pilkington, T. R. E. (1968). *Proc. Nutr. Soc.,* **27,** p. 2A.
68. Dunnigan, M. G., Fife, T., McKiddie, M. T. and Crosbie, S. M. (1970). *Clinical Science,* **38,** p. 1.
69. Chambers, R. A. and Pratt, R. T. C. (1956). *Lancet,* **2,** p. 340.
70. Froesch, E. R., Prader, A., Labhart, A., Stuber, H. W. and Wolf, H. P. (1957). *Schweiz. Med. Wschr.,* **87,** p. 1168.

71. Froesch, E. R., Prader, A., Wolf, H. P. and Labhart, A. (1959). *Helv. Paediat. Acta,* **14,** p. 99.
72. Froesch, E. R. (1970). In *International Symposium on Clinical and Metabolic Aspects of Laevulose,* Calmic Limited, Crewe, pp. 9–20.
73. Schapira, F., Schapira, G. and Dreyfus, J. C. (1961). *Enzymol. Biol. Clin.,* **1,** p. 170.
74. Nikkila, E. A., Somersalo, O., Pitkanen, E. and Perheentupa, J. (1962). *Metabolism,* **11,** p. 727.
75. Morris, R. C. Jr, Ueki, L., Loh, D., Eanes, R. Z. and McLin, P. (1967). *Nature,* **214,** p. 920.
76. Levin, B., Snodgrass, G. J. A. I., Oberholzer, V. G., Burgess, E. A. and Dobbs, R. H. (1968). *Amer. J. Med.,* **45,** p. 826.
77. Froesch, E. R., Wolf, H. P., Baitsch, H., Prader, A. and Labhart, A. (1963). *Amer. J. Med.,* **34,** p. 151.
78. Lieber, C. S. (1967). *Ann. Rev. Med.,* **18,** p. 35.
79. Pawan, G. L. S. (1967). *Biochem. J.,* **106,** p. 19P.
80. Pawan, G. L. S. (1967). *New Scientist,* **36,** p. 539.
81. Pawan, G. L. S. (1968). *Nature,* **220,** p. 374.
82. Pawan, G. L. S. (1970). *Nutrition,* **24,** p. 77.
83. Pawan, G. L. S. (1972). *Proc. Nutrit. Soc.,* **31,** p. 83.
84. Patel, A. R., Paton, A. M., Rowan, T., Lawson, D. H. and Linton, A. L. (1969). *Scottish Med. J.,* **14,** p. 268.
85. Lowenstein, L. M., Simone, R., Boulter, P. and Nathan, P. (1970). *J. Amer. Med. Assoc.,* **213,** p. 1899.
86. Dalton, M. S. and Duncan, D. W. (1970). *Med. J. Australia,* **57,** p. 659.
87. Frostell, G., Keyes, P. H. and Larson, R. H. (1967). *J. Nutrition,* **93,** p. 65.
88. Davis, P. S. and Deller, D. J. (1967). *Gut,* **8,** p. 200.
89. Reynafarje, B., Oyola, L., Cheesman, R., Marticorena, E. and Jimenez, S. (1969). *Amer. J. Physiol.,* **216,** p. 1542.
90. Mehnert, H. (1971). In *Handbuch des Diabetes Mellitus,* Vol. 2, Ed. E. F. Pfeiffer, J. F. Lehmanns Verlag, Munchen, p. 1069.
91. Thoren, L. (1964). *Acta. Chir. Scand.,* Supplement 325, p. 75.
92. Aitken, J. M., Dunnigan, M. G. and Ford, J. A. (1970). In *International Symposium on Clinical and Metabolic Aspects of Laevulose,* Calmic Limited, Crewe, pp. 81–90.
93. Gibson, R. M., Fitch, W. and MacDowall, G. (1970). In *International Symposium on Clinical and Metabolic Aspects of Laevulose,* Calmic Limited, Crewe, pp. 97–103.
94. Stone, H. and Oliver, S. M. (1969). *J. Food Sci.,* **34,** p. 215.
95. Froesch, E. R. (1965). In *Handbook of Physiology*, Section V, Adipose Tissue, Eds. A. E. Renold and G. F. Cahill Jr, American Physiological Society, Washington, pp. 281–293.
96. Hers, H. G. and Kusaka, T. (1953). *Biochim. Biophys. Acta,* **11,** p. 427.

DISCUSSION

Hollingsworth: Most of the things Dr Pawan has said about fructose this afternoon seem to suggest that the consumption of fructose is a good thing. Can he tell us about its effects on blood triglycerides?

Pawan: As our Chairman has shown it seems that fructose taken in certain quantities in both sexes and all ages does produce an increase of triglycerides. Some have decried this but I feel it is a perfectly valid conclusion. Whether this would be harmful or produce problems of arteriosclerosis I don't know. It certainly has the effect of increasing the phosphate content. It seems also to have an effect on the gut acids and to inhibit lypolysis from the liver. In these circumstances I would certainly say it seems to have some slight ability to increase lipids.

Green: Leading on from that question can you tell us at what point in the metabolic pathway the body converts to triglycerides? Does it come from glycerol, glycerol aldehyde or glycerol phosphate?

Pawan: The glyceride can be produced from fructose.

Chairman: It is suspected that there is an alternative pathway which is now being investigated.

Radley: Is there a significant effect shown on higher alcohol content? With the legal limit of 80 quite a lot of people are interested in getting it down. There are a number of things on the market to eliminate alcohol quickly before the police stop you. Have you tried experiments?

Pawan: Our experiments were not planned to beat the breathalyser, but we have found even with quite high tests of blood alcohol—150 mg in the severely intoxicated—it does have a certain effect. It varies between individuals but on average the alcohol is eliminated much faster.

McMichael: I hesitate to question Dr Pawan on the metabolism of fructose but I think it is now clearly established that insulin *is* necessary for the later stages of fructose metabolism (although not necessary for its entry into cells). This is particularly important when fructose is used for intravenous feeding in sick patients. I have observed in one patient lactic acidosis so induced successfully treated by insulin on two occasions.

Pawan: I meant to imply not that it is absolutely insulin independent but that it does not require insulin levels that one would require with glucose. I think this is a very important point. I agree that insulin is required but in much smaller amounts than glucose. There are very few diabetics without any insulin. The point about lactic acid is extremely important but in our tests of fructose given parenterally, and in oral doses, I did not see much severe lactic acidosis. Problems raised are the increase in the uric acid level and the possibility of precipitate attacks. The problem is one many people have been arguing from the use of fructose infused intravenously. Results so obtained have been transferred to taking it by mouth. I think one must be careful not to associate the two.

Chairman: I would like to support the dangers of intravenous fructose, and particularly after an operation. It is convenient for the surgeon but not the patient, particularly many sufferers with gout. I have one patient who was given a large dose of fructose which precipitated an attack of gout.

Spence: Do large oral doses of fructose induce nausea in normal people when ingested in the quantities being discussed?

Pawan: Yes, this is why we used doses of 30 g. Marks used much larger doses, 100 to 90 g at one go. He tells me there were very little side effects, but I imagine if you used larger than that some people would have gastric pain and some would have diarrhoea.

da Rocha-Afodu: You have talked of fructose administration producing the elimination of ethanol from the blood in alcoholism. It is known that smokers studied with respect to atheroma have raised blood lipids. Do you think that fructose would relieve smokers of high level of blood lipids?

Pawan: Certainly fructose has been used in certain types as an anti-ketogenic agent, where effects would cause a rise in blood lipids and this would be involved in the production of atheroma. I don't think anyone has suggested that fructoses themselves are a causal agent of atheroma. Certainly fructose has an anti-effect on adipose tissue but at the same time it tends to increase the triglycerides. The whole question is quite open.

Parker: With respect to the effect of fructose on the rate of metabolism of alcohol when compared with its effect when taken as the equivalent amount of sucrose, is it possible that one mode of action of fructose is by increasing the relative equilibrium concentration of ethanol in the digestive tract by forming the diethyl ketal, a reaction which takes place very rapidly at low pH with fructose? Fructose is less rapidly absorbed than sucrose, and published evidence exists suggesting that fructose has no significant effect in reducing the levels of blood alcohol under practical conditions.

Pawan: That is a possibility. We find that by giving sugar some time after alcohol we lower the alcohol level. We still find fructose not as effective as sucrose.

Questioner (not clearly audible): (Referred to taking of fructose and the paper of Sir Francis Camps).

Pawan: With due respect to Sir Francis Camps, there is a great deal of evidence in many countries of its use intravenously, and in glucose form as a treatment for casualties brought in with head injuries and smelling of alcohol. The evidence seems to support it, and I am convinced because I have done it on myself—if you go to a party and have a little honey or fructose you can go on drinking.

6

Honey

Douw G. Steyn

Emeritus Professor of Pharmacology, Medical Faculty, University of Pretoria, Republic of South Africa

ABSTRACT

The composition and physiological actions of honey and queen-bee jelly (royal jelly, 'Gelée Royale') and their uses in the prevention and treatment of diseases are discussed.

The composition, taste and health-giving and therapeutic properties of honey depend on the following factors: age (spring, unripe or winter honey), source (kind of nectar), natural or sugar-fed honey, whether commercially processed or not, period and method of storage, percentage of pollen present, pH, type of container and place of storage.

It is obvious that, depending on the above factors, the composition of honey, especially the vitamin content, varies considerably.

The coronary dilatory and inotropic action of honey depends on its acetylcholine content and honey also determines the degree of its vasodilatory (hypotensive) effect. It has laxative properties, and owing to the presence of various enzymes in honey it favourably affects certain processes of metabolism.

Honey and royal jelly are used medicinally in the treatment of diabetes mellitus*; hypertension; diseases of the liver; chronic constipation; disturbances of carbohydrate and other processes of metabolism; and infected sores and wounds.*

Honey constitutes an excellent source of energy. Honey poisoning is discussed.

Probably owing to the presence of oestrogenic and androgenic substances in royal jelly, it is of value in the treatment of certain female disorders and in impotence.

INTRODUCTION

In 1970, Steyn[1] reviewed the composition of different types of honey and royal jelly (also known as 'queen-bee jelly' or 'Gelée Royale') and their physiological actions and medicinal uses in the prevention and treatment of diseases. Honey poisoning in different parts of the world was discussed.

Honey, an age-old food also used in the prevention and treatment of disease in man and animal, could be defined as a sweet substance prepared (processed) by honey-bees from nectar and other sweet juices of plants by passing these through their bodies and enriching, and then storing, the product in combs in which the honey matures.

The ancients believed that honey prolonged life. It was used as a conditioner for strenuous activity by the athletes of ancient Greece. Even today it is used for this purpose by mountain climbers and long-distance runners and swimmers, for whom the excellent nutritional value of a honey–milk diet is stressed.[2] Before the introduction of cane sugar into Europe, honey was the only agent used for the sweetening of foods.[3]

Honey[4] has been, and still is, used in the preparation of alcoholic beverages, one of the oldest and most well-known being 'mead'.[3] In Article 348 of Latin American Legislation it is stated: 'Mead, formed by alcoholic fermentation of honey, may contain citric, lactic or tartaric acid (2·5 g/litre), potassium bitartrate (250 mg/litre), clarifiers (albumin, casein, gelatin, isinglass, tannin), caramel and sulphur dioxide, or pure alkaline bisulphites (retained sulphur dioxide, 300 ppm). Volatile acids (expressed as acetic) must not exceed 2·5 %'.[3]

COMPOSITION OF HONEY

In 1956, Husing[5] made a most valuable contribution to our knowledge of the different types of honey, their origin, composition, nutritive qualities, adulteration and medicinal uses. He also discussed bee poison, its origin, composition, relationship to other animal poisons, immunity problems, idiosyncrasy and anaphylaxis.

Herold[2] has provided us with one of the most comprehensive reviews on all aspects of honey covering its history (commencing with primitive man), nectar, composition, value to pregnant mothers, infants, juveniles and in geriatrics, its effects on the different organs and systems of man, and allergy. He discussed the collection of pollen and clinical experiences with it. Attention was also given to royal jelly and bee poison.

Kandos[4] studied the reducing power of honey towards chloramine as a possible means of distinguishing between different classes of honey. He stated that the degree of reduction was slight and not due to the presence of sugars but to minute quantities of an unknown substance. Honey contains up to 20% sucrose. Unripe honey (fresh spring honey) has very low reducing power. In general, the sucrose content of sugar-fed honey is higher than that of normal honey of the same kind and, on standing, the sucrose content falls more slowly than that of normal honey.

Ellewood and Fischer[6] analysed four samples of honey prepared from the nectar of *Epilobium angustifolium* and other species of *Epilobium*. The water content varied from 13·91 to 17·56%, invert sugar from 69·85 to 74·62%, sucrose from 2·65 to 8·50%, ash from 0·49 to 0·99%, and free acid (as formic acid) from 0·03 to 0·05%. Honey also contains other sugars like maltose, isomaltose, erlose, kestose, raffinose and melezitose.[2] Undetermined materials varied from 3·27 to 9·60%.

In the summary and conclusions of their investigations of USA and foreign honeys, Haydak *et al.*[7] state: 'Microchemical and microbiological determinations showed the presence in honey of thiamine, riboflavin, ascorbic acid, pyridoxine, pantothenic acid and nicotinic acid. The amounts are extremely variable, depending probably on the source of the honey and the number of pollen grains present in the

TABLE 1

Vitamins in honey

Vitamin	Quantity per 100 g honey	Ref.
Nicotinic acid	4·0 to 92·0 mg	7,8
	63·0 to 590·0 μg	9
Pantothenic acid	25·0 to 190·0 μg	7,8
	9·0 to 360·0 μg	9
Pyridoxine (B_6)	227·0 to 480·0 μg	7,8
	0·0 to 27·7 μg	9
Riboflavin (B_2)	35·0 to 145·0 μg	7,8
	7·0 to 60·0 μg	9
Thiamine (B_1)	2·1 to 9·1 μg	7,8
	1·4 to 12·0 μg	9
Biotin	0·066 μg (average)	7,8
Folic acid	3·0 μg (average)	7,8
Ascorbic acid (Vitamin C)	0·5 to 6·5 mg	7,8

product. The most pronounced variation found was in the nicotinic acid and ascorbic acid content'. Table 1 reflects the extreme variation in the vitamin content of different samples of honey.

Haydak and his associates assayed clarified and unclarified honey for the above vitamins and found a general decrease in the vitamin concentration of the clarified samples, ranging from 8 to 45%. In contrast they found no perceptible reduction in the anti-haemorrhagic activity of the clarified honeys compared with the unclarified controls. This suggests that the anti-haemorrhagic factor is due, not to the pollen present in honey, but to substances dissolved in it. Husing[5] states that certain types of honey contain 400 mg% ascorbic acid and 22 mg % aneurin (Vitamin B_1).

According to Kitzes *et al.,*[9] honey is naturally acid with a pH range of 4 to 5; this may facilitate slow destruction of vitamins, especially pantothenic acid, on storage. Commercial processes for clarifying honey reduce the vitamin content to 33 to 50% of the original values, probably due to removal of pollen, as the vitamin content largely depends on the percentage of pollen present. These authors compared the vitamin content with that of pollen and royal jelly (Table 2).[10,11]

From Table 2 it is clear that pollen and royal jelly are much richer than honey in the B-complex vitamins. Several workers have reported the presence of acetylcholine (2·5 mg/kg) and choline (at least 60·0 mg/kg) in honey. On storage an acid pH may facilitate slow destruction of vitamins, especially pantothenic acid.

Herold[2] states that honey contains hydrochloric acid and phosphoric acid, but chiefly the organic acids: acetic acid, malic acid, citric acid, lactic acid, butyric acid and traces of formic acid. These acids originate, to a small degree, in the plant itself, but are mainly formed in the salivary glands of the bees or from glucose through enzymic action. They contribute to the odour and taste of honey and favourably influence appetite and digestion. Marguardt and Vogg,[12] referring to the cholinergic factor in honey, state that: 'this factor in honey is heat-stable unlike acetylcholine in pure solution, and may be explained by the presence of choline in honey, since acetylcholine solutions are also stabilised to heat by choline'.[13–16]

Marguardt and Vogg[12] and Herold[2] also reported the presence of diastase in honey.

König[17] stated that owing to the small size of samples of imported honey it is often difficult to ascertain whether they satisfy the demands

TABLE 2

Vitamins (in μg/g) in honey, pollen and royal jelly

	No. of samples	Pantothenic acid	Ribo-flavin	Nicotinic acid	Thiamine	Pyridoxine	Biotin	Folic acid
Honey	19	0·55	0·26	1·1	0·044	0·10	0·001	0·03
Pollen	2	27·0	16·7	100·0	6·0	9·0	0·25	—
Royal jelly	1	320·0	28·0	111·0	18·0	10·2	3·1	0·5

of the 'Lebensmittelgesetz'. Honey samples were judged by their taste and especially by their 'diastase count'. König explored the possibility of a simpler method of analysis which could be rapidly executed on a small specimen of honey. He found that the Zeiss-photometer lent itself well to rapid tests on the quality of honey and royal jelly.

Helvey[18] found that there was a natural abundance of deuterium in honey and that the concentration varied in different samples.

By means of paper chromatographic investigations, Chemnitius and Engel[19] demonstrated the presence of fourteen different saccharides in nine samples of honey. There were, among others, fructose, glucose, saccharose, maltose, lactose, melezitose and raffinose. They were unable to classify the remaining seven saccharides. The different samples of honey varied in the number of saccharides present. The authors found a direct relationship between the number of saccharides present in the honey and its pharmacological activity. The coronary dilatory and inotropic action of honey depends on its qualitative sugar content.

Sherpaz[20] continued previous investigations by himself and his co-workers on glucose-oxidase (β-D-glucose: O_2 oxido-reductase, EC 1.1.3.4.) in honey. He determined the effect of fructose, hydrogen peroxide, L-glucose and ascorbic acid on glucose-oxidase.

Smith and McCaughey[21] identified some trace lipids in honey and Lampitt and Bilham[22] reported on the absorption spectra of honey. Smith[23] reviewed the literature on the composition of honey and studied the extractable long-chain fatty acids. He definitely showed that methyl laurate, myristeolate, palmitate, stearate, oleate and lineolate were present in cotton honey. He states[23] that: 'Dörrscheidt and Friedrich (1961) recently separated the odorous substances of several honeys by gas–liquid chromatography and identified, by retention time, methyl propionate, methyl butyrate, methyl valerate and methyl caproate.' Other tests conducted by Smith indicated the presence of triglycerides, sterols, and possibly phospholipids, in cotton honey.

Duisberg[24] and his associates have examined thousands of honey samples from many countries. He has reviewed the literature on honey and Table 3 is reproduced from his article.

The valuable trace elements iron, copper, manganese and silicon have been repeatedly shown to be present in honey.[2] Iron and copper are indispensable in the formation of haemoglobin and certain important enzymes, whilst manganese is indispensable in the synthesis of several enzymes, and in the utilisation of vitamin B_1 (thiamine). Silicon plays a role in the synthesis of lipoids.

Natural honey contains saccharase (invertase) which is added by the bee in order to transform nectar into honey, and also diastase[2] which breaks up starch. Other enzymes present in honey are catalase,

TABLE 3

Some constituents of honey

Constituents of honey per 100 g			
Protein	0·3 g	Copper	0·07 mg
Fat	0·0 g	Manganese	0·2 mg
Cholesterin	0·0 g	Phosphate	16·0 mg
Carbohydrates	79·5 g	Sulphate	5·0 mg
Water	21·0 g	Vitamin A	0·0 IU
Uric acid	0·0 mg	Vitamin B_1	trace
Purin bases	0·0 mg	Vitamin B_2	40?
Sodium chloride	0·0 mg	Vitamin C	—
Potassium	10·0 mg	Vitamin D	—
Sodium	5·0 mg	Nicotinic acid	0·2 mg
Calcium	5·0 mg	Vitamin E	—
Magnesium	6·0 mg		
Iron	0·2 mg		

phosphatase and glucose-oxidase.[2] Bergner and Körömi (Herold[2]) reported the presence of small amounts of protein and amino acids in honey—alanine, asparagine, arginine, glutamic acid, glycine, histidine, leucine, isoleucine, lysine, phenylalanine, serine, threonine, valine, cystine, proline—the total amount being 34·96 μg in 5 g of honey.

COMPOSITION OF ROYAL JELLY

Herold[2] recently described the production of royal jelly, its composition and mode of action. Ammon and Zoch[15] studied the chemical constitution of royal jelly (nutritive substance of the queen-bee). They found:

1. Eleven amino acids: lysine, arginine, asparagine, glycine, serine, glutamic acid, β-alanine, γ-aminobutyric acid, proline, methionine and leucine.

2. Five sugars, four of which have been identified as sucrose, glucose, fructose and ribose.
3. That royal jelly possessed the ability to split acetylcholine, benzoylcholine, methyl-*n*-butyrate and tributyrine, said to be due probably to a non-specific cholinesterase. When stored over a long period the jelly loses its esterase action. An acid phosphatase action was also observed.

Kitzes *et al.*[9] showed how many more times queen-bee jelly is richer in B-complex vitamins than pollen and honey. Forster[16] states that its composition is well-known; amongst others, it contains (all figures are in mg/kg): thiamine (B_1), 1·2 to 18·0; riboflavin (B_2), 6 to 28; pyridoxine (B_6), 2·2 to 50; biotin (H), 1·2 to 4·1; nicotinic acid, 48 to 125; pantothenic acid, 110 to 320; folic acid, 0·16 to 0·5; and inositol, 80 to 400.

The acetylcholine content of royal jelly is 20 to 30 times higher than that of honey. The composition of food juices for drones and worker-bees is similar to that of royal jelly but with the difference that the relative quantities differ and biopterin is not generally found in the feeding juices of female workers. Forster states that, in general, the vitamin concentrations of queen-bee jelly are too low to exert any effect in man (the quantities are homeopathic).

In collaboration with the Max-Planck Institute in Munich, and with other institutions, Forster,[16] who is associated with a large bee-breeding industry and pharmaceutical factory, has conducted large-scale investigations into royal jelly and the food juices of drones and workers. He found that, in general, it is essential to fortify its chief constituents to achieve a significant action in man. As a result of the above investigations, 'Apifortyl' is being marketed. In this preparation, the vitamins have been fortified 10 times and in addition Vitamin A (2000 IU), Vitamin D_3 (500 IU), Vitamin E (5 mg), 10-hydroxy(2)-decenic acid[16] (0·27 mg), biopterin (1 μg) and trace elements (Cu, Mg, Fe, Co) have been added to each capsule.

According to Hadhanyi,[25] there are methods (paper chromatography, high frequency electrophoresis, etc.) by which both the composition and the value of royal jelly preparations can be estimated. In the last five years there has been a considerable increase in the number of these preparations on the market. Their value varies according to the royal jelly content and the method of preparation. König[17] describes a method of determining the comparative purity of different samples of royal jelly. According to Dayan,[26] it contains proteins, lipids, carbohydrates, fatty acids (one of which is unique) and vitamins.

HONEY AND ROYAL JELLY IN THE PREVENTION AND TREATMENT OF DISEASE

The possible value of honey as a health-giving food has been briefly referred to in a recent chemical treatise.[27] However, like overconsumption of sugar, the daily consumption of excessive quantities of honey may play an important role in the genesis of cardiovascular and other diseases.[28]

Nevertheless, excessive quantities of honey are thought to be much less harmful than white sugar because, in contrast to processed sugar, honey contains B-complex vitamins and enzymes which play an important role in the metabolism of sugar and other carbohydrates.

Beckmann (Hiller[29]) reported favourable results with honey injections in heart patients. However, urticaria, asthmatic conditions and even oedema of the lungs may follow such injections. Beckmann believed that this was due to idiosyncrasy and that anti-histaminics should be kept in readiness. Nissen, who had seen severe attacks of asthma after honey injections, advised against the use of such injections, whilst Hiller[29] reports a case of most severe general shock, apart from reactions, after intravenous administration of honey.

In the course of extensive honey injections, Hiller found that many patients reacted with a sensation of warmth, nausea, retching, dizziness, pressure in the head and typical reactions of an allergic nature, such as conjunctivitis and itching of the skin. These symptoms were mostly not very pronounced; however, some patients showed, apart from asthma, a state of collapse, and in one case pronounced shock associated with a deep coma resulted. In order to prevent or inhibit reactions of an allergic nature, Hiller used substances which inhibited anaphylaxis. Calcium appeared to counteract allergic reactions, although this depended on the sensitivity of the patient and the speed of injection, and there was a fair degree of success with phenobarbitone. In animal experiments, injections of honey induced allergic responses in guinea-pigs only after many injections. In rabbits it was found that honey protein did not lead to antibody production. Hiller is in general agreement with other authors that the administration of honey may induce undesirable reactions; however, by applying precautionary measures, such as the preparation of special solutions of honey and administering these in dilute form, to a large extent these could be prevented.

Chemnitius *et al.*[30] determined the action of sugars and varying concentrations of different samples of honey on the isolated homothermal heart, papillary muscle and atrium of guinea-pigs and cats. They found that solutions of honey were generally superior to invert sugar. The various samples of honey showed differences in their action on the heart. Every one of the eight different kinds of honey showed a pronounced, if varying, effect on the heart in that they markedly stimulated the contractile force and induced dilation of the coronary vessels. The authors presumed that the effects of honey on the heart are due to the presence of a cholinergic substance. Deproteinated honey retained its cholinergic effect. On the other hand, Helvey[18] states that the coronary dilatory action of honey depends on its qualitative sugar content. This subject is now of interest to carbohydrate chemists.[31]

Hammerl and Pichler (Ref. 32) were able to show that royal jelly ('Gelée Royal Holzinger (GRH)') caused a fall in the total cholesterol content, an increase in phospholipids and a fall in the arteriosclerotic elevated C/P quotient.

Other workers[32] injected GRH into 16 female and 4 male patients. The cytological changes in the females pointed to oestrogenic action in the vagina and on the cervix. There were no changes in the endometrium. In the males, cytological changes suggested androgenic action. The patients showed pronounced improvement in vegetative conditions (insomnia, dysmenorrhoea, increased blood flow). Unpleasant side-effects (slight headache, dizziness) rarely appeared. In two of the patients *impotentia coeundi* was successfully treated. Proliferation in vaginal epithelium set in 24 hr after injection of GRH into patients with senile atrophy. There was also improvement in primary and climacteric ovarial insufficiency. Herold[2] described the use of honey in pregnancy, infants, juveniles, geriatrics and its beneficial effects on the kidneys, liver, heart, nerves, skin, respiratory apparatus, digestive organs, wounds, eyes, diabetics, radiation sickness and drunkenness.

Forster[16] reported favourable effects of 'Apifortyl' (*see* p. 88) in the prophylaxis of exhaustion and the treatment of diseases of old age (atherosclerosis, vitamin deficiencies and anorexia).

Stadler[33] administered orally, to normal subjects and patients suffering from various diseases, 25 g of invert sugar and honey. The results were inconsistent in that sometimes the blood sugar was higher after honey than after invert sugar and sometimes it was lower. In diabetics, there was little difference, while in patients with liver disease, honey often produced a higher blood sugar level than did invert sugar. According to Stadler[33] there seem to be no therapeutic indications for the administration of honey in *diabetes mellitus*.

Tobiasch and Killian[34] administered equivalent amounts of honey and glucose to healthy individuals and diabetics and found that:

1. 'In healthy subjects, blood sugar values after honey rose somewhat faster and fell somewhat sooner than after glucose. The peaks reached after both (taking initial values as zero) were about equal after honey and glucose. In diabetics, there was a striking difference in the behaviour of the blood sugar curves after honey and glucose, a difference far greater than could be explained by the margin of error inherent in the method. In single instances, in fact, the blood sugar rise after honey was only half that after glucose. Often the rise was faster after honey, and there was a more rapid decline in the curve. In 9 out of the 17 cases, the blood sugar fell after 180 min to below the initial value. Among diabetics who regularly excreted a slight amount of sugar in the urine, there was generally no increase in glucosuria on honey days. Often, in fact, there was a *decrease* in sugar excretion on these days. In no case was any lasting disturbance of carbohydrate metabolism (extending to the next day) observed after honey had been given.

   After these preliminary experiments it was decided to add small amounts of honey to the regime of diabetics, without otherwise altering the strictly dietary or insulin-aided control of the patients. Since it was difficult to ensure strict clinical control of the subjects, the authors offer no final opinion on this phase of their study. However, their short-term experiments indicate that small amounts of honey in the diabetic diet are well tolerated. The addition of 20 g of honey in the morning and 20 g in the afternoon had practically no effect on the blood sugar curve (the peak was no higher than that reached without honey). In older diabetics, 20 g of honey every second day did not disturb the control previously achieved. (This amount of honey would, of course, supply no more than 60 to 120 calories.)'

2. 'Of great importance is that pure summer honey is much better tolerated than winter honey (from bees fed cane sugar). Winter sugar-produced honey caused a much higher elevation in the blood sugar level than summer honey, though in neither case was the contrast as striking as that between the rises following honey and sugar.'
3. 'These short-term experiments require confirmation by long-term studies, but they seem to show that pure summer honey in small amounts (10–20 g/day) does not interfere with carbohydrate metabolism in controlled cases of mild– and medium–severe diabetes.'

In a personal communication, dated 14th May, 1970, Dr G. D. Campbell, Durban (co-author with T. L. Cleave of the book *Diabetes, Coronary Thrombosis and the Saccharine Diseases*) stated: 'In insulin-dependent diabetics I would certainly allow them to take a teaspoon in a cup of tea, once a day.' Herold[2] discusses the use of honey in diabetes and states that it can be taken with beneficial effects. He rightly recommends that diabetics should take honey only under medical supervision in order that the urinary sugar content can be controlled.

Goldschmidt *et al.*[10] state that the physiological and therapeutic effects of honey are due to the presence of a cholinergic factor, which is probably acetylcholine (2·5 mg/kg). Honey also contains at least 60 mg/kg choline. Goldschmidt *et al.*[35] confirmed the results of investigations made by Koch and Baumgarten that intravenous transfusion of honey solutions (4 mg/kg/min) into anaesthetised rabbits induces a lowering of blood pressure due to the presence of acetylcholine. The increase in blood pressure with higher concentrations of honey is brought about by the high concentration of sugar in the honey markedly raising the sugar content of the blood, thus preventing the action of acetylcholine.

Herold[2] also discusses the value of honey in drunkards. Martensen-Larsen of Copenhagen (Foreign Letters),[36] who has a wide experience in the treatment of cases of acute alcohol poisoning, reported that fructose promotes the metabolism of alcohol, has a sobering and sedative effect corresponding to that of Vitamin B_6 and tends to rid the patient of any desire for more alcohol. As a substitute for pure fructose, Martensen-Larsen used Danish honey, half the sugar content of which is fructose, administering two doses (each 125 g) at 30-min intervals.

Artner[37] reported on experiences with GRH iontophoresis on 1438 patients in 7 outpatient departments of the Austrian Health Service. All these patients had previously been treated by physical methods and had received drug treatment, mostly without success. Of 1135 patients suffering from epicondylitis, arthrosis, arthritis, intermittent claudication, vascular diseases, neuralgia, sciatica and myalgia, 238 showed no response to the GRH therapy. However, many of the patients showed significant improvement in their conditions, while many were completely cured. In almost all cases of hypertension there was a return to normal blood pressure.

Referring to the work done by Rückl and Klein, Artner regards it as feasible that the action of GRH could be explained by its activating and regulating action in the mid-brain. Such a mode of action, Artner states, would also explain the favourable results achieved by him in the treatment of his cases with GRH.

Treatment of 25 cases of seborrhoea and *effluvium capitis* with a GRH hair lotion, in combination with ultraviolet radiation, met with complete success and increased growth of hair.

It is stated: 'The biological effects of the jelly are disputed. It is reported to have antibiotic power, to affect the adrenal cortex, to cause hyperglycaemia, and to have an anti-tumorigenic effect in mice which appears to be due to 10-hydroxy decanoic acid. There is no good evidence of its oestrogenic activity, or that it affects the growth, longevity or fertility of animals. Clinically it has been used as a general tonic to ward off the effects of old age and to ease sufferers from chronic degenerative disease. It seems likely that the novelty of the treatment, and not the substance, has been responsible for whatever successes it has had in these conditions.'[26]

Referring to royal jelly, Kreze and Toman[38] state: 'After 3 weeks administration of Vita-Apinol, in daily doses corresponding to 150 mg of neutral royal jelly, no significant increase in the urinary excretion of total and individual 17-hydroxycorticosteroids has been found in 10 patients. The results indicate that royal jelly is incapable of activating steroidgenesis by the adrenal gland (20 references).'

Grad *et al.*[39] injected 1 ml of royal jelly subcutaneously into mice. Seventeen out of 27 animals died within 48 hr. Histologic examination showed many haemorrhages in the brain of the mice. They proved that the toxicity of the royal jelly was due neither to its acidity nor to an osmotic effect. Mice which received 0·1 ml of royal jelly daily for 27 days gained more in weight than the controls, while others treated daily with 0·1 or 0·01 ml of royal jelly for 14 days showed increased weight of the adrenals and histologically large and pale cells were seen in the *Zona fasciculata*. After treatment with 0·1 ml of royal jelly for 15 to 18 days the lymph nodes showed an increase in weight.

Duisberg,[24] Director of the Institute for Honey Research, Bremen, Germany, reviewed the literature on the composition and on the physiological and therapeutic action of honey. In the review he reported on the extensive research on honey done at the Institute. He stated that the favourable action of honey on man's health has been known for ages:

1. Acetylcholine present in the honey induces increased coronary blood flow, and a decrease in the heart-rate, and lower blood pressure. Honey also regulates cardiac arrhythmias.
2. Administration of hypertonic sugar and honey solutions is followed by:

   (*a*) diffusion of fluid from the tissues into the blood stream resulting in diuresis. The degree of diuresis depends on the dose, the concentration and the rate of excretion;

   (*b*) an increase of blood sugar concentration followed by increased insulin production. After fructose administration, the blood sugar content rises to a lesser degree. Intravenous administration of honey is followed by a fall in blood pressure, probably because of acetylcholine.

3. After administration of honey, glycogen formation is stimulated, especially by the cholinergic factor.
4. Honey has a favourable effect on parenchymatous liver damage (reducing the absorption of bile acids into the blood which in turn counteracts itching of the skin), gastro-duodenal ulcers,

hyperemesis gravidarum, disturbances of peripheral circulation and vegetative dystonias.

5. In contrast to sugar, honey increases gastric secretion, probably due to the cholinergic action of the latter. The slight laxative action of honey is probably also due in part at least to the presence of acetylcholine.
6. It is known that sugar and honey have an effect on the vegetative nervous system and that especially fructose has a favourable action on intoxication with alcohol, barbituric acid and in cases of decompensated *diabetes mellitus*.
7. It is known that for the metabolism of sugar in the human body fair amounts of the B-complex vitamins are required. These vitamins are lacking in artificial honeys. Natural honey is not rich in vitamins but it does help to increase vitamin intake and hence plays a part in the vitamin balance of metabolism.

Duisberg[24] and his associates have examined thousands of samples of honey from almost all honey-producing countries and found that the enzyme content of natural honey is sufficiently high to ensure a significant action in human digestive processes. Honey saccharase is more resistant to hydrochloric acid and pepsin than honey diastase and it is also fairly heat resistant (little inactivation occurring after heating at 50°C for 10 hr). Barmstedt (Duisberg[24]) drew attention to the fact that in caries-prone individuals the saccharase content of the saliva is very low with the result that acid formation from sugar in the mouth (especially between the teeth) is enhanced. Honey, which contains fair amounts of saccharase, will serve to raise the lowered saccharase content of the buccal cavity.

Duisberg[24] affirmed that, apart from sugars, honey contains other biological factors: a plant-rooting hormone (Oliver); an oestrogenic substance (Dingemanse); a guinea-pig anti-stiffness factor (Church); a bactericidal factor (inhibine) (Dold); a permeability stimulatory factor (Klotzbücher).

Apparently there is also present in honey a growth factor. Vignec and Julia (Herold[2]) reported that in trials with honey on 387 infants and babies up to 4 months of age they found, in comparison with the controls, not only a higher haemoglobin content of the blood, but also increased rate of growth.

HONEY AS A BACTERICIDAL AGENT AND IN THE TREATMENT OF WOUNDS

Zaiss,[40] who apparently had extensive experience with honey used as a medicant applied externally, reviewed the literature and quoted his personal experience in the treatment of wounds and other afflictions of the skin and the buccal mucous membrane. He stressed the importance of honey as an agent for the prevention of infection of fresh wounds and he compared the healing effect of honey with that of other preparations used in the treatment of wounds and found it superior to all other medications in general use at the time, especially in the cleansing and treatment of necrotic and 'dirty' wounds. He described his very successful method of treatment of thousands of infected wounds, some in great detail, and his great success in the treatment of burns, oral infections, furunculosis and carbuncles. He also stressed that he used only ordinary honey centrifuged from the combs, and not any specially prepared type, and that it should not be heated above blood temperature. Zaiss stated that it is as yet not clear what is the mode of action of honey on wounds. Lührs[41] confirmed the favourable results obtained by Zaiss[40] in the treatment of lacerated and infected wounds with honey, reporting it to be superior to other methods. He also referred to Straub's successful treatment of fistulous and other wounds in military horses with a paste prepared from honey, rye meal and olive oil.

Bahr[42] stated that honey is of great nutritional value, and that lime-tree and clover honey and other natural honeys are of great value in the prevention of infections in white mice with the ratin-bacillus group (paratyphoid enteritidis group). The active principle, which is heat-labile, was unknown. Artificial honeys were much less effective in prevention of infections.

Müller [43] stated that, since honey is recorded in the 'Deutsches Arnzneibuch', purity tests are prescribed. Honey has a cleansing and healing effect on wounds. It is said to stimulate the formation and flow of lymph. The resins and terpenes dissolved in colloidal form and the organic acids and higher alcohols act partly as irritants and partly as resorptive agents, and in this way support antiseptic and anti-inflammatory action. Vitamin A and riboflavin also have a healing effect on wounds. He studied the effect of honey on lesions on the ears of rabbits induced by mustard gas and other war gases, and found that it had an antiseptic and healing effect. It also counteracted secondary infections, reduced the period of healing and reduced the size of the cicatrix.

In experiments embracing bacterial counts on agar dishes and in tests on white mice, Prica[44] found that natural honey from different sources, as well as mixed samples of honey, had a pronounced bactericidal action on both gram-positive and gram-negative bacteria. The samples of honey were diluted with tap water (1:1, 1:2 1:3 and 1:5). The bactericidal action was due not to the normal acidity of the honey nor to its sugar content, but apparently to the presence of a specific bactericidal agent. This substance may be present in the nectar or may be a secretory product of the bees. The bactericidal agent is filterable, thermolabile, susceptible to high acidity and almost unaffected by diffuse daylight. Prica stated that the bactericidal agent may be the inhibine described by Dolds and also referred to by Herold.[2]

According to investigations conducted by Marienburg,[45] a honey–cod liver oil preparation marketed by the firm Atarost yielded favourable results in the treatment of wounds and other skin diseases in cats, dogs, cattle and horses.

Yang[46] reported marked success in the employment of an ointment consisting of 80% honey in a base of vaseline or lard in the treatment of 50 cases of chilblains, chilblain ulcers and small wounds. He thought 'that honey might be bacteriostatic because of its high sugar content and that it might contain Vitamin A because its yellow pigment is derived from various yellow flowers.

Yang noted the following effects:

1. 'Rapid subsidence of passive congestion and edematous swelling.'
2. 'Rapid stimulation of epithelisation and granulation.'
3. 'In some cases rapid diminution of local pain.'
4. 'The presence of a moderate amount of seropulent discharge did not interfere with its effectiveness.'

It should be added that such a high sugar content in the ointment would exert a marked osmotic pressure which would 'draw' toxins and bacteria out of the wound and hence have a cleansing and detoxicating effect.

Quadratullah[47] urges the wider therapeutic use of honey in poor and backward areas where sulphonamides and antibiotics are unobtainable, as it has antiseptic, analgesic and sedative properties.

The bactericidal properties of honey have been stressed,[48] and honey is an excellent source of energy;[49] one ounce supplying 320 calories. The following nine characteristics of honey render it superior to other sources of sugar:

1. it does not irritate the mucous membranes of the digestive organs;
2. it is quickly and easily assimilated;
3. as a source of energy it releases energy quickly;
4. it induces quick recovery of sportsmen and others who expend much energy after their exertions;
5. of all sugars it is best tolerated by the kidneys;
6. it has a slight and natural laxative action;
7. it has a sedative effect—the calming effect of a glass of hot milk with a teaspoonful of honey is well known;
8. the mineral components of honey do not occur in the free state but are bound organically and hence are easily assimilable;
9. it contains many enzymes.

According to L.J.B.[50] royal jelly is an excellent general tonic. Rubin *et al.*[51] discuss honey as a vehicle for medicinal preparations.

POLLEN AND POLLEN HONEY

Herold[2] describes the gathering, purification, storage and medicinal uses of honey to which pollen has been added. He warns, however, that pollen may be poisonous if attacked by fungi.

HONEY POISONING

Honey prepared from the nectar of poisonous plants has been responsible for many cases of poisoning in man. Apparently the most ancient report of honey poisoning is that described by Xenophon at the Black Sea in 401 BC. After the battle of Xunaxa many soldiers who had eaten honey developed severe gastro-intestinal symptoms and lay as if intoxicated on the ground. Similar cases were described by Diodorus, Strabon and Plinius.[52] It is advisable to suspect honey of being poisonous if prepared from any poisonous plant. Plants are well-known to have poisoned bees and their larvae, and to have produced poisonous honey. Certain species of *Rhododendron,* (*Ericaceae*) *R. ponticum L., R. Javanicus* Benn., *R. maximum* L. (great laurel, North America), *R. barbatum* Don (East India), *R. Falconeri* Hook f., *R. fulgens* Hook, *R. grande* Wight, *R. punctatum* Andr. (North America), *R. Cinnabarium* Hookf., *R. indicum* Siv. (China) (*Azalea amoena* Lindl) contain andromedotoxin (*R. ponticum* contains 0·05 to 0·1 %) (Wehmer[53]).

Andromedotoxin, also poisonous to fish, occurs in species of *Andromeda, Azalea* and *Kalmia.* It is a bitter substance which induces drunkenness, salivation, a burning sensation in the throat, vomiting, diarrhoea, pronounced sweating, severe weakness, slow pulse and spasms. Death is due to respiratory paralysis. Dogs have died after 0·3 mg of andromedotoxin per kg of body weight (Wehmer[53]). Moeschlin,[54] Wirth *et al.*[55] and Carey *et al.*[56] investigated the toxicity of honey prepared from *Rhododendron* species and their hybrids which are regarded as poisonous to bees. They showed that the nectar from different species of *Rhododendron,* especially from the flower of *Rhododendron thomsoni* and its hybrids, was very toxic to bees and mice, and they were able to isolate a substance identical to andromedotoxin (acetylandromedol).

The following is an abstract of the results of investigations conducted by Scott *et al.*[57] into honey poisoning:

'A toxic honey sample from Grouse Mountain, British Columbia, was shown to contain Grayanotoxin II and Grayanotoxin III compounds closely related to Grayanotoxin I (andromedotoxin), together with desacetyl pieristoxin B. Identification was by thin-layer chromatography and mouse bio-assay. No Grayanotoxin I was detected in the honey. Intraperitoneal LD50 values for Grayanotoxin I and III were 1·28 and 0·908 mg/kg, respectively, in mice: Grayanotoxin II was not toxic at low intraperitoneal dose level.'

Apart from other aspects of honey, Husing[5] also discussed honey poisoning with special reference to the collection by bees of nectar from species of *Rhododendron Kalmia, Azalea* and *Andromeda.* The symptoms of poisoning are nausea, abdominal pain, diarrhoea, disturbances of consciousness and eyesight.

He also referred to the fact that bees are at times themselves poisoned if they collect nectar from *Colchicum autumnale* L., *Aesculus californica* N. and *Tilia argentea* Dest. Poisoned bees became paralysed and unconscious and often died under the poisonous plants from which they had collected the nectar. According to Dayton[58] (p. 102), Vansell reported fatal poisoning among Californian bees and their larvae from the nectar, pollen and sap of *Aesculus californica* N. (California buckeye). Grubb[59] describes cases of poisoning with honey prepared from the nectar of flowers of the mountain laurel (mountain ivy), *Kalmia latifoloa.* The symptoms were vomiting, slow pulse and weakness at the wrist. Moeschlin[54] states that it is known that honey from certain areas causes poisoning by virtue of atropine-like substances. Hodges and White[60] developed a thin-layer chromatographic technique for the detection of hyaenanchin (previously called mellitoxin) and tutin in honey. From one honey sample the authors also isolated (+) 2-hydroxy-3-phenylpropionic acid. They state: 'Tutin and hyaenanchin have now been isolated from three toxic honey samples and recognised in 15 others by their RF's on silica gel plates. Together they account for most of the toxicity which can be extracted from honey by organic solvents. A method for the detection of tutin and hyaenanchin in 5-g samples of honey is given.' Rabbits dosed with the outer soft portion of the fruit of *Hyaenanche globosa* Lamb, which contains hyaenanchin, developed strychnine-like convulsions and died within 15 min (Steyn[61]).

Swanson[62] has shown that tutin (the toxic principle of *Coriaria ruscifolia* (toot-plant of New Zealand) very closely resembles coriamyrtin in its toxic effects. The prominent symptoms in man are giddiness, stupor, loss of memory, and coma with or without delirium or convulsions. The delirium may resemble alcoholic intoxication. There may be violent convulsions and acute mania.

Rausching[63] detected up to 365 ppm of zinc in artificial honey prepared in zinc vessels. The question of prohibiting the use of zinc vessels in the preparation of honey is raised.

Numerous investigations (Schuette and Ihde[64]) have reported on the presence of lead in various raw and canned foods and drinks. They reviewed the literature concerned and proceeded to determine lead in various samples and brands of honey. In 2 out of 16 samples of honey in the comb they detected 0·03 and 0·05 mg Pb/kg respectively; in 4 out of 11 samples of honey sold in glass containers they found from 0·05 to 6·80 mg Pb/kg; and in 9 out of 19 samples of honey in tinned containers they detected from 0·02 to 4·26 mg Pb/kg. The authors state that the source of the lead in honey is probably not connected with lead-containing insecticidal sprays on fruit trees and flowers as the bees which visit such flowers would be fatally poisoned. It is possible that in the process of extraction of the honey, lead-containing apparatus was used. Kerin and Kerin[65] refer to contamination of honey with lead-containing aerosols used in industry.

There is also a possibility that honey may be contaminated with herbicides. Courtney *et al.*[66] refer to 2,4,5-trichlorohenoxyacetic acid (2,4,5-T).

ALLERGY

Beekeepers may develop contact dermatitis caused by *propolis* (Burney[67]), a brownish resinous substance of waxy consistency, collected by bees from the buds of trees and used as a cement.

CONCLUSIONS

Honey is the product of the processing of nectar by the honey-bee. According to information collected from an extensive literature, honey and royal jelly have the properties listed below.

Composition of Honey

(*a*) Vitamins—ascorbic acid (Vitamin C), B-complex vitamins.
(*b*) Proteins.
(*c*) Minerals (potassium, sodium, calcium, magnesium, iron, copper, manganese, phosphate and sulphate).
(*d*) An anti-haemorrhagic factor.
(*e*) Enzymes—diastase, glucose-oxidase, saccharase.
(*f*) Deuterium.
(*g*) Saccharides—sucrosc (saccharose), glucose, fructose, maltose, lactose, melezitose, raffinose and seven unclassified saccharides.
(*h*) Traces of lipids.
(*i*) An oestrogenic substance.
(*j*) A guinea-pig anti-stiffness factor.
(*k*) A bactericidal (antibiotic) factor (inhibine).

The composition, taste, health-giving and therapeutic properties of honey depend on the following factors: age (spring, unripe or winter honey), source (kind of nectar), natural or sugar-fed honey, whether commercially processed (clarified) or not, period of storage, percentage of pollen present (removal of pollen reduces the vitamin content), pH, type of container, and place of storage (diffuse light decreases the vitamin content of honey). There is a considerable variation in the composition, especially the vitamin content, of honey.

Honey is naturally acid with a pH range of 5 to 7.

Physiological Actions of Honey

(*a*) The coronary-dilatory and inotropic (affecting the force or energy of muscular contractions) action of honey depends on its acetylcholine and qualitative sugar content. It was found that honey markedly stimulated the contractile force of the heart.

(*b*) Owing to the presence of acetylcholine, honey induces a lowering of blood pressure. This effect is antagonised by atropine.

(*c*) It is an excellent energy and protective food.

(*d*) It has laxative properties.

(*e*) It has a favourable effect on processes of metabolism probably chiefly due to the presence of various enzymes (saccharase, glucose-oxidase, diastase, etc.).

Composition of Royal Jelly

(*a*) Eleven amino acids—lysine, arginine, asparagine, glycine, serine, glutamic acid, β-alanine, γ-aminobutyric acid, proline, methionine and leucine.

(*b*) Five sugars, four of which have been identified as sucrose, glucose, fructose and ribose.

(*c*) Much higher concentrations of all the B-complex vitamins than in honey.

(*d*) Acid-phosphatase.

(*e*) Proteins, lipids and fatty acids.

(*f*) A non-specific cholinesterase capable of splitting acetylcholine, benzoylcholine, methyl-*n*-butyrate and tributyrine. When stored for long periods, it loses its esterase action.

Royal jelly has a significant influence on fat metabolism. It reduces the cholesterol and increases the phospholipid content of the blood and induces a fall in the arteriosclerotic elevated C/P quotient.

Oestrogenic and androgenic actions have been ascribed to royal jelly.

It is necessary to fortify the chief constituents of royal jelly in order to improve its medicinal properties.

Medical Uses of Honey

According to reports in the literature, it appears that honey and royal jelly are of value in the prevention and treatment of diseases.

Diabetes mellitus. Pure summer honey in small amounts does not seem to interfere with carbohydrate metabolism in controlled cases of mild and medium–severe cases. However, the short-term experiments require confirmation.

Hypertension. Acetylcholine in the honey is responsible for increasing coronary blood flow, a decrease in the heart rate and lowering of blood pressure. Honey also regulates cardiac arrhythmias, supplies energy to the heart muscle and improves peripheral circulation.

Diseases of the liver, including poisoning.

Vomiting during pregnancy.

Chronic constipation.

Disturbances of carbohydrate, and processes of metabolism.

Infected wounds and sores. Honey has a bactericidal action due to inhibine; cleanses wounds and sores, stimulates epithelisation and reduces the size of the cicatrix; increases the subsidence of passive congestion and oedematous swelling, and reduces local pain.

Sexual disorders and general. It appears that owing to the presence of oestrogenic and androgenic substances in royal jelly, it is of value in the treatment of dysmenorrhoea, senile atrophy of the vaginal epithelium, primary and climateric ovarial insufficiency, and impotence. It also induces pronounced improvement in vegetative dystonia (insomnia, lack of energy, depressive states, retarded blood flow).

A fortified royal jelly preparation was of value in the prevention and treatment of old age (exhaustion, atherosclerosis, lack of appetite, etc.).

By means of GRH (*see* p. 90) many patients suffering from hypertension, epicondylitis, arthrosis, intermittent claudication, vascular diseases, neuralgia, sciatica and myalgia showed improvement and some were completely cured.

A hair-lotion, containing GRH, applied together with ultraviolet radiation, completely cured cases of seborrhoea and increased hair growth.

Cautionary Note

Many cases of honey poisoning are described. It is wise not to eat any off-flavour honey. The toxicity of honey may be due to the nectar having been collected from the flowers of poisonous plants and/or flowers sprayed with insecticides. Cases of zinc and lead poisoning have been described as a result of the use of zinc- or lead-containing apparatus and utensils in the extraction and storing of honey.

REFERENCES

1. Steyn, D. G. (1970). 'Honey as a Food and in the Prevention and Treatment of Disease, Publications of the University of Pretoria, South Africa, New Series No. 52 (Brochure). (Also published in *Internat. J. Vitalstoffe* (Germany), **14** (1969) p. 201.)
2. Herold, E. (1970). *Heilwerte aus dem Bienenvolk,* Ehrenwirth Verlag, München, Germany, 226 pp.
3. Editorial (1967). *Food and Cosmetic Toxicology,* **5,** p. 73.
4. Kandos, R. F. (1940). *Zeitschrift für Untersuchung der Lebensmittel,* **79,** p. 258. (Abstract in *Analyst,* **65** (1940) p. 363.)
5. Husing (1956). *Honig, Wachs, Bienengift,* Die Neue Brehm, Bucherei, A. Ziemsen Verlag, Witteberg Lutherstadt, Germany.
6. Ellewood, J. A. and Fischer, L. (1941). *Food Research,* **5,** p. 559.
7. Haydak, M. H., Palmer, L. S., Tanguary, M. C. and Vivino, A. E. (1942). *J. Nutrition,* **23,** p. 581.
8. Haydak, M. H., Palmer, L. S., Tanguary, M. C. and Vivino, A. E. (1943). *J. Nutrition,* **26,** p. 319.
9. Kitzes, G., Schuette, H. A. and Elvehjem, C. A. (1943). *J. Nutrition,* **26,** p. 241.
10. Goldschmidt, S., Burkert, H. and Helmreich, E. (1952). *Zeitschrift Naturforschung,* **7b,** p. 365. (Abstracted in *Berichte über die gesamte Physiologie und experimentele Pharmakologie,* **157** (1953) p. 330.)
11. Marguardt, P. and Vogg, G. (1952). *Arzneimittel-Forschung,* **2,** p. 152.
12. Marguardt, P. and Vogg, G. (1952). *Arzneimittel-Forschung,* **2,** p. 446.
13. Marguardt, P. and Vogg, G. (1953). *Arzneimittel-Forschung,* **3,** p. 446.
14. Schuler, R. (1957). *Arzneimittel-Forschung,* **7,** p. 330.
15. Ammon, R. and Zoch, E. (1957). *Arzneimittel-Forschung,* **7,** p. 699.
16. Forster, K. A. (1957). *Deutsche Apotheker-Zeitung,* **97,** p. 1162.
17. König, R. (1959). *Deutsche Apotheker-Zeitung,* **99,** p. 28.

18. Helvey, T. C. (1953). *Science,* **177,** p. 276.
19. Chemnitius, K. H. and Engel, C. H. (1961). *Deutsche Apotheker-Zeitung,* **101,** p. 691.
20. Sherpaz, A. I. (1966). *Acta Biochemica et Biophysica* (Enzymes and Biological Oxidations), **118,** p. 637.
21. Smith, M. R. and McCaughey, W. F. (1966). *J. Food Sci.,* **31,** p. 902.
22. Lampitt, L. H. and Bilham, P. (1936). *Analyst,* **720,** p. 192.
23. Smith, M. R. (1963). *Identification of Some Trace Lipids in Honey.*
24. Duisberg, A. (1962). *Internat. J. Vitalstoffe* (Germany), **7,** p. 122.
25. Hadhanyi, A. L. (1958). *Vitalstoffe Konventbericht,* 4 Internationale Vitalstoffe und Ernährungs-Konvent, 8–12 October, Essen, Germany, p. 46.
26. Dayan (1960). *Pharmaceutical J.,* Fourth Series, **131,** p. 35.
27. Siddiqui (1969). 'Der Wendepunkt', Medical Publication, Bircher–Benner Clinic, Zurich, Switzerland, p. 33.
28. Cleave, T. L., Campbell, G. D. and Painter, N. S. (1969). *Diabetes, Coronary Thrombosis and the Saccharine Disease,* 2nd Edition, John Wright and Sons, Ltd, Bristol.
29. Hiller, E. (1951). *Medizinische Monatschrift,* **5,** p. 626.
30. Chemnitius, K. H., Pilz, H. and Prufer, H. (1959). *Arzneimittel-Forschung,* **9,** p. 151.
31. Siddiqui (1970). *Advances in Carbohydrate Chemistry,* **25,** p. 285.
32. Editorial (1958). *Medizinische Monatschrift,* **12,** p. 727.
33. Stadler, A. (1954). *J. Clinical Nutrition,* **12,** p. 69. (Abstracted from *Deutsche Zeitschrift für Verdauungs-und Stoffwechselkrankheiten,* **12** (1952) p. 108.)
34. Tobiasch, V. and Killian, P. (1953). *J. Clinical Nutrition,* **1,** p. 410. (Abstracted from *Deutsche Zeitschrift für Verdauungs-und Stoffwechselkrankheiten,* **13** (1953) p. 401.)
35. Goldschmidt, S., Burkert, H., Gloxhuber, C., Gramms, H. and Anders, C. (1955). *Hoppe-Seylers Zeitschrift für Physiologiese Chemie,* **300,** p. 201.
36. Martensen-Larsen (1954). *Jour. Amer. Med. Assoc.,* **156,** p. 733.
37. Artner, F. (1958). *Münchener Medizinische Wochenschrift,* **100,** p. 1968.
38. Kreze, A. and Toman, A. (1969). *International Pharmaceutical Abstracts,* **6,** No. 22, p. 869. (Abstracted from *Vnitrni Lekar,* **15** (1969) p. 341, Czechoslovakia.)
39. Grad, B., Kral, V. A. and Berenson, J. (1961). *Canadian J. Biochemistry,* **39,** p. 461.
40. Zaiss (Dr.) (1934). *Münchener Medizinische Wochenschrift,* **8,** p. 1891.
41. Lührs, B. (1935). *Jahresbericht Veterinäre Medizin,* **57,** p. 295. (Abstracted from *Zeitschrift Veterinärkunde,* **47** (1935) p. 57.)
42. Bahr, L. (1934). *Berliner Tierarztliche Wochenschrift,* **4,** p. 321.
43. Müller, W. (1938). *Berichte über die gesamte Physiologie und experimentele Pharmakologie,* **105,** p. 678. (Abstracted from *Medizinische Welt,* 1937, p. 1981.)
44. Prica, M. (1938). *Zeitschrift für Hygiene und Infektionskrankheiten,* **120,** p. 437.

45. Marienburg, M. (1939). 'Bienenhonig-Lebertransalbe bei der Wundbehandlung', Dissertation: Hanover, Germany. Reviewed in *Jahresbericht Veterinäre Medizin*, **66** (1939) p. 108.
46. Yang, K. L. (1944). *American J. Pharmacy,* **116,** p. 479. (Abstracted from *Chinese Medicine*, **62** (1944) p. 55.)
47. Quadratullah, M. D. (1953). *Excerpta Medica,* Section II, **6,** p. 461. (Abstracted from *The Medicus* (Karachi), **3** (1952) p. 201.)
48. Editorial (1962). *De Natuurgeneeswyze,* June, p. 150.
49. Editorial (1962). *De Natuurgeneeswyze*, July/August, p. 173.
50. L.J.B. (Dr.) (1958). *De Natuurgeneeswyze,* **10,** p. 288.
51. Rubin, N., Gennaro, A. R., Sideri, C. N. and Osol, A. (1959). *American J. Pharmacy,* **131,** p. 246.
52. Diodorus, Strabon and Plinius. (1967). *Medizinische Monatschrift,* **21,** p. 77.
53. Wehmer, C. (1931). *Die Pflanzenstoffe,* Vol. 2, Gustav Fisher, Jena, p. 909.
54. Moeschlin, S. (1959). *Klinik und Therapie der Vergiftungen,* Georg Thieme Verlag, Stuttgart.
55. Wirth, W., Hect, G. and Gloxhuber, C. (1967). *Toxikologie-Fibel,* Georg Thieme Verlag, Stuttgart, p. 263.
56. Carey, F. M., Lewis, J. J., MacGregor, J. L. and Martin-Smith, M. (1959). *J. Pharmacy and Pharmacology*, **II,** p. 269T.
57. Scott, P. M. *et al*. (1970). *BIBRA Bull.*, 9**,** p. 552.
58. Dayton, W. A. (1931). 'Important Western Browse Plants', United States Dept. Agric., Miscellaneous Publication No. 101.
59. Grubb, A. B. (1948). *Excerpta Medica*, Section II, **1,** p. 426. (Abstracted from *Virginia Medical Monthly*, **74** (1947) p. 86.)
60. Hodges, R. and White, E. P. (1966). *New Zealand J. Sci.,* **9,** p. 233.
61. Steyn, D. G. (1949). *Vergiftiging van Mens en Dier,* J. L. van Schaik, Ltd., Pretoria, South Africa.
62. Swanson (1947). *The Dispensatory of the United States of America,* 25th Edition, p. 541.
63. Rausching, S. (1944). *Brit. Chem. and Physiol.,* **8,** III, p. 163. (Abstracted from *Zeitschrift für Untersuchung der Lebensmittel,* **84** (1942) p. 30.)
64. Schuette, H. A. and Ihde, A. J. (1939). *Food Research*, **4,** p. 555.
65. Kerin, D. and Kerin, Z. (1971). *Protectio Vitae,* **16,** p. 61. (*International J. Vital Substances and Civilisation Diseases.*)
66. Courtney, K. *et al.* (1970). A taste of honey (flavoured with 2, 4, 5-T), *BIBRA Bull.,* **9,** p. 363. (Abstracted from *Science,* New York, **168** (1970) p. 363.)
67. Burney, M. H. (1968). *Berufsdermatosen* (Germany), **14,** p. 244.

DISCUSSION

Birch: I should like to raise the general point of the balance of minerals and the complex sugar mixture present in honey. For example, the absorption of carbohydrate, as Dr Barnett will mention tomorrow, depends on an intraluminal sodium content and there is much current work on this subject in the literature. Apart from this there is the intrinsic effect of minerals on sugar conformation, *e.g.* Angyal and Pickles have shown that 5% concentrations of some minerals can indeed alter the conformation of sugars from favoured to unfavoured forms, and hence possibly their absorptive properties. Has Professor Steyn or anyone else any information on these questions?

Steyn: I do believe it is possible and when we go into food processing we seem to attach so much value to vitamins that we have lost sight of the trace elements that play such a role in enzymes. As far as changes in the sugar moiety are concerned I would not venture an opinion for I have no information.

Hollingsworth: We have all heard of myths about honey. Has any experimental work been done on the physiological effects of honey?

Steyn: As a so-called scientist and pharmacologist interested in scientific proof, I would say that not all the claims made by laymen are proved scientifically but enough has been done. We know of inhibine. I believe there is such a possible cause of the anti-bacterial action of honey—it may be due to the high quantity of sugar, but I believe there is something like inhibine, because in experiments it has been proved that there is an anti-bacterial effect.

Pawan: The professor mentioned ascorbic acid. What was the amount?

Steyn: 400 mg %.

Pawan: Was the pollen from any particular plant?

Steyn: No, unfortunately not.

Bender: One of our foremost writers in this field is Barbara Cartland and she makes it plain that the honey must be from bees that were fed on honey during the winter. Is there any major difference in chemical composition between honey from bees fed or not fed sugar in winter?

Steyn: I think it would be fair to accept that honey from the flower-fed bee is better. We can't control or compare results because I don't know any two jars of honey where the composition is the same, especially processed honey and clarified honey. It depends on how long it has been stored.

Chairman: You say in your abstract that honey is used in the treatment of impotence, and that the old need it. Are these two things connected?

Steyn: I am taking honey, but not for that purpose! I believe you will find in many publications that honey is very beneficial, especially in geriatrics—it reduces blood pressure, improves digestion and is more absorbable than other sugars, and it also protects against arteriosclerosis. Whether the claims are true or not I don't know. There are claims from Germany for honey injected intravenously. I think that very dangerous.

Chairman: I just wondered what it was about the physiology of the old that they need honey and the young do not.

Steyn: There is a very widespread use of honey in athletics. The Greek athletes used it.

da Rocha-Afodu: It is said that honey contains a spreading factor and is anti-bacterial. These are two connected things, because people who have been trying to take honey and whose blood contains a high level of spreading factor are candidates for heart disease.

7

Biological Specificity of L-Xyloascorbic Acid (Vitamin C)

R. E. HUGHES

Department of Applied Biology, University of Wales Institute of Science and Technology, Cardiff, Wales

ABSTRACT

The biological specificity of a nutrient may refer to its specificity either in an isolated system (biochemical specificity) or as a dietary component (nutritional specificity). Differences in gastro-intestinal absorption and in the tissue retention of the nutrient frequently account for the lack of agreement between the two specificities. Nutritional studies on the antiscorbutic potencies of ascorbic acid analogues usually involve simple dosing techniques and should not be interpreted in terms of biochemical specificity.

The antiscorbutic potency of D-*araboascorbic acid* (iso*ascorbic acid,* iso*AA*) *has been widely reported to be one-twentieth of that of the natural isomer,* L-*xyloascorbic acid* (*Vitamin C, ascorbic acid, AA*). *This is in marked contrast with its known ability to replace AA in a number of well-characterised biochemical systems.*

Recent work has indicated that this discrepancy is probably attributable to the low tissue levels of iso*AA that result from its oral administration. Absorption of* iso*AA from the gastro-intestinal tract and its abstraction and retention by the tissues are very much lower than for similar oral doses of AA. Guinea-pigs whose tissue levels of* iso*AA have been raised by a special dosing technique to correspond to those of AA-sufficient animals do not develop scurvy, and their growth and other characteristics are indistinguishable from those of the AA-maintained guinea-pigs.*

In comparing iso*AA and AA, it would appear that AA does not possess any marked biochemical specificity; there are, however, important differences between the behaviour of the two isomers at biological membranes and in their retention by tissues.*

The elucidation of the structure of ascorbic acid (Vitamin C, Fig. 1A) in 1933[1] and the demonstration the following year that synthetic L-xyloascorbic acid was identical with the naturally occurring form of the vitamin[2] were followed by a series of nutritional studies designed to examine the biological potency of a wide range of ascorbic acid isomers and related compounds. A recent article summarised this early work and compared the antiscorbutic potencies of some sixteen compounds structurally related to L-xyloascorbic acid.[3] Of the compounds tested a number, such as D-xyloascorbic acid (Fig.

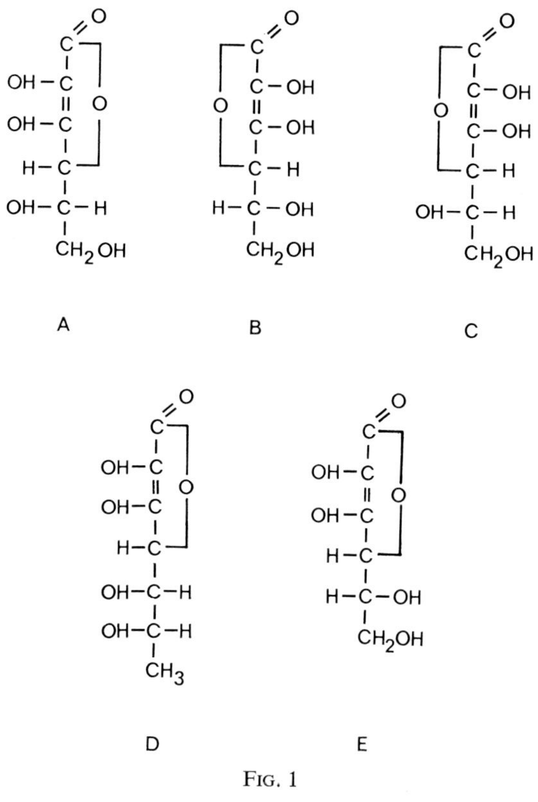

FIG. 1

1B) and L-araboascorbic acid (C), were found to be inactive, whereas others such as L-rhamnoascorbic acid (D) and D-araboascorbic (E) acid had biological potencies of 0·20 and 0·05 respectively (L-xyloascorbic acid = 1·0). These, and other results, led to the suggestion that a compound would possess antiscorbutic activity only if the five-atom lactone ring lay to the right of the carbon chain when the

Fischer convention for carbohydrate structure was followed. Of the sixteen or so compounds examined in the 1930s for antiscorbutic potency some ten showed no activity at all and in none of the others did it exceed 0·3. The reports of many of these early nutritional studies are lacking in much essential experimental detail, but it would appear that in most cases the test compound was administered orally as a single daily dose.[4–6] Recent studies (to be discussed later in this paper) have demonstrated that the mode and frequency of administration of an ascorbic acid are of critical importance in determining its apparent nutritional specificity. The results of these early, and somewhat uncritically designed, experiments should therefore be interpreted with caution.

IN VITRO STUDIES

This apparent lack of antiscorbutic activity on the part of ascorbic acid isomers and related compounds is in marked contrast with their behaviour in a number of *in vitro* enzyme systems involving ascorbic acid. Ascorbate oxidase (EC 1.10.3.3.) was examined in detail by Dodds who reported that its specificity was dependent upon the presence of a dienol grouping adjacent to a carbonyl group and closed ring system; L-xyloascorbic acid and D-araboascorbic acid were oxidised with equal facility.[7] A similar lack of specificity characterises the enzyme glutathione dehydrogenase (EC 1.8.5.1.) which catalyses the formation of L-xyloascorbic acid from its immediate oxidation product, dehydro-L-xyloascorbic acid, reduced glutathione acting as a hydrogen donor. A preparation of this enzyme made from pea cotyledons was equally active towards both dehydro-L-xyloascorbate and dehyro-D-araboascorbate (R. E. Hughes, unpublished observations). A functionally similar enzyme identified in animal tissues showed a 50% greater activity towards dehydro-D-araboascorbate than towards dehydro-L-xyloascorbate.[8,9]

More recent enzyme studies have centred on the role of ascorbic acid in biological hydroxylation.[10] A preparation of dopamine-β-hydroxylase (EC 1.14.2.1.) (necessary for the conversion of 3,4-dihydroxyphenylethylamine to norepinephrine) from bovine adrenal medulla showed comparable activities in the presence of L-xylo-ascorbic acid, D-xyloascorbic acid and D-araboascorbic acid and a slightly reduced activity in the presence of glucoascorbate.[11] L-xyloascorbic, D-araboascorbic and glucoascorbic acids possessed equivalent activity in stimulating *p*-hydroxyphenylpyruvate hydroxylase (EC 1.14.2.2.) which is responsible for the enzymic conversion of *p*-hydroxyphenylpyruvic acid into homogentisic acid, an obligatory step in the normal metabolic breakdown of phenylalanine.[12] It has also been shown that D-araboascorbic acid and L-xyloascorbic acid have similar potencies in activating γ-butyrobetaine hydroxylase which hydroxylates 4-trimethylaminobutyrate to 3-hydroxy-4-trimethylaminobutyrate (carnitine).[13] It is likely, however, that in the last two examples the ascorbic acids act not as electron donors, but by maintaining other essential factors in the reduced state,[14] in which case the question of their biological specificity becomes less relevant.

Probably the most significant recent development in the field of biological hydroxylation has been the characterisation of the mechanism whereby proline and lysine are hydroxylated in the biosynthesis of collagen;[10] hydroxylation occurs after their incorporation into protocollagen, the collagen precursor. A defect in this system, with a consequent impairment of collagen formation, would account for most, if not all, of the characteristics of classical scurvy. *In vitro* studies have indicated that with highly purified samples of proline hydroxylase, D-araboascorbic acid can completely replace L-xyloascorbic acid as a co-factor;[15] a separate study showed that in a cell-free proline hydroxylase system, L-xyloascorbic acid, D-xyloascorbic acid, D-araboascorbic acid and L-araboascorbic acid all had comparable activities.[16]

Available evidence would therefore appear to indicate that in animals the requirement of *in vitro* systems for ascorbic acid is not a rigidly defined one in terms of biochemical specificity. The only apparent exception to this is the finding that D-xyloascorbic acid is metabolised to carbon dioxide more rapidly than the L-isomer.[17]

The ascorbic acid-stimulated enzymic hydrolysis of mustard oil glucosides would appear to fall into a quite different category of reactions.[18] Six substances structurally related to L-xyloascorbic acid had similar upper limiting velocities for the rate of hydrolysis of sinigrin under standardised conditions. Glucoascorbate and D-xyloascorbate, however, were inactive—a finding in marked contrast with the activity of D-xyloascorbate in the proline hydroxylase system. Amongst the compounds active in the sinigrin system is

2-*O*-methyl-L-ascorbate, thus indicating that the ascorbate does not function in a reducing capacity. Furthermore, this is a system that would appear to be characteristic of the plant kingdom alone and as such has little bearing on the biological specificity of the ascorbic acids in animal systems.

BIOCHEMICAL AND NUTRITIONAL SPECIFICITIES

It would therefore appear that the same substance may possess a high nutritional specificity but a low biochemical one. This emerges clearly when L-xyloascorbic acid (Vitamin C, ascorbic acid, AA) is compared with D-araboascorbic acid (D-*iso*ascorbic acid (*iso*AA), erythorbic acid). The remainder of this discussion will centre on the behaviour of these two isomers; they have been extensively used in recent years as a model system in studies of nutritional and biochemical specificity. *Iso*AA differs from AA in the position of the —H and —OH groups on carbon 5; in some countries it has been used as an antioxidant in place of the more expensive AA and this is probably one reason why its physiological behaviour and metabolic fate have attracted attention over the last decade. It will be recalled that although *iso*AA can fully replace AA in biochemical systems where the vitamin is believed to be important, its antiscorbutic potency when measured by standard nutritional tests is only one-twentieth that of AA.[5,6]

It is possible to explain this apparent discrepancy in two ways. The first possibility is that AA has biochemical involvements other than those currently characterised in *in vitro* terms and that its role in these hitherto unrevealed systems is a highly specific one. The second possibility is that differences between the two isomers exist at the physiological level; these could be differences in membrane transport or in tissue retention or in renal threshold. Recent studies have indicated that the second of these possible explanations is probably the correct one. There is evidence that in respect of both its behaviour at membranes and its retention by tissues, *iso*AA behaves differently from AA. The results of nutritional tests are therefore a measure of the extent to which dosed *iso*AA is made available to the tissues; they should not be interpreted in terms of biochemical specificity.

THE PASSAGE OF *iso*AA ACROSS BIOLOGICAL MEMBRANES

There is considerable evidence that AA crosses biological membranes in the oxidised form, *i.e.* after conversion to dehydroascorbic acid.[19–21] Within the tissues the dehydroascorbic acid is quickly converted back to AA by glutathione in the presence of a glutathione reductase shown to be present in erythrocytes, liver and stomach.[8,9] Using the isolated erythrocyte to provide a model physiological membrane system, Hughes and Maton showed that there was virtually no uptake of dehydro*iso*AA under conditions that permitted a rapid uptake of dehydroAA (Fig. 2).[21] Furthermore, the presence of dehydro*iso*AA did not appear to impair the uptake of dehydroAA.

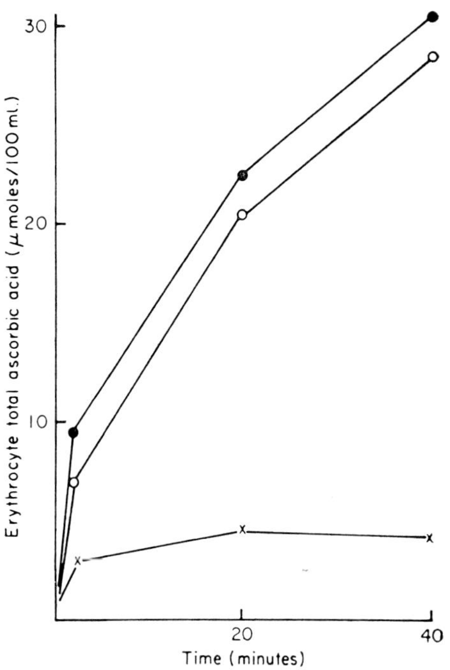

FIG. 2. Uptake of dehydro*iso*AA and dehydroAA by washed sheep erythrocytes.[21] ×, 1 ml erythrocytes incubated with 5 μmoles dehydro*iso*AA in 9 ml buffer pH 6·6; ○, 1 ml erythrocytes incubated with 5 μmoles dehydroAA in 9 ml buffer; ●, 1 ml erthyrocytes incubated with 5 μmoles dehydro*iso*AA and 5 μmoles dehydroAA in 9 ml buffer.

Subsequent work indicated that a similar state of affairs existed in the gastrointestinal tract. Guinea-pigs on a maintenance dose of 0·3 mg AA/100 g body weight/day were given a daily oral supplement of 1·5 mg/100 g body weight of AA or *iso*AA. The AA was deposited in the tissues, the *iso*AA was not (Table 1).[22] Intramuscularly

TABLE 1

Tissue concentrations of AA and iso*AA resulting from single daily doses of each isomer.*[22]

Group	Daily supplement (mg/100 g body wt) AA	*iso*AA	Tissue concentration of 'total ascorbic acid' (mg/100 g) Adrenals	Spleen
A (6)	0·3	0	27·0 ± 0·69	10·2 ± 0·98
B (8)	0·3	1·5	26·8 ± 1·63	8·6 ± 0·81
C (6)	1·8	0	64·3 ± 3·18	19·6 ± 1·10

A maintenance dose of 0·3 mg AA was given to all animals; mean values with standard errors are given and the number of animals present in each group at the end of the experiment is given in brackets.

administered *iso*AA was deposited in the tissues but not to the same extent as equivalent amounts of intramuscularly administered AA.[22] Thus there would appear to be a considerable barrier to the absorption of *iso*AA from the gastrointestinal tract. The existence of this low 'absorption ceiling' implies that only a very small proportion of a single dose of *iso*AA would ultimately reach the tissues. Tissue concentrations of substances with a low 'absorption ceiling' may be increased in two ways—by parenteral administration of the substance or by allowing it to 'trickle in' to the blood by continuous dietary presentation. This latter procedure was applied to guinea-pigs by providing them with 1% *iso*AA in their drinking water daily. In this way tissue concentrations of *iso*AA similar to saturation levels for AA were obtained;[23] these concentrations could not be attained by the single-dose technique of the standard nutritional test.

*iso*AA AND THE PREVENTION OF SCURVY IN GUINEA-PIGS

An experiment was designed to determine whether guinea-pigs saturated with *iso*AA by the 'trickle dosing' technique were fully protected against scurvy in the absence of AA. Two groups of male guinea-pigs were given a scorbutogenic diet supplemented with either AA or *iso*AA (1 % in drinking water) for 53 days. The AA intake (1 mg/100 g body weight/day) was sufficient to maintain maximum growth rate; at the end of the experiment the tissue concentrations of the two isomers were determined (Table 2*a*). There was no significant difference between the biochemical and physiological characteristics of the two groups or between their growth rates (both groups increased in mean body weight from 300 g to 650 g over the 53 days) (Table 2*b*).

TABLE 2*a* (cf. Table 1)

Deposition of AA (single daily dose of 1 *mg*/100 *g body weight) and* iso*AA* (1 *mg/ml drinking water) in tissues of guinea-pigs* (*there were seven animals in each group*)

	AA group (mg AA/100 g)	*iso*AA group (mg *iso*AA/100 g)
Aqueous humour	3·5 ± 0·3	8·9 ± 0·7
Vitreous humour	3·2 ± 0·3	7·8 ± 0·9
Lens	7·7 ± 0·2	8·6 ± 0·6
Adrenal glands	43·4 ± 2·4	110 ± 15·1
Spleen	18·7 ± 0·9	26·1 ± 3·1
Brain	11·3 ± 1·5	18·1 ± 1·3
Testes	9·3 ± 0·4	11·6 ± 1·2

Of especial significance were the weights of the kidneys and adrenal glands—organs which undergo a significant hypertrophy in chronic hypovitaminosis C.[24] Fabianek and Herp had already indicated that a single daily dose of 10 mg *iso*AA protected guinea-pigs against scurvy (a dose of 2 mg is sufficient in the case of AA) but a normal growth rate was not maintained.[25] Pelletier and Godin also maintained guinea-pigs on a scorbutogenic diet by supplementing them with *iso*AA (40 mg/day); their animals, however, gained only ca. 150 g over a 53-day period.[26]

Earlier studies had indicated that there was no conversion of *iso*AA to AA in the guinea-pig.[22] It would therefore appear that provided the tissue concentrations are not limiting *iso*AA can completely replace AA as an antiscorbutic factor; whether there is a complete equivalence between the two compounds in terms of tissue concentrations has yet to be demonstrated. Previous reports that *iso*AA

TABLE 2*b*

Physiological characteristics of guinea-pigs maintained for 53 days with either AA or iso*AA* (see *Table 2a*)[23]

	Group 1 (AA)		Group 2 (*iso*AA)	
Body weight (g)				
Initial	290 ± 11		302 ± 8	
Final	684 ± 19		659 ± 29	
Organ weights[a]				
Liver	27·5 ± 1·1	(3·91 ± 0·10)	25·3 ± 2·7	(3·69 ± 0·19)
Testes	2·85 ± 0·24	(0·406 ± 0·034)	2·97 ± 0·25	(0·442 ± 0·031)
Brain	3·76 ± 0·08	(0·536 ± 0·016)	3·72 ± 0·13	(0·559 ± 0·026)
Kidney	4·44 ± 0·17	(0·631 ± 0·017)	4·28 ± 0·19	(0·640 ± 0·024)
Spleen	0·82 ± 0·03	(0·117 ± 0·005)	0·67 ± 0·06	(0·099 ± 0·007)
Adrenal glands	0·27 ± 0·02	(0·039 ± 0·004)	0·27 ± 0·02	(0·040 ± 0·003)
Eye lens	0·14 ± 0·004	(0·020 ± 0·001)	0·14 ± 0·002	(0·022 ± 0·002)
Packed cell volume (ml)	41·8 ± 0·98		41·3 ± 1·93	
Serum cholesterol (mg/100 ml)	45·1 ± 3·1		48·7 ± 2·6	
Serum transaminase (GPT mU/ml)	28·6 ± 4·7		29·0 ± 3·8	

[a] Absolute weights (g) are given for all organs; the values in parentheses are the percentage body weights.

possessed an antiscorbutic potency one-twentieth that of AA were therefore essentially a reflection of different rates of transport by biological membranes, operating primarily at the gastrointestinal tract.

THE RETENTION OF *iso*AA BY TISSUES

A second factor which may influence the antiscorbutic properties of a compound is the degree to which it is retained by the tissues. A low tissue retention capacity would mean that at low dietary intakes tissue concentrations sufficiently high to protect against scurvy might never be attained. In 1963 Rivers, Huang and Dodds showed that daily doses of 50–100 mg *iso*AA taken orally by human volunteers produced no change in the leucocyte concentrations, although plasma and urinary measurements indicated that substantial amounts of the isomer were being absorbed and excreted.[27] These authors concluded: 'that the uptake or "tissue fixation" of L-ascorbic acid is structurally specific for the L-configuration about C5' and that: 'The rejection of erythorbic acid (*iso*AA) by the white cells explains the high urinary excretion of this isomer and its apparent lack of antiscorbutic activity'.

These conclusions are based on the assumption that the behaviour of the leucocytes *vis-à-vis iso*AA is representative of the body tissues in general. If this is true, then the findings reported by Rivers, Huang and Dodds are at a variance with more recent studies in guinea-pigs indicating that absorbed *iso*AA is retained by body tissues (but not necessarily by leucocytes) and that it possesses antiscorbutic properties.[23]

TABLE 3

Half-life (days) of AA and iso*AA in tissues of guinea-pigs*[28]

	AA	*iso*AA
Brain	20·0	4·5
Liver	2·2	0·5
Heart	2·0	0·5
Kidneys	2·5	0·6
Adrenals	3·2	0·7
Spleen	3·0	0·6

TABLE 4

Loss of AA and iso*AA from tissues of male guinea-pigs placed on a scorbutogenic diet—values are percentage of original concentration remaining* (cf. *Fig.* 3)[29]

Time after last dose (days)	Adrenals		Spleen		Brain		Eye lens	
	AA	*iso*AA	AA	*iso*AA	AA	*iso*AA	AA	*iso*AA
2	69	18	69	14	84	73	79	61
6	29	2	33	<2	45	47	57	32
9	12	<1	13	—	27	29	43	19
14	4	—	5	—	24	—	27	—
20	1	—	<2	—	15	—	18	—

However, there can be little doubt that the capacity of tissues to retain *iso*AA is much less than their capacity to retain AA. Pelletier has shown that the rate of turnover of *iso*AA in guinea-pig tissues is much more rapid than that of AA;[28] in the same paper he compared the rates of loss of AA and *iso*AA from the tissues of guinea-pigs previously saturated with the two isomers respectively and showed that the *iso*AA was retained to a much smaller extent than the AA (Table 3). He concluded that: 'the lower activity of *iso*AA is not due so much to its inability to be transported in the organs, but rather to the ability of the organ to retain *iso*AA'. Hughes, Hurley and Jones in a similar study obtained results essentially in agreement with those of Pelletier.[29] They found that, irrespective of sex, and with the possible exception of the brain, all organs lost *iso*AA much more rapidly than AA (Table 4, Fig. 3). As a corollary to this experiment AA-saturated guinea-pigs were given a scorbutogenic diet and the survival times compared with those of an *iso*AA-saturated group similarly treated; the AA-saturated animals survived for 24–27 days and the *iso*AA-saturated ones for 12–14 days.[23] This indicated that the capacity of a tissue to retain ascorbic acid is an important factor in determining antiscorbutic potency. It brings to mind Zilva's prophetic statement that 'the antiscorbutic activity of this class of compounds is correlated with their "fixation" in the tissues'.[5]

SPECIFICITY OF THE RETENTION MECHANISM

Stereospecific requirements for membrane transport of nutrients have been well characterised and the different rates of transport of dehydro*iso*AA and dehydroAA across biological membranes can, conceptually at least, be accommodated within a system similar to those believed to operate in the case of sugars and amino acids. The marked difference in the retentions of the two isomers by tissues, however, poses an interesting biochemical problem. Virtually nothing is known of the fine mechanics of the system whereby an ascorbic acid is retained by a tissue. It is conceivable that intracellular binding to a second molecule occurs, the resulting complex being retained within the cell. It would presumably be a feature of such a binding that certain molecular structures amongst the ascorbic acids would be preferred to others and this could explain the existence of different

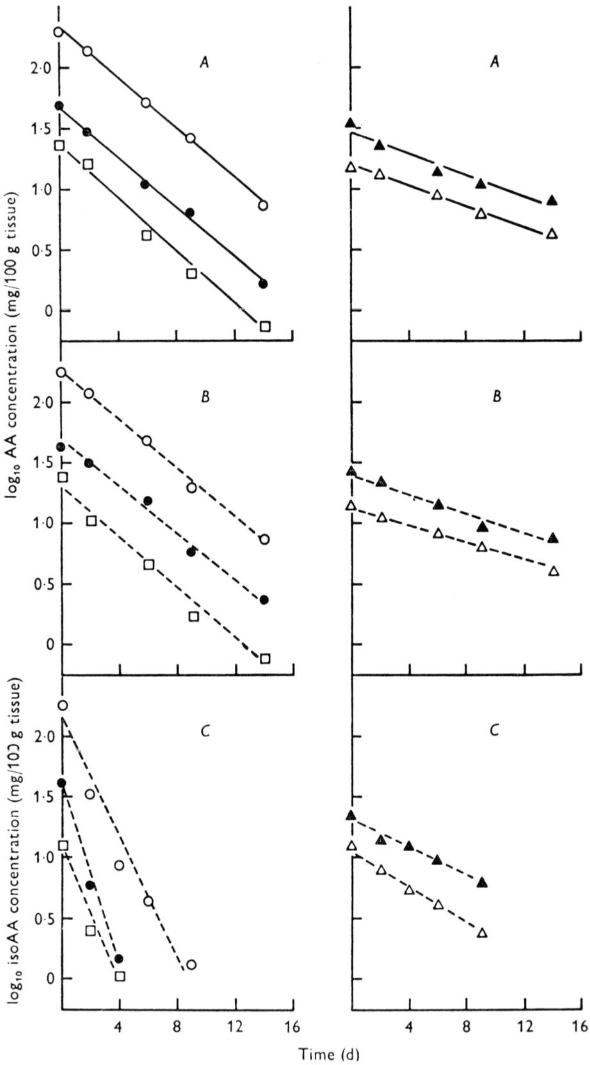

FIG. 3. Loss of L-xyloascorbic acid (AA) (*A, B*) and D-araboascorbic acid (*iso*AA) (*C*) from adrenal glands (○), spleen (●), aqueous humour (□), brain (▲) and eye lens (Δ) in male (– – –) and female (——) guinea-pigs when placed on a scorbutogenic diet.

degrees of retention. A number of workers have claimed that bound forms of ascorbic acid exist; Fiddick and Heath indicated that in the rat adrenal glands up to 40% of the ascorbic acid is present in a bound form in association with a larger molecule.[30] On the other hand, studies using Sephadex gel filtration techniques to separate bound and free ascorbic acids have so far produced no evidence for the presence of bound AA in guinea-pig tissues (Hurley, R. J. and Hughes, R.E., unpublished work). If a bound form of AA exists it must be of a very labile nature.

A second possibility is that the retention mechanism is in some way linked to the overall energy potential of a tissue, an increased capacity for retention on the part of a tissue being, in general, associated with a raised metabolic index.[31] This would imply that the system partakes of the characteristics of an endergonic process and would offer at least a partial explanation of the finding that tissue AA concentrations show a negative correlation with age (and therefore with metabolic activity).[32,33] This second theory, however, presents little opportunity for any type of explanation of the stereospecificity of tissue retention. A further possibility involves both theories. A constant availability of biochemical energy could be a condition of the formation of bound ascorbic acid. This would accommodate both the apparent relationship between metabolic index and tissue retention on the one hand and stereospecificity requirements on the other; it would also explain the difficulties in detecting bound ascorbic acid in tissue extracts.

CONCLUSION

In comparing AA and *iso*AA it must be borne in mind that AA is the naturally existing isomer and, as far as is known, the form biosynthesised by living systems. Assuming that systems of membrane transport and tissue retention of ascorbic acid have evolved, primarily in response to the existence of the natural isomer, it is not entirely unexpected to find that a considerable difference exists between the behaviour of the isomers in these two systems. One would perhaps expect these differences to be more marked in species unable to synthesise AA (and therefore possessing a correspondingly greater need to conserve the vitamin) than in species able to produce their own supply of AA.

The existence of such physiological differences means that 'nutritional specificity' (in this case, antiscorbutic potency) as determined by the standard single-daily-dose technique is little more than a measure of adaptational inadequacies in terms of membrane transport and/or tissue retention capacity. Such observations should never be equated with 'biochemical specificity'. In a nutritional context terms such as 'biological potency' very frequently lack precision; in the case of the ascorbic acids they are quite meaningless.

REFERENCES

1. Herbert, R. W., Hirst, E. L., Percival, E. G. V., Reynolds, R. J. W. and Smith, F. (1933). *J. chem. Soc.*, p. 1270.
2. Haworth, W. N., Hirst, E. L. and Zilva, S. S. (1934). *J. chem. Soc.*, p. 1155.
3. Hay, G. W., Lewis, B. A. and Smith, F. (1967). In *The Vitamins*, 2nd ed., eds. W. H. Sebrell and R. S. Harris, Academic Press, New York and London, p. 307.
4. Demole, V. (1934). *Biochem. J.*, **28,** p. 770.
5. Zilva, S. S. (1935). *Biochem. J.*, **29,** p. 1612.
6. Yourga, F. J., Esselen, W. B. Jr and Fellows, C. R. (1944). *Fd. Res.*, **9,** p. 188.
7. Dodds, M. (1948). *Archs. Biochem.*, **18,** p. 51.
8. Hughes, R. E. (1964). *Nature*, **203,** p. 1068.
9. Grimble, R. F. and Hughes, R. E. (1967). *Experientia*, **23,** p. 362.
10. Barnes, M. J. and Kodicek, E. (1972). *Vitamins and Hormones*, **30,** p. 1.
11. Levin, E. Y., Levenberg, B. and Kaufman, S. (1960). *J. biol. Chem.*, **235,** p. 2080.
12. La Du, B. and Zannoni, V. (1961). *Ann. N.Y. Acad. Sci.*, **92,** p. 175.
13. Lindstedt, G. and Lindstedt, S. (1970). *J. biol. Chem.*, **245,** p. 4178.
14. Lindblad, B., Lindstedt, G. and Lindstedt, S. (1970). *J. Amer. chem. Soc.*, **92,** p. 7446.
15. Hutton, J. J., Tappel, A. L. and Udenfriend, S. (1967). *Archs. Biochem. Biophys.*, **118,** p. 231.
16. Kutnink, M. A., Tolbert, B. M., Richmond, V. L. and Baker, E. M. (1969). *Proc. Soc. exp. Biol. Med.*, **132,** p. 440.
17. Dayton, P. G. and Burns, J. J. (1958). *J. biol. Chem.*, **231,** p. 85.
18. Ettlinger, M. G., Dateo, G. P. Jr., Harrison, B. W., Mabry, T. J. and Thompson, C. P. (1961). *Proc. natn. Acad. Sci. U.S.A.*, **47,** p. 1875.
19. Raiha, N. (1958). *Acta physiol. Scand.*, **45,** Suppl. 155, p. 24.
20. Martin, G. R. (1961). *Ann. N.Y. Acad. Sci.*, **92,** p. 141.
21. Hughes, R. E. and Maton, S. C. (1968). *Br. J. Haemat.*, **14,** p. 247.
22. Hughes, R. E. and Hurley, R. J. (1969). *Br. J. Nutr.*, **23,** p. 211.

23. Hughes, R. E., Hurley, R. J. and Jones, P. R. (1971). *Nutr. Rep. int.*, **4,** p. 177.
24. Hughes, R. E. (1965). *Br. J. Nutr.*, **19,** p. 307.
25. Fabianek, J. and Herp, A. (1967). *Proc. Soc. exp. Biol. Med.,* **125,** p. 462.
26. Pelletier, O. and Godin, C. (1969). *Can. J. Physiol. and Pharmacol.,* **47,** p. 985.
27. Rivers, J. M., Huang, E. D. and Dodds, M. E. (1963). *J. Nutr.,* **81,** p. 163.
28. Pelletier, O. (1969). *Can. J. Physiol. and Pharmacol.,* **47,** p. 993.
29. Hughes, R. E., Hurley, R. J. and Jones, P. R. (1971). *Br. J. Nutr.,* **26,** p. 433.
30. Fiddick, R. and Heath, H. (1967). *Biochim. biophys. Acta,* **136,** p. 206.
31. Williams, R. S. and Hughes, R. E. (1972). *Br. J. Nutr.,* **28,** p. 167.
32. Brook, M. and Grimshaw, J. J. (1968). *Am. J. clin. Nutr.,* **21,** p. 1254.
33. Hughes, R. E. and Jones P. R. (1971). *Br. J. Nutr.,* **25,** p. 77.

DISCUSSION

Grenby: Are we likely to encounter *iso*AA? Does it occur in any foods, or is it cheaper to produce than ascorbic acid?
Hughes: It isn't listed now but apparently it is used, I think, in Canada.
Weir: In the determination of tissue levels are you determining total ascorbic acid or are you differentiating between L-xyloascorbic acid and D-araboascorbic acid?
Hughes: We determine only total ascorbic acid but have carried out experiments to show that there is no conversion of D-araboascorbic acid to L-xyloascorbic acid within the tissues.
da Rocha-Afodu: We have followed the metabolism of the *iso*AA. I wanted to ask if the tissue does use *iso*AA if it is converted to ascorbic acid. Would you detect *iso*AA in the tissues, *i.e.* in the tissues but not necessarily in the pathway that ascorbic acid takes?
Hughes: I don't think I suggested that, did I?
da Rocha-Afodu: You spoke only about the way the ascorbic acid is used.
Hughes: You are suggesting *iso*AA is not really a substitute for it, it is being converted into AA. There is no evidence of this.
Parker: Is there any physiological objection to the use of *iso*AA as an anti-oxidant or preservative in foodstuffs?
Hughes: The only one I have seen is that it could give a falsely high value, so I assume from this there is some feeling you get a falsely high value when analysing the food. From the physiological point it does substitute completely. The only disadvantage is that it takes a long time to get into the tissues, so you could argue it is less use than ascorbic acid, but in foodstuffs I can't see there is going to be any difference.
Hollingsworth: If I remember one of your slides correctly there is a different behaviour in the brain. Can you comment?

Hughes: We have always found the brain has always behaved peculiarly both with *iso*AA and AA. An animal can die of scurvy and still have amounts of it in the brain. The brain is abnormal with regard to this.

Shallenberger: Would you comment briefly on the suspected metabolic function?

Hughes: Nothing has been established.

Shallenberger: Wasn't there some work not too long ago related to the sense of smell?

Hughes: The most recent comment was in *The Times*, bnt these are what I call peripheral effects—just acting as a biological reductive. The theory is if you give massive doses of Vitamin C to guinea-pigs you lower the cholesterol.

Chairman: I thought that had been disputed.

Hughes: We find if we give large doses of cholesterol to guinea-pigs they normally die off in a short period and if we give a large dose of ascorbic acid they don't die off. In other ways there is no relation, but Gunter produced work to show that if you give high doses to guinea-pigs you can lower the cholesterol. Whether it works or not I don't know. Sokolov started it off but he worked with rabbits and from very small doses.

Fallon: As regards ascorbic acid and its retention in the tissues, is *iso*AA actually degraded in the tissues or is it excreted intact in the urine? If the latter, does its anti-oxidant activity remain undiminished?

Hughes: I would not know. We never measured whether it comes off as ascorbic acid. I don't know. I haven't done any measures of that type. It is very difficult to do with guinea-pigs. You rarely get a measurable amount of ascorbic acid in guinea-pig urine. Dodds had a certain number of volunteers and measured ascorbic acid coming out in urine, but other than that I don't know.

Barnett: Is the reduction of biological half-life of *iso*AA due to excretion or metabolism?

Hughes: The latter is the possible explanation, that it is being used up more quickly, in terms of capacity, than the rate at which it vanishes from the tissues.

da Rocha-Afodu: The question I wish to ask is related to that of the last questioner. The identification of *iso*AA as such in the tissues does not mean that an enzyme which converts it to AA does not exist. To follow the metabolic pathway of AA which does exist, it seems there is an isomerase or deisomerase necessary for its conversion to AA. Was your study of the rates of disappearance of AA and *iso*AA from tissues carried out at the early stage of the establishment of scurvy or at the chronic stage? The stage at which the experiments were carried out would probably throw light on the metabolic pathways of both *iso*AA and AA and on whether an isomerase or deisomerase is necessary for the conversion of *iso*AA into AA before it is metabolised.

Hughes: We started one group of animals with AA with a similar group started to the same level with *iso*AA. Then we measured the rate at which it vanished from the tissues. We removed all sources of Vitamin C so had conditions of acute scurvy.

8

Polysaccharide Conformation as a Basis of Food Structure

E. R. Morris

Unilever Research, Unilever Limited,
Sharnbrook, Beds., England

ABSTRACT

Being extremely hydrophilic giant molecules, polysaccharides can radically change the physical properties of many times ($\simeq 10^2$) their own weight of water, and are therefore widely used in the food industry as thickeners, texture modifiers and emulsion stabilisers. Their water binding properties are shown even more dramatically in gel formation where, for example, 1% calcium alginate can hold 99% water in a firm, crisp structure.

Maintenance of shape in such gels cannot be accounted for by point cross-linking between the polysaccharide molecules, but arises from the co-operative association of long, structurally regular regions of the chains, in ordered conformations. We have characterised two different types of linking. In the uronic acid polymers alginate and pectin, the junction zones are microcrystalline regions where several chains align, with divalent counterions sandwiched between them, with the geometrical regularity of macroscopic crystals. In carrageenan, on the other hand, structurally regular junctions are formed by chains intertwining into double helices, which then aggregate by co-operative attractions.

In both cases the junctions are terminated by structural irregularities which, by destroying the necessary geometric repeat, prevent complete aggregation and consequent precipitation of the polysaccharide. Small changes in the number of such 'junction breaking' groups can radically alter gel texture. Geometric fitting of structurally regular regions of two different polysaccharides is also possible, a notable example being the formation of strong gels by locust bean gum and the bacterial polysaccharide Keltrol, neither of which will gel on its own.

These concepts allow us to explain many aspects of the texture of natural foods, providing a basis for the intelligent and novel use of polysaccharides as food additives, and may be extended to synergistic interactions between polysaccharides and other molecules, particularly proteins, indicating a powerful future technique for the food technologist.

The unique solution properties of polysaccharides have been known and exploited for many centuries, and are so widely utilised in present day food technology that there must be few products marketed which do not contain a polysaccharide additive of some sort. Their usefulness in extremely low concentrations ($\simeq 1\%$) as thickeners, texture modifiers, emulsion stabilisers, and so on arises from two general properties shared by all polysaccharides: their great molecular length (extending to hundreds or even thousands of sugar units) and their extremely hydrophilic composition which allows them to tie down the surrounding water lattice to their own sluggish translational time-scale.

Although of immense practical importance, these aspects of polysaccharide behaviour are well known at least in broad outline. The gelation properties of polysaccharides and their structural role in naturally occurring foodstuffs, however, are less widely understood, and it is on these that I wish to concentrate, outlining in particular the unifying concepts developed by Professor Rees and my colleagues at Unilever Research. I will first illustrate our approach with one group of polysaccharides, the alginates, and then discuss its broader application to other systems.

Sodium alginate, a mannuronate/guluronate copolymer, shows typical polysaccharide solution properties, and is widely used, for example, to improve the texture of ice cream. In the presence of calcium ions, however, it forms firm crisp gels at concentrations of 1% or less, and these may be used as a matrix to impart texture to food products. Until recently it was widely believed that the gel network was held together by 'calcium bridges' between carboxylate groups on different polymer chains. This model, however, is totally incapable of explaining the rigidity of such gels: if it were, the properties of, for example, a solution of calcium sulphate would, to say the least, be intriguing.

Recently, however, we have demonstrated by circular dichroism the specific involvement of uninterrupted polyguluronate sequences in network formation, reinforcing less direct evidence from studies of ion binding to alginates of different composition. This suggests that calcium ions are bound, not between isolated pairs of carboxylate groups, but between long, structurally regular homopolymeric chain segments, forming 'junction zones' with ordered crystal-like geometry. Although the total binding energy may not be increased by co-operative association of this type, the stability may be vastly increased, since before the two chains involved can come apart and alter their relative orientations in the gel, all the individual links in the junction zone must be severed simultaneously (*e.g.* if the probability of a single link coming apart and staying apart over a given time interval is 1 in 2, the probability of dissociation of a junction zone 20 units long is 1 in 2^{20}: about one chance in a million!).

Computer model building, reinforced by X-ray diffraction studies of oriented alginate fibres, shows that polyguluronic acid chains can readily adopt a buckled or 'zig-zag' shape with hydrophilic 'nests' of the right size to accommodate a calcium ion, and with two-fold symmetry permitting the association of further chains into a 'microcrystalline' bundle. Association is, of course, terminated when the end of the homopolymeric region is reached, preventing complete

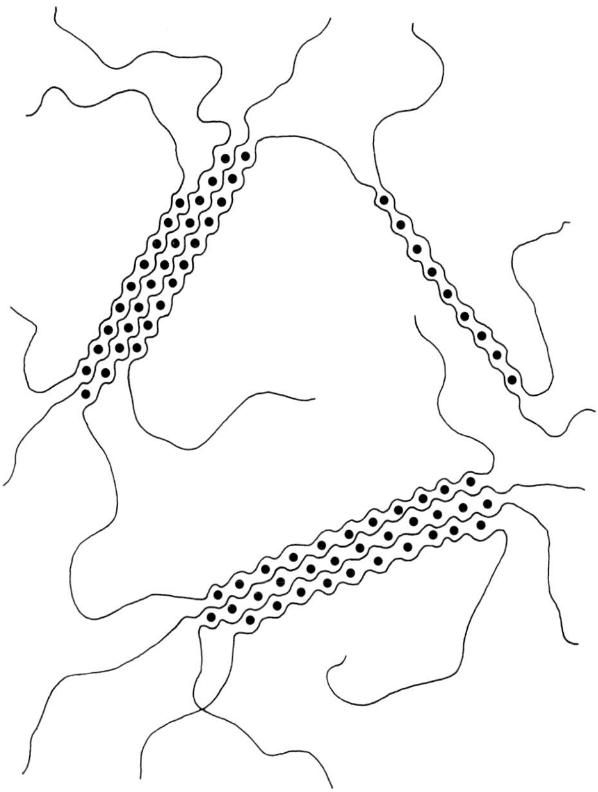

FIG. 1. Alginate gel structure.

aggregation and consequent precipitation of the polysaccharide. We thus picture the calcium alginate gel structure as being held together principally by crystalline calcium polyguluronate junction zones, linked by heteropolymeric or polymannuronate segments in the normal random solution conformation, and immobilising approximately a hundred times it own weight of water (Fig. 1).

We believe that pectic acid forms gels in the same way, with crystalline calcium polygalacturonate junctions. In this case, however, complete aggregation is prevented by the presence of rhamnose as a structural irregularity, causing 'kinking' of the polysaccharide chain, or by chain branching.

This general principle of gel network formation by the co-operative association of long, structurally regular chain segments is shown by many other polysaccharide systems, although the nature of the

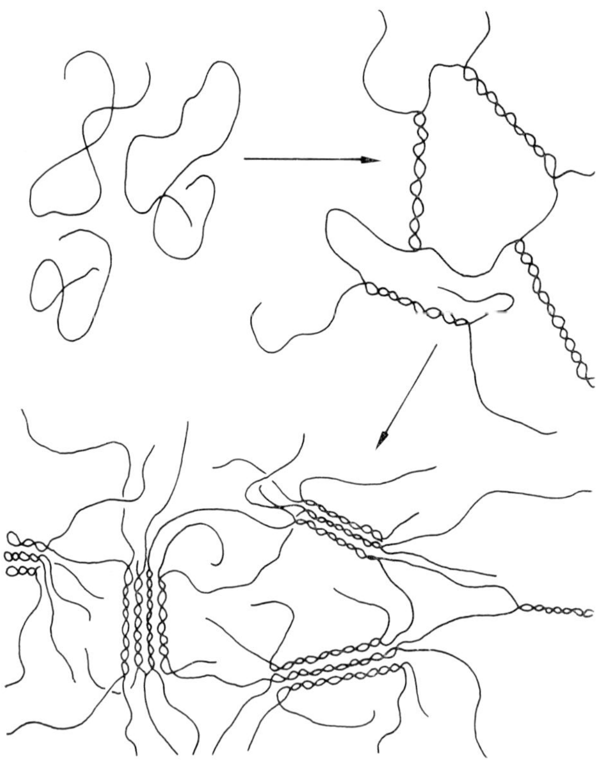

FIG. 2. Carageenan gelation.

cohesive forces involved may be very different. In carrageenan, ordered junctions are formed by chains intertwining into double helices which then aggregate by co-operative attractions (Fig. 2). Although ionic forces no doubt contribute, binding is probably predominantly due to van der Waal attractions and hydrogen bonding. The junction zones, therefore, once more have a regular microcrystalline structure, but this time essentially of the 'organic crystal' type, which is reflected in the different properties of the two types of gel. For example, while carrageenan gels may be melted by heating and reform on cooling, alginate gels show considerable resistance to heat, but any breakdown which does occur is irreversible.

Although the existence of the carrageenan double helix in the solid state was established by X-ray diffraction, its occurrence in solutions and gels is shown by studying changes in optical rotation with temperature. As the more highly disymmetric helical structure is adopted, there is a marked rise in optical activity which can be quantitatively related to chain conformation. Application of the same technique to the extracellular bacterial polysaccharide from *Xanthamonas campestris*, sold under the trade name 'Keltrol', shows that it too adopts an ordered conformation on cooling, and reverts to the normal 'random coil' on heating. This understanding allows us to explain one of the puzzling, but extremely useful, properties of this material, which makes it so attractive in the food industry: Keltrol solutions show virtually no decrease in viscosity on heating, which must obviously be due to the increase in effective hydrodynamic volume as the ordered structure unravels, offsetting the usual drop in solution viscosity with temperature.

Although not itself a gelling polysaccharide, Keltrol forms firm mixed gels with another non-gelling polysaccharide, locust bean gum. Chemically, locust bean gum is a galactomannan: it has a linear backbone of β-1,4-linked mannose units, extremely similar in shape to the cellulose chain, but substituted with blocks of 1,6-linked galactose units over about a quarter of its length. We can thus picture the molecule as being made up of 'smooth', regular, cellulose-like sections separated by substituted 'hairy' regions (Fig. 3). The synergistic gel network formation with Keltrol can now be explained by association of 'smooth' regions with the ordered Keltrol structure, with the 'hairy' regions acting as junction terminators in the same way as mannuronate-containing regions in alginates and 'kinks' in carrageenan and pectin. *Xanthamonas campestris* is a plant pathogen, and this association probably mimics the role of its extracellular polysaccharide in providing an anchor to the wall of the plant vascular system. Exactly the same type of geometric association to the 'smooth' regions of galactomannans occurs with the helical forms of carrageenan and agar (Fig. 4).

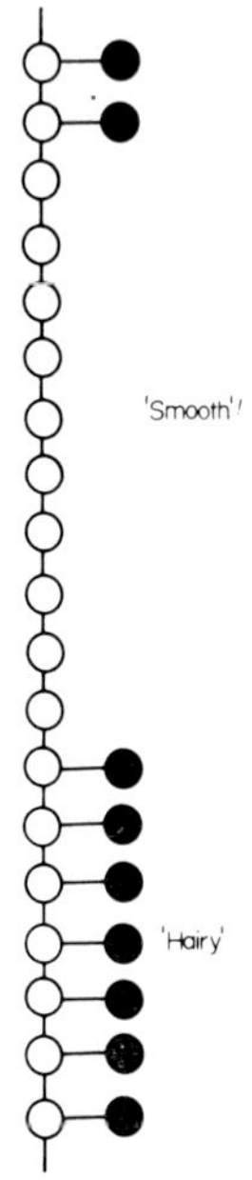

FIG. 3. Galactomannan block structure.

The general unifying concept central to all these interpretations is that polysaccharides do not gel by 'point cross-linking' of tangled chains in random conformations, but by the co-operative association of long, structurally regular regions in ordered conformations, the extent of association being critically controlled by irregularities in primary structure.

Although so far we have characterised only associations between polysaccharide molecules, the same principles may well be relevant to the association of polysaccharides with other substances, particularly proteins, and this points the way to a whole new field of texture manipulation by the food technologist, and provides a conceptual framework for interpretation of naturally occurring food textures.

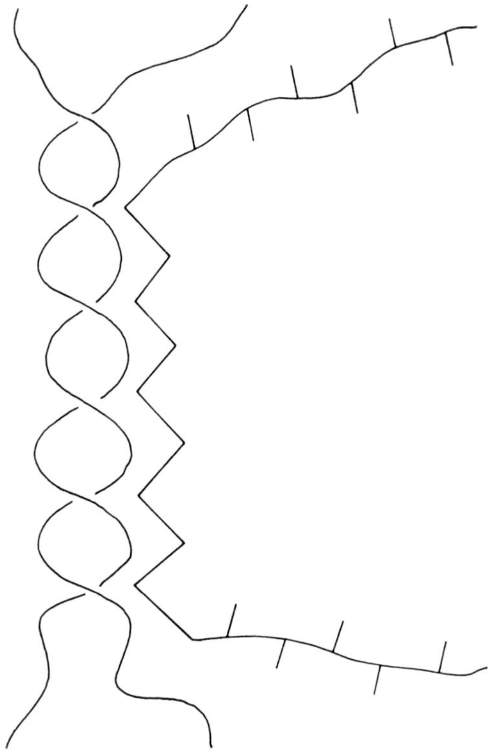

FIG. 4. Synergistic gelation.

DISCUSSION

Hood: It is known that carrageenan and protein react in a unique way and I wonder if you would speculate as to how protein in particular cases might act in double helices in a spatial way. Carrageenan reacts with the milk protein, casein. Would you speculate on how this interaction may affect the formation of the double coil or where the casein micelle or molecule might be positioned in the helix?

Morris: I am not familiar with the geometry of the structure of proteins, but I imagine that they are in regular repeating helical structure. If the geometric repeat is right between protein and polysaccharide, there seems to be no reason why we should not have some structure with hydrogen bonding between the two.

Hood: Are you suggesting then it would become part of the helix internally?

Morris: No. If this is possible geometrically it would be an aggregation of helices one with the other rather than a mixed helix.

Fallon: Would homogenisation of a solution containing Ca^{2+} alginate cause permanent disruption of the formed gel structure?

Morris: In the presence of calcium I would imagine so.

Fallon: Are these structures large enough to be taken down to the level of 2 microns?

Morris: I really don't know. This is something it would be easier to find out experimentally by looking at the gel before homogenisation and afterwards. I haven't tried this idea of breaking up the gel structure in a cell by sonication; unfortunately there are experimental difficulties, so it is a bit difficult to put this to a practical test. I think it is really more a question of the process of the breaking up mechanism rather than the gel structure. Certainly if the process is capable of breaking up the gel structure, once it is broken up it will stay broken up.

Parker: Referring to the structure of alginate gels, which depend on the interaction of homopolar blocks of L-guluronic acid for their formation, what interaction may be expected between similar homopolar D-mannuronic acid blocks?

Morris: I was guilty of over-simplification there. Almost certainly, acid blocks will be associated in some way to some extent but this is undoubtedly a much less strong association probably where there is competition, geometric competition. We certainly have evidence that, where there is no such competition, acid blocks can come together with calcium.

Parker: Since alginate gels are stable to high temperatures but do not reform on cooling the solution, does this imply that thermal degradation of the polymer chain has occurred?

Morris: There are probably two possibilities. I don't know anyone who has checked this.

Parker: It sounds rather drastic to me that the temperature must be high.

Morris: Alginate gels can withstand fairly drastic treatment without breakdown. Chemical degradation is surely possible. Although this type of association must be very much more stable, certainly if you put enough energy in it will come apart eventually.

Halek: Referring to the synergistic gel formation between xanthomonas polysaccharide and locust bean gum, do other galactomannans, particularly guar gum, interact in the same way?

Morris: This is quite interesting because it doesn't in fact gel, but there is an interaction and the viscosity of the mix solution is much higher, so it looks as if there is some association but not enough to produce a microscopic link. This is quite an interesting observation. It is a pathogen in fact and Keltrol is an extracellular polysaccharide. It is quite likely that this association can be seen in galactomannans.

9

Thermal Degradation of Carbohydrates

YORAM HOUMINER

Department of Organic Chemistry, The Hebrew University, Jerusalem, Israel

ABSTRACT

The thermal degradation of solid and/or molten carbohydrates is reviewed and classified according to types of reactions. The process is complex and for various mono-, oligo- and polysaccharides it has been shown to consist of many competitive and consecutive reactions. Primary transformations which do not include cleavage of the carbohydrate carbon skeleton, such as anomerisation, aldose–ketose isomerisation, inter- and intramolecular transglycosylation and inter- and intramolecular dehydration, are followed by a complex set of reactions yielding volatile products by fragmentation of the carbohydrate carbon skeleton. Mechanistic routes for the formation of some of the major volatile products by use of ^{14}C*-labelled carbohydrates have been established. Data obtained for* ^{14}C*-labelled glucose by us and for* ^{14}C*-labelled* 1,6-*anhydro-β-*D*-glucopyranose by Shafizadeh's group indicated that the same volatile products may originate from different parts of the glucosyl carbon skeleton by parallel routes, although for some volatiles one preferential pathway could be observed.*

The formation of glucosidic anhydro-sugars, which are the main products from various glucose-containing mono-, oligo- and polysaccharides, is discussed in relation to the structure of the carbohydrate. The different proposed mechanisms for the formation of 1,6-*anhydro-β-*D*-glucopyranose as well as for the corresponding furanose isomer, either by a direct route (intramolecular* S_N1 *or* S_N2*) or via a* 1,2-*anhydro or* 1,4-*anhydro intermediate, are reviewed and discussed in detail. A high* 1,6-*anhydro-β-*D*-glucofuranose/*1,6-*anhydro-β-*D*-glucopyranose ratio* (0·8–1·0) *is characteristic of glucose whereas different glucopyranose as well as oligo- and polysaccharides give a low value* (0·1–0·3). *A high* 1,6-*anhydro-hexofuranose/*1,6-*anhydro-hexopyranose ratio is also characteristic of other aldohexoses such as* 2-*deoxyglucose mannose and galactose. These data, as well as other differences in the thermal behaviour of monosaccharides compared to their glycosides as well as to their oligo- and polysaccharides, are discussed in detail.*

Some special aspects of the thermal degradation of starch and cellulose are reviewed with respect to the importance of these carbohydrates as the major components and structural units in foodstuffs, wood, etc.

Very small amounts of organic and inorganic compounds have been shown to affect strongly the degradation process for both mono- and polysaccharides. Acidic and basic salts show different catalytic behaviour. The effect of the different catalysts on the degradation process is discussed, and the very important problem of the influence of impurities in the starting material on the rates and direction of the various processes is considered.

INTRODUCTION

The study of the thermal behaviour of solid and/or molten carbohydrates is important for its many practical applications in addition to being a fertile field for basic research. Cellulose[1,2] and starch[3] have been most widely investigated because of their importance as the major components in wood and foodstuff respectively. The thermal decomposition of cellulose is of special interest and is significant in relation to the problem of wood combustion.[1,4] The thermal degradation of starch and other carbohydrates is important in the food industry, for instance, in the preparation of some commercial products such as 'pyrodextrines' which are used industrially as gums.[3] Reviews on the thermal degradation of cellulose[1] and starch[3,5] have appeared in the literature.

Various mono-, oligo- and polysaccharides undergo similar thermal reactions.[1,3,6] Therefore, D-glucose and its derivatives such as glucosides and oligosaccharides have often been used as model compounds for the more 'complex' polysaccharides, cellulose and starch.[1,3] The thermal degradation of carbohydrates has been shown to consist of many competitive and consecutive reactions.[7,8] Primary transformations without cleavage of the carbon skeleton, such as isomerisations and dehydrations, are followed by reactions yielding volatile products as a result of fragmentation of the carbon skeleton. Characterisation of the primary reactions is of vital importance in understanding the much more complex fragmentation reactions. This paper aims to describe the thermal degradation of carbohydrates in terms of reaction types as well as pointing out the importance of each reaction in the overall degradation process. Glycosidic anhydro-sugars are the major products from the thermal degradation of various carbohydrates.[9,10] This paper also presents data regarding the formation of 1,6-anhydro-hexopyranoses and 1,6-anhydro-hexofuranoses from aldohexoses such as D-glucose, 2-deoxyglucose and D-mannose and discusses the possible mechanistic routes through which they are formed.

EXPERIMENTAL METHODS

The most common method for studying the thermal degradation is in a closed system and under reduced pressure.[8] Under these conditions various volatile products evaporate from the heated zone and, as a consequence, many possible secondary reactions, which could make the overall process much more complex, are eliminated. Usually[8] under reduced pressure, three main fractions are isolated. (i) The residue which remains in the heated zone and consists of non-volatile products as well as unreacted starting material. (ii) The tar which contains products volatile at high temperatures but practically none volatile at room temperature. Anhydro-sugars are mainly found in the tar. (iii) An aqueous fraction which consists mainly of water but also of a variety of volatile organic products. This fraction is usually trapped in liquid air and can be separated into other fractions of varying volatilities. Characterisation of each of the above fractions with respect to their amounts and constituents at different stages of the degradation process is of vital importance in understanding the whole process.

Thermal gravimetric analysis (TGA) and differential thermal analysis (DTA) have been widely used for studying the thermal degradation of sugars.[1–4,11] However, the TGA and DTA methods measure weight loss and heat changes respectively, which are the sum of many reactions taking place simultaneously, and therefore this information is limited and does not yield details.

Many physical factors such as temperature, pressure size of the sample, geometry of the pyrolysis tube and the type of glass used, as well as chemical factors such as the purity of the starting materials, are important and affect the thermal degradation process.[1,3,8,12] These factors must be considered when a comparison is made between results obtained by different research groups. It is rather disappointing to note that in many works some of the above factors are not even reported.

REACTIONS WITHOUT CLEAVAGE OF THE CARBOHYDRATE CARBON SKELETON

Anomerisation (α,β-Equilibrium)

D-Glucose undergoes a fast anomerisation on melting,[13] and an equilibrium mixture is obtained when starting from either the α- or the β-D-glucose. This primary thermal transformation is very fast and proceeds with almost no competing reactions.[13] A mechanism involving the acyclic form has been proposed[13] (Scheme 1). Through the acyclic form, pyranose–furanose isomerisation might also take place[10] (*see* below). The anomerisation of molten glucose is catalysed both by acids and bases.[13] Reports relating to the thermal behaviour of α- and β-D-glucose seem to indicate similar or slightly

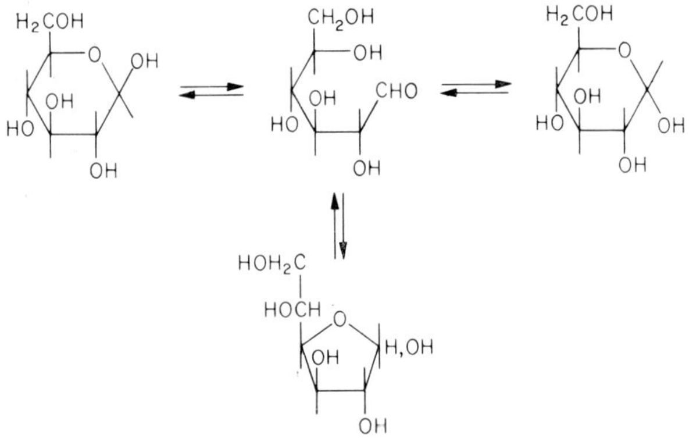

SCHEME 1

differing reactivities of the two anomers.[14] However, we believe that the existence of primary rapid anomerisation excludes the study of differences in the thermal behaviour of the two anomers. Shafizadeh *et al.*[15] recently reported that D-xylose also undergoes anomerisation and that equilibrium of the sugar takes place on melting. We have recently investigated the thermal anomerisation of several molten aldohexoses such as D-mannose, 2-deoxyglucose and D-galactose and found that anomerisation is completed before other reactions take place to any appreciable extent. In preliminary tests we have observed that α,β-equilibrium also occurs with disaccharides such as cellobiose (at their reducing glycosyl unit).

The thermal α,β-equilibrium of free sugars seems to be a general phenomenon which takes place on melting without the need for solvent or catalyst.[9,13,15,16] We believe that when differences in the thermal behaviour of two anomers of the same sugar are observed this may be attributed to differences in the purity of the two samples.[8,12]

Aldose–Ketose Isomerisation

Sugisawa *et al.*[17] reported that D-fructose was produced from D-glucose by heating at 150°C. Similarly, at 150° maltose was partially converted into maltulose.[16] Houminer and Patai[12] observed that isomerisation at 160° of D-glucose to D-fructose and vice versa occurred only in the presence of basic catalysts, and not when pure sugars were used, but even 0·04% (w/w) of $NaHCO_3$ is sufficient to effect the isomerisation.

The glucose–fructose isomerisation in the presence of basic catalysts competes with various degradation reactions of the two sugars and as a result equilibrium is not reached.[12] We found also that D-fructose is thermally much less stable than D-glucose.[12] D-Mannose, which is also formed in basic aqueous solutions, could not be detected in the thermal glucose–fructose isomerisation.[12]

Inter- and Intramolecular Dehydrations

The major volatile product from the thermal degradation of various mono-, oligo- and polysaccharides,[1,2,8,14] based on molar ratio, is water. Free monosaccharides undergo polycondensation[8,14,18] above their melting point to give polysaccharides with the formation of a maximum of 1 mole of water from 1 mole of sugar (Scheme 2). This reaction is reversible but reduced pressure favours

$$n\text{-}C_6H_{12}O_6 \rightleftharpoons C_6H_{11}O_5\text{—}(C_6H_{10}O_5)_{n-2}\text{—}C_6H_{11}O_6 + (n-1)H_2O$$

SCHEME 2

the polymer.[18] The reaction is also catalysed by various acidic catalysts.[18] In oligo- and polysaccharides the reverse reaction, *i.e.* depolymerisation via hydrolysis, has been observed.[10] It proceeds to a small extent even under reduced pressure.[10] The polycondensation of monosaccharides has been reviewed by Goldstein and Hullar.[18]

Sugisawa and Edo[19] have shown that glucose at 150° undergoes polymerisation to give disaccharides and oligosaccharides with all possible glucosidic linkages, but with preferential formation of (1 → 6) glucosidic bonds. Higher polymers were shown to be highly branched[18] and to consist of D-glucofuranosyl units either at the reducing end group or inside the chain.[20] Polycondensation is also characteristic of disaccharides which give similar polymers.[17]

The formation of ethers (other than acetalic ones) is not an important thermal dehydration route since it is known that the polymers, for instance from glucose, do not contain such ether linkages.[18] However, some water may be produced via this route, as for example in the formation of 1,4-3,6-dianhydro-D-glucopyranose[9] from glucose-containing carbohydrates, where the 3,6-anhydro bond is an ether linkage.

The formation of water from monosaccharides such as D-glucose, and in particular from polysaccharides such as starch and cellulose, also proceeds via an intramolecular dehydration process[2,8] (Scheme 3). This process is also an intramolecular oxidation–reduction

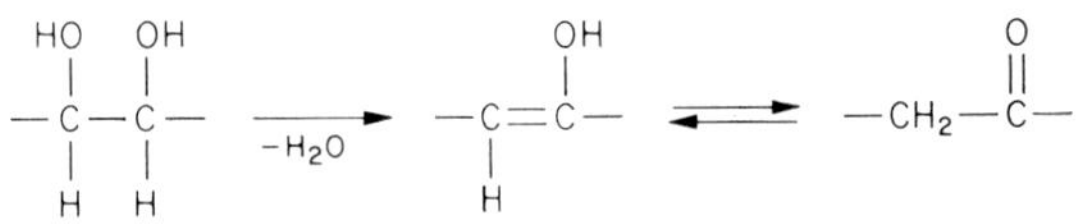

SCHEME 3

reaction.[8] Houminer and Patai[8] have shown that in glucose the intramolecular elimination of water at 175° proceeds in parallel to the polycondensation from the beginning of the reaction, although the polycondensation is faster. At higher temperatures, *e.g.* 250°, the intramolecular dehydration becomes more important.[8] Elimination of water can occur at different parts of a glucosyl unit, as shown for example in Scheme 4 for the case of glucose,[8] from which 5-hydroxymethylfurfural and 2-furyl hydroxymethyl ketone are formed. Elimination from other sites is probably also possible.

However, in oligo- and polysaccharides, where at least one of the hydroxyl groups at one glucosyl unit is blocked, elimination at this blocked position would be more difficult. Nevertheless, starch and cellulose also produce furan derivatives,[9] probably either through internal elimination of ROH (R being another carbohydrate unit) or through preliminary glucosidic bond cleavage[7] (*see* below).

There is some evidence that the intramolecular double-bond forming dehydration is the first step through which the carbon skeleton of the glucose molecule[8] as well as glucosyl units in polymers[2,7,9] are decomposed to a variety of volatile organic substances. Indeed most of the volatile products are furan derivatives and carbonyl compounds.[1,3,21] Houminer and Patai[8] have shown that intramolecular elimination of water from glucose is faster than from non-reducing glucosyl units in polyglucose. It has been suggested

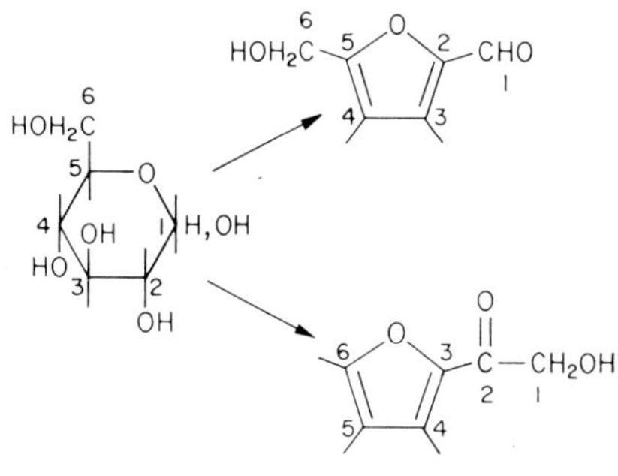

SCHEME 4

that the enhanced internal dehydration in free glucose is due to its ability to exist in the acyclic form.[8] Such a form is not obtained from non-reducing glucosyl units. These arguments might explain the observation[22] that the formation of furan derivatives is greater in the thermal decomposition of glucose than in that of different di- and polysaccharides.

Transglycosylation and Hydrolysis

Thermal transglycosylation in which a glycosyl residue bonded to one aglycone is transferred to another was first reported by Wolfrom *et al.*[23] who found that when pure starch is heated at 200° a very rapid reaction occurs in which the normal α-D(1 → 4) glucosidic bonds tend to disappear and the pyrodextrines obtained contain many α- and β-D(1 → 6) and β-D(1 → 2) glucosidic linkages. A similar phenomenon has been previously observed under acid catalysis.[24]

Houminer and Patai[10] reported that intermolecular transglycosylation is a relatively rapid reaction characterising the thermal degradation at 250° of various glucosides, and glucose-containing di- and higher oligosaccharides. This results in both cleavage and isomerisation of the glucosidic bonds as demonstrated in Scheme 5 for the case of cellobiose. ROH represents another sugar molecule, one of the hydroxyl groups attacking C-1 of a non-reducible glucosyl unit in the cellobiose. It has been shown[10] that a parallel cleavage route in disaccharides is by hydrolysis, even *in vacuo*, utilising water formed in the dehydration processes (in this case, $ROH=H_2O$).

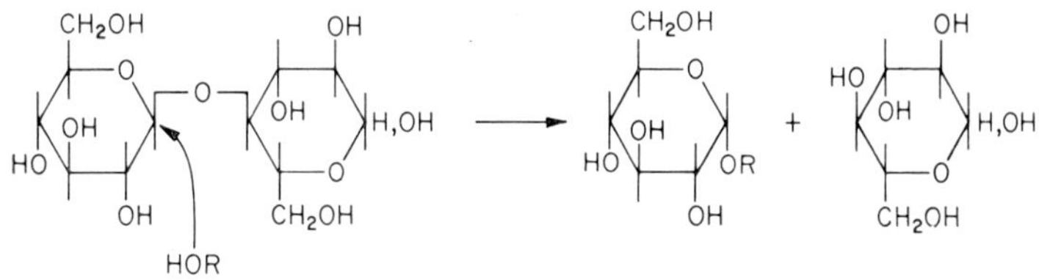

SCHEME 5

Different glucosides[10] and xylopyranosides[15] undergo polycondensation via transglycosylation with the release of aglycone. Scheme 6 demonstrates this reaction for the case of α-D-methyl glucopyranoside.[10] The reaction is presented with the sterically least hindered primary hydroxyl group at C-6 as the nucleophile. The expulsion of the aglycone can continue with the formation of higher oligomers.

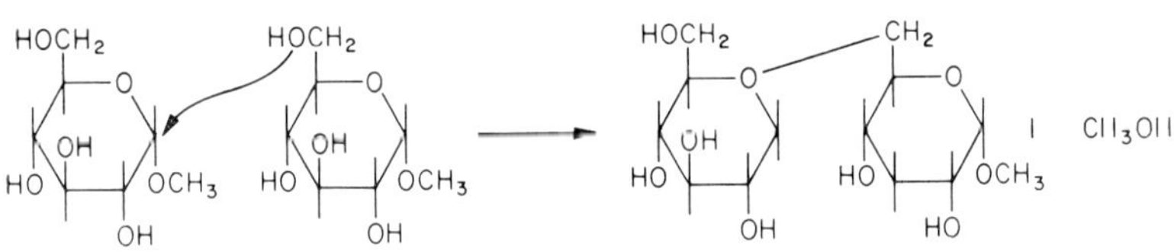

SCHEME 6

The relative thermal stability of glucosides depends both on the nature of the aglycone and on the configuration of the glucosidic bond.[10] For instance, β-D-phenyl glucopyranoside is much more reactive than β-D-methyl glucopyranoside and the latter is less reactive than α-D-methyl glucopyranoside. In contrast to oligosaccharides, no hydrolysis has been observed in glucosides.[10] This is probably due to the relatively small amount of water formed from glucosides[10] by the time the polycondensation has terminated.

Schemes 5 and 6 represent only one possible mechanism of an S_N2 type for the transglycosylation. However, both transglycosylation and hydrolysis may proceed also via an S_N1 type mechanism, *i.e.*

via heterolysis of the glycosidic bond[15] as shown in Scheme 10 for the case of a glucoside. Not very much is known about the existence of carbonium ions in molten sugars, and in the absence of solvent, stabilisation of carbonium ions is probably slight. Therefore, concerted mechanisms are generally favoured.[9,10] It should be noted, however, that molten sugars might solvate carbonium ions by their many hydroxyl groups and the heterolytic mechanism may therefore operate as well.[15] There is some evidence[15] that, at least at temperatures of up to 300°, homolytic cleavage of glucosidic bonds is not important.

The data so far collected[10,15,23] clearly indicate that transglycosylation, whether acid catalysed or not, is an important and relatively fast primary reaction in the thermal degradation of glucosides, oligo- and polysaccharides at 200–300°. However, no transglycosylation has been found in the case of cellulose,[25] the very rigid solid structure of which may inhibit such a reaction.[26]

Formation of Glycosidic Anhydro-sugars

Glycosidic anhydro-sugars are formed in the thermal degradation of various mono-, oligo and polysaccharides.[1,3,9,10,25] From glucose-containing carbohydrates, four anhydro-sugars have been isolated and characterised: 1,6-anhydro-β-D-glucopyranose I (laevoglucosan),[27] 1,6-anhydro-β-D-glucofuranose II,[28] 1,4-3,6-dianhydro-D-glucopyranose III,[29] and 1,6-anhydro-3,4-dideoxy-Δ^3-β-D-pyranosen-2-one IV (laevoglucosenone).[30]

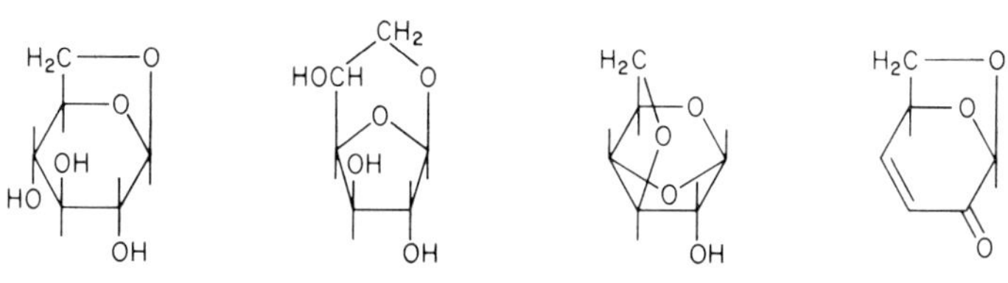

I II III IV

Carbohydrates derived from other aldohexoses also produce the corresponding anhydro-sugars. From mannose-containing carbohydrates, 1,6-anhydro-β-D-mannopyranose, 1,6-anhydro-β-D-mannofuranose and 1,4-3,6-dianhydro-D-mannopyranose have been isolated.[9] Galactose-containing carbohydrates give 1,6-anhydro-β-D-galactopyranose and 1,6-anhydro-α-D-galactofuranose.[9] We have recently investigated the thermal degradation of aldohexoses such as D-glucose, 2-deoxyglucose and D-mannose and some of the results regarding the formation of their corresponding 1,6-anhydrohexoses are listed in Table 1. These results indicate that 2-deoxyglucose also produces the corresponding 1,6-anhydro derivatives during its thermal degradation.

TABLE 1

Thermal decomposition of $2 \cdot 10^{-3}$ *mole of various aldohexoses at* 212° in vacuo (10^{-1} *mm Hg*)

Starting material	Time (min)	Residue[a] (%)	Yield of 1,6-anhydro-β-D-hexopyranose (%)	Yield of 1,6-anhydro-β-D-hexofuranose (%)	1,6-anhydro-β-D-hexofuranose/1,6-anhydro-β-D-hexopyranose[b]
D-glucose	60	74	2·2	1·5	0·68
	130	65	3·1	2·7	0·87
2-Deoxyglucose	60	33	3·8	3·2	0·84
	120	25	4·6	3·6	0·77
D-Mannose	60	64	0·9	1·0	1·11
	120	61	1·2	1·3	1·08

[a] No starting material has been detected in the residue after 20 min in the case of D-glucose and D-mannose and after 8 min in the case of deoxyglucose.

[b] D-Galactose gives a ratio of 1·50 at a temperature of about 400°C.[9]

Since most of the carbohydrates investigated are derived from glucose, we shall mainly discuss the formation of I–IV from different glucose-containing sugars. Laevoglucosenone (IV) has been isolated only recently by Halpern *et al.*[30] in the acid catalysed thermal degradation of glucose, cellulose and laevoglucosan. Since I is converted into IV in almost quantitative yield under acid catalysis, it has been suggested that the formation of IV in the acid catalysed thermal degradation of glucose and cellulose may proceed via I.[30] The 1,4-3,6-dianhydro-D-glucopyranose is formed in small amounts from D-glucose and glucose-containing di- and polysaccharides.[9]

Gardiner[9] reported that a high yield of III is obtained in the thermal degradation of 3,6-anhydroglucose.

The relative yields of the 1,6-anhydro-sugars I and II depend strongly on the structure of the starting material (*see* below) and on the experimental conditions, *e.g.* temperature, pressure and time of heating.[10] Usually the yields increase with increasing temperature and time of heating but decrease with increasing pressure.[10]

The structure of the starting material is very important since the formation of anhydro-sugars competes with various other degradation reactions. For instance, α,α-trehalose produces relatively high yields of I and II, whereas from reducing disaccharides the yields are lower,[10] probably because of competing reactions in which the reducing glycosyl units are decomposed faster via intramolecular dehydration reactions.[10,12] Houminer and Patai[10] have shown that various other factors related to the structure of the starting material affect the yields of both I and II. Some of these factors are discussed below in relation to the reaction mechanism.

The formation of the 1,6-anhydro linkage in a glucopyranosyl unit can be regarded in general as an intramolecular transglycosylation.[10] This may proceed via different mechanisms.

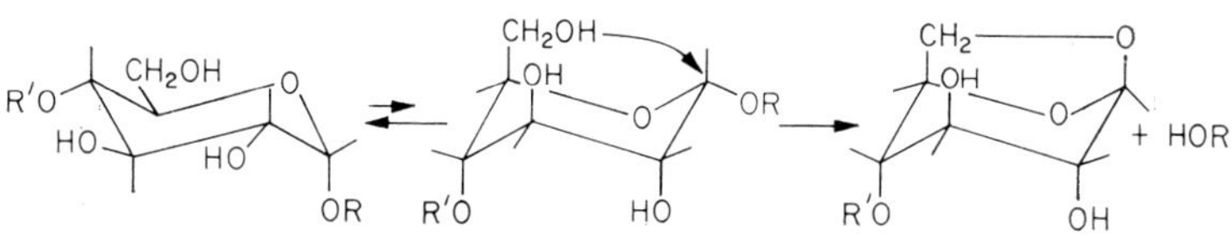

SCHEME 7

(i) Scheme 7 represents a generally accepted mechanism for the formation of a 1,6-anhydro linkage from a glucosyl unit having the α-configuration at C-1.[9,10] To enable the formation of a 1,6-anhydro bond, the glucopyranosyl unit has first to change from the C-1 to the 1-C conformation.[10] The reaction may then proceed via nucleophilic attack by the primary hydroxyl group on C-1. R′ may be either hydrogen or another carbohydrate unit. It may also be linked to the hydroxyl groups at the 2 and 3 positions. When R′ = H, laevoglucosan will be formed, while if it is another carbohydrate unit a 1,6-anhydro-glucopyranosylic end group will be formed from which I may be formed in a subsequent step. The nature of R (hydrogen, alkyl, aryl or carbohydrate unit), its bulk and its ability to stabilise the leaving group, can affect the rate of the reaction.[10]

(ii) In glucosyl units having β-configuration at their C-1 atom, and in particular in those cases where glucosidic bond anomerisations do not occur, such as in cellulose,[25] the above mechanism (Scheme 7) cannot operate since the attacking and the leaving groups are *cis* to each other. For this sytem, a mechanism operating via the 1,2-anhydro intermediate has been proposed[9,10,31] (Scheme 8).

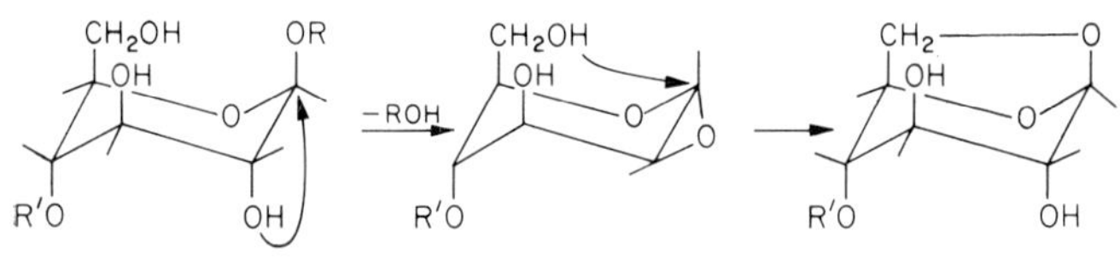

SCHEME 8

Wollwage and Seib[32] have recently shown that in the thermal degradation of 2-*O*-methyl cellulose a large amount of 2-*O*-methyl laevoglucosan is formed. Moreover, the thermal degradation of β-D-(1 → 4) linked mannan gives 1,6-anhydro-β-D-mannopyranose.[33] These data were taken as evidence against a 1,2-anhydro intermediate[32] and consequently a different mechanism was suggested[32] (*see* below). Our results (Table 1) do not support the above mechanism either since both 2-deoxyglucose and mannose give 1,6-anhydro-sugars. However, in our cases the 1,6-anhydro-hexopyranoses can be formed from glycosyl units having the α-configuration at their C-1 atom. Moreover, it should be noted that no information regarding the existence of glycosidic bond anomerisation via intramolecular transglycosylation is available for the cases of 2-*O*-methyl cellulose and β(1 → 4) linked mannans. If such isomerisation occurs in these systems, the formation of 1,6-anhydro-hexopyranoses could very well proceed from those glycosyl units which isomerise to the α-configuration at their C-1 atom (Scheme 7) as a result of the intermolecular transglycosylation.[10]

(iii) Broido *et al.*[11] as well as Wollwage and Seib[32] suggested that the formation of 1,6-anhydro-β-D-glucopyranose from cellulose or from 2-*O*-methyl cellulose proceeds through a 1,4-anhydro-α-D-glucopyranose which then rearranges to I (Scheme 9). This is possible only at a non-reducing glucosyl unit in which the hydroxyl group linked to C-4 is free. 1,4-Anhydro-α-D-glucopyranose has not yet been isolated in the thermal degradation of glucose-containing carbohydrates. However, recently it has been prepared by Michael and Kreutzer,[34] although no direct evidence for its structure has been given. It would be most interesting to investigate its thermal behaviour in order to establish the above mechanism.

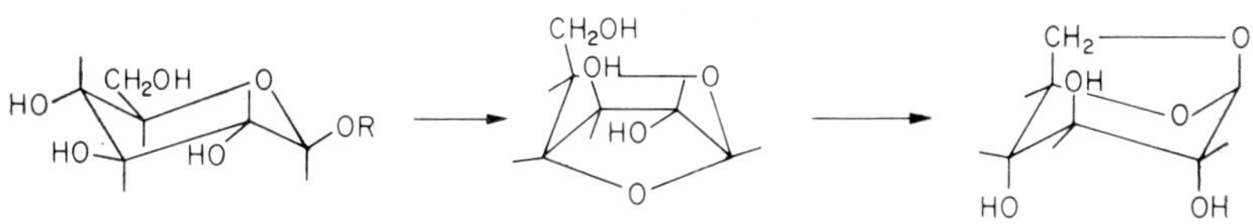

SCHEME 9

(iv) The formation of both I and II is strongly catalysed by acids.[12] Therefore, we do not exclude the possibility of a heterolytic mechanism involving a carbonium ion (Scheme 10), as in the case of the intermolecular transglycosylation. Although such a mechanism is not favoured in solventless systems,[9,10,32] it may take place in molten sugars[15] for the reasons given above. Such a mechanism may explain the formation of 1,6-anhydro linkage in glucopyranosyl units having either α- or β-configuration at their C-1 atom.

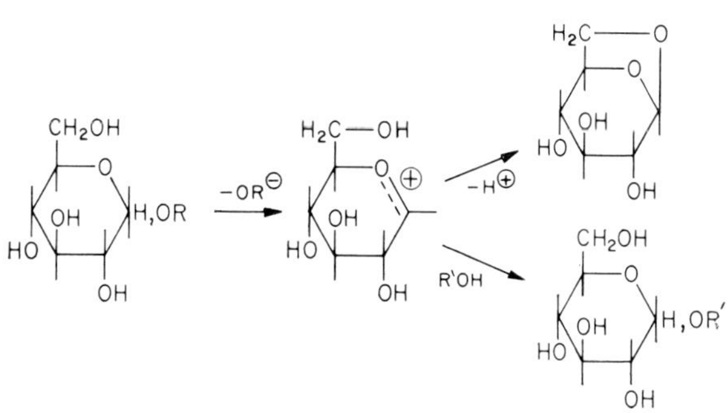

SCHEME 10

The formation of 1,6-anhydroglucofuranose (II) from glucose-containing carbohydrates always accompanied the formation of I.[9,10] The formation of a 1,6-anhydro linkage in a glucofuranosyl unit may proceed through mechanisms similar to those shown above, and various factors affecting the yield of I (*see* above) will also affect the yield of II. The relative yields of II and I are determined by two factors: (i) the rate of formation of the 1,6-anhydro linkage in the glucopyranosyl unit compared to that of the 1,6-anhydro linkage formation in a glucofuranosyl unit; (ii) the relative 'concentration' of glucopyranosyl and glucofuranosyl units in the substrate.

The formation of a 1,6-anhydro linkage in a glucopyranosyl unit requires a preliminary transformation of the unit from its normal C-1 conformation to the energetically unfavoured 1-C conformation.[9,10] However, the formation of a 1,6-anhydro linkage in a glucofuranosyl unit has no similar energy requirements.[9,10] Therefore, it has been suggested[10] that the formation of the 1,6-anhydro linkage is more favoured in a glucofuranosyl unit than in a glucopyranosyl one.

The formation of a 1,6-anhydro-β-D-glucofuranose (II) from carbohydrates consisting exclusively of glucopyranosyl units requires an additional pyranose–furanose isomerisation step. This poses a problem, since various glucose-containing carbohydrates, although consisting exclusively of glucopyranosyl units, give different II/I ratios.[10] Isomerisation of 1,6-anhydro-β-D-glucopyranose (I) to 1,6-anhydro-β-D-glucofuranose (II) is known in aqueous solution.[35] However, no similar isomerisation has been detected in melts under atmospheric pressure at temperatures up to 210°,[36] nor under reduced pressure where both I and II evaporate rapidly at temperatures above 175°.[8,10,37] Therefore, the pyranose–furanose isomerisation takes place before the formation of I, II or even the 1,6-anhydro linkage.

It has been shown that glucose undergoes fast polymerisation and both I and II are formed mainly from the polyglucose.[8,10] It is therefore rather interesting that the ratio of II/I in the thermal degradation of glucose is much higher[10] (0·8–1·0, *see* also Table 1) than that obtained from glucose-containing polysaccharides or from any other glucoside, di- and oligosaccharide[10] (0·1–0·3). This indicates that in the thermal degradation of glucose a pyranose–furanose equilibrium, which probably proceeds via the acyclic form,[10] (Scheme 1) is established before polymerisation occurs. While in aqueous solution the glucopyranose–glucofuranose equilibrium favours overwhelmingly the pyranose form,[38] there are no data on the position of the equilibrium in molten glucose. Nevertheless, thermally prepared glucose polymers have been shown to consist of a considerable proportion of glucofuranosyl units.[39] This may represent[10] either a freezing of the glucopyranose/glucofuranose ratio at the time of polymerisation or, probably more important, a preferential polymerisation of the furanose form with a displacement of the equilibrium in the melt. We recently observed that the II/I ratio (0·4–0·5) at the initial stages of the reaction, where the residue still contains about 50% of unreacted glucose, was lower than the ratio in the latter stages (0·8–1·0), where all the glucose reacted. Once the polymer, in which the anomeric positions are blocked, is formed, subsequent pyranosyl–furanosyl isomerisation will be more difficult and hence the II/I ratio reaches a constant value.

The situation differs basically in the thermal polycondensation[10] of glucopyranosides. Here the anomeric hydroxyl group is blocked and the pyranose–furanose isomerisation via the acyclic form is strongly hindered. Indeed, these substrates give a much lower II/I ratio (0·1–0·2),[10] as do polysaccharides such as starch,[9] cellulose[2] and oligosaccharides.[10]

The formation of II from different oligosaccharides does not necessarily involve a pyranosyl to furanosyl isomerisation and II may originate from glucose formed from these substrates by transglycosylation or by hydrolysis,[10] as discussed above. It is also possible that in oligosaccharides,[10] II originates from reducing glucosyl units which may undergo pyranose–furanose isomerisation via their acyclic form. However, such isomerisation is possible only if the hydroxyl group at C-4 in the same unit is free. In cellulose, II cannot be formed by either of the above two routes and Kilzer and Broido[11] have suggested that the 1,4-anhydro-α-D-glucopyranose may be a common intermediate for both I and II. Such a mechanism may operate also in methyl- and phenylglucosides.[10]

The thermal degradation of 2-deoxyglucose and D-mannose resembles that of glucose in that it has similar high 1,6-anhydrohexofuranose/1,6-anhydro-hexopyranose ratios (Table 1). The factors affecting the relative rate of formation of II compared to that of I from glucose exist also in 2-deoxyglucose and D-mannose. We observed that these aldohexoses also undergo fast polymerisation and the corresponding 1,6-anhydro-sugars are formed mainly from the polysugar. In addition, the ratio of 1,6-anhydro-hexofuranose/ 1,6-anhydro-hexopyranose is lower at the initial stages of the reaction and reaches a constant value at the latter stages, as in the case of glucose.

There is no information regarding the position of the furanose–pyranose equilibrium in molten 2-deoxyglucose or D-mannose. In aqueous solution both sugars exist preferentially in the pyranose form[40] and this resembles the situation in glucose.[38] We believe, therefore, that at least in part the 1,6-anhydro-hexofuranose–1,6-anhydro-hexopyranose ratio, obtained in the thermal degradation of molten aldohexoses, is affected by the position of the pyranose–furanose equilibrium in these molten sugars. This assumption is supported by the high ratio obtained[9] in the thermal degradation of D-galactose (1·5). This aldose contains in aqueous solution more of the furanose form than any of the above aldohexoses.[40]

FRAGMENTATION OF THE CARBOHYDRATE CARBON SKELETON

Volatile Products

Secondary thermal reactions lead to carbon–carbon bond cleavage with the formation of low-molecular-weight volatile products. Various mono- and polysaccharides produce similar volatile products.[6,19,21,22,41]

Therefore, it has been suggested that all carbohydrates undergo similar degradative reactions.[6,41] The relative amounts of the various volatile products are strongly affected by heating time, pressure, temperature and the structure of the starting materials.[6,22] By the use of GC and combined GC–MS, over a hundred products from glucose-containing carbohydrates have been identified and in some cases separated quantitatively.[21,41,42] The volatile products generally are: carboxylic acids, ketones, diketones, aldehydes, unsaturated ketones and aldehydes, furan derivatives, alcohols, hydrocarbons and aromatic compounds as well as carbon monoxide and dioxide. Obviously the fragmentation of the carbohydrate carbon skeleton is a very complex process. Some of the volatile products may arise from secondary reactions between other volatile products, in particular when the thermal degradation takes place under atmospheric pressure. The formation of carboxylic acids and carbon dioxide indicates that oxidation reactions occur even in the absence of oxygen or other oxidising agents.[8] Many mechanisms have been proposed for the various fragmentation processes, however, invariably on insufficient evidence.[22,41]

It has been suggested that the characteristic aroma of glucose caramels and other thermally processed carbohydrates arises from the various volatile products.[42]

Mechanistic Elucidation Using ^{14}C-Labelled Carbohydrates

The use of ^{14}C-labelled carbohydrates is of value in clarifying the mechanistic routes through which the major volatile products are formed. A study of the thermal degradation of ^{14}C-labelled D-glucose has been carried out by Houminer *et al.*[8,12,43,44] and some of their data, at 225°, are shown in Table 2.

TABLE 2

Contribution (%) of the different carbon atoms in D-*glucose to the formation of several volatiles*

Product	C-1	C-3	C-6
CO	67	16	9
CO_2	57	12	7
HCHO	15	5	65
HCOOH	mainly from C-1		
CH_3COOH	mainly from C-1 and C-2		
Furfural	80% with the expulsion of C-6		
	20% with the expulsion of C-1		
	100% retention of C-2		

Furfural is formed by two distinct pathways,[8] as shown in Table 2. It has been suggested that 5-hydroxymethyl furfural and 2-furyl hydroxymethyl ketone are the precursors (Scheme 11).

Other fragmentation schemes based on the above labelling experiments have been proposed.[8] The data in Table 2 show that the same volatile products may originate from different parts of the carbon skeleton, thus indicating the existence of many parallel reactions, although for some volatile products one pathway operates preferentially. Shafizadeh and Lay[7] recently obtained similar results from

^{14}C-labelled 1,6-anhydro-β-D-glucopyranose. They have carried out the degradation at 600° and the selectivity of the volatile products formed from the various carbon atoms was low.

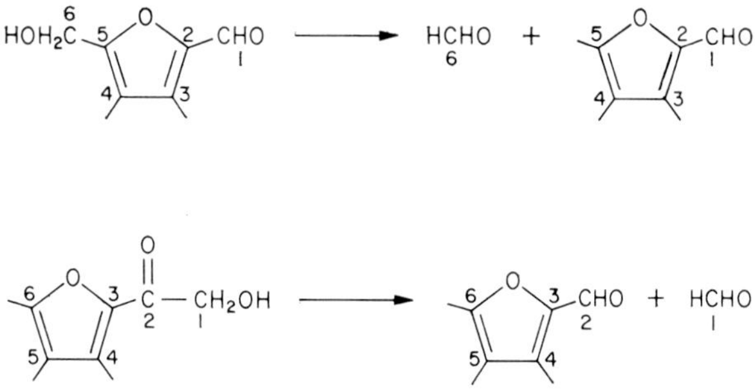

SCHEME II

CATALYSED THERMAL DEGRADATION

Effect of Organic and Inorganic Additives

Small amounts of various organic and inorganic additives catalyse strongly the thermal decomposition of mono-, oligo- and polysaccharides.[1-3] In a study of the catalysed thermal degradation of D-glucose, Houminer and Patai[12] have shown that neutral inorganic salts do not affect the degradation process, whereas acidic and basic salts affect it strongly. Similar results were obtained for cellulose.[1,2] Acidic catalysts such as NaH_2PO_4, $NaHSO_4$, H_3BO_3, etc. strongly catalyse the polycondensation of D-glucose but have no significant catalytic effect on the fragmentation.[12] They also catalyse the formation of anhydro-sugars from D-glucose[12] and cellulose,[2] and intermolecular transglycosylation in starch.[24] Basic additives such as Na_2CO_3, Na_3PO_4, etc. strongly catalyse both the intramolecular dehydration and the fragmentation processes in D-glucose,[12] cellulose[2] and starch.[3] In the presence of basic additives, anhydro-sugars are not formed either from glucose[12] or from cellulose.[2] Studies of the catalysed thermal degradation of ^{14}C-labelled D-glucose[12,43] have shown that acidic additives do not significantly affect the fragmentation pathways, whereas basic additives affect them strongly and there is much less selectivity in the formation of the same volatile product from the different carbon atoms. Similarly, the fragmentation pattern of the uncatalysed thermal degradation of ^{14}C-labelled 1,6-anhydro-β-D-glucopyranose resembles that of the acid catalysed rather than the base-catalysed one.[7]

The Problem of Impurities

Even as small an amount of 0·04% w/w of $NaHCO_3$ already strongly catalyses the isomerisation, dehydration and fragmentation of D-glucose.[12] Such small amounts of inorganic salts are often found in 'commercially pure' or even in 'analytical' grade carbohydrates. These impurities must be considered when a study of the thermal degradation of carbohydrates is made. It is also essential to consider the above problem when comparing results obtained by different research groups on the same sugar, since it has been shown [12,43] that the amount and the nature of the contaminations affect both the rate and the nature of the thermal degradation routes.

This may be of vital importance in the industrial thermal processing of carbohydrates since the reproducibility and even the pathway of various processes may be dependent on the impurity of the starting material.

SUMMARY AND CONCLUSIONS

The thermal degradation of mono-, oligo- and polysaccharides is a complex process, although for various carbohydrates some of the main reactions have been clarified. Physical factors, as well as chemical ones, in particular the purity of the starting material, are important and affect the process.

Additional research is still required in order to obtain detailed understanding of the whole degradation process. Although many volatile products are known, there are still many more to be identified. More information about the structure and composition of the non-volatile residue is also necessary since very little work has been done in this direction. The mechanisms of the various fragmentation pathways are not known and further study with the aid of ^{14}C-labelled carbohydrates may be very useful.

A detailed study of the effect of different catalysts on the degradation process may have very important practical applications, *e.g.* it may allow one to control and direct an industrial process in a desired direction.

In starch and cellulose, more work is needed in order to understand the primary structural changes occurring in materials which remain solid up to relatively high temperatures.

ACKNOWLEDGEMENTS

I wish to thank Professor S. Patai for his many helpful comments. Much of the above work was carried out in collaboration with Dr Y. Halpern and I wish to thank him for his useful contribution.

REFERENCES

1. Shafizadeh, F. (1968). *Adv. Carbohyd. Chem.,* **23,** p. 419.
2. Halpern, Y. and Patai, S. (1969). *Israel J. Chem.,* **7,** pp. 673, 685, 691 and references included therein.
3. Greenwood, C. T. (1967). *Adv. Carbohyd. Chem.,* **22,** p. 483.
4. Shafizadeh, F. and McGinnis, G. D. (1971). *Carbohyd. Res.,* **16,** p. 273.
5. Janos, H. (1968). *Zesj. Probl. Postepow Nauk Rolu,* **80,** p. 169.
6. Heyns, K. and Klier, M. (1968). *Carbohyd. Res.,* **6,** p. 436.
7. Shafizadeh, F. and Lai, Y. Z. (1972). *J. Org. Chem.,* **37,** p. 278 and references included therein.
8. Houminer, Y. and Patai, S. (1969). *Israel J. Chem.,* **7,** p. 513.
9. Gardiner, D. (1966). *J. Chem. Soc.,* C, p. 1473.
10. Houminer, Y. and Patai, S. (1969). *Israel J. Chem.,* **7,** p. 535.
11. Kilzer, F. J. and Broido, A. (1965). *Pyrodynamics,* **2,** p. 151; Patai, S., Halpern, Y., Esterman, L. and Weinstein, M. (1968). *Israel J. Chem.,* **6,** p. 445; Morita, H. (1956). *Anal. Chem.,* **28,** p. 64.
12. Houminer, Y. and Patai, S. (1969). *Israel J. Chem.,* **7,** p. 525.
13. Broido, A., Houminer, Y. and Patai, S. (1966). *J. Chem. Soc.,* B, p. 489.
14. Hurd, C. D. and Edwards, O. E. (1949). *J. Org. Chem.,* **14,** p. 680; Liskowitz, J. W. (1962). *Diss. Abs.,* **23,** p. 1945; Liskowitz, J. W. and Carroll, B. (1967). *Carbohyd. Res.,* **5,** p. 245.
15. Shafizadeh, F., McGinnis, G. D., Susott, R. A. and Tatton, H. W. (1971). *J. Org. Chem.,* **36,** p. 2813.
16. Pincock, R. E. and Kiovsky, T. E. (1966). *Chem. Commun.,* p. 864; Pincock, R. E., Wilson, K. R. and Kiovsky, T. E. (1967). *J. Amer. Chem. Soc.,* **89,** p. 6890.
17. Sugisawa, H., Usuki, R., Sasaki, M. and Komura, T. (1966). *Chem. and Ind.,* p. 812.
18. Goldstein, I. J. and Hullar, T. L. (1966). *Adv. Carbohyd. Chem.,* **21,** p. 431.
19. Sugisawa, H. and Edo, H. (1964). *Chem. and Ind.,* p. 892; *ibid.* (1966). *J. Food Science,* **31,** p. 561.

20. Dutton, G. G. S. and Unrau, A. M. (1964). *Can. J. Chem.*, **42,** p. 2048.
21. Heyns, K., Stute, R. and Paulsen, H. (1966). *Carbohyd. Res.*, **2,** p. 132.
22. Kato, K. (1967). *Agri. Biol. Chem.* (Tokyo), **31,** p. 657.
23. Thompson, A. and Wolfrom, M. L. (1958). *J. Amer. Chem. Soc.*, **80,** p. 6618; Wolfrom, M. L., Thompson, A. and Ward, R. B. (1959). *ibid.*, **81,** p. 4623.
24. Christensen, G. M. and Smith, F. (1957). *J. Amer. Chem. Soc.*, **79,** p. 4492.
25. Halpern, Y. (1969). PhD Thesis, The Hebrew University, Jerusalem.
26. Bryce, D. J. and Greenwood, C. T. (1965). *Starke*, **17,** p. 275.
27. Pichet, A. and Sarasin, J. (1918). *Helv. Chim. Acta*, **1,** p. 87; *ibid.* (1918). *Comptes Rend.*, **38,** p. 166.
28. Dimler, R. J., Davis, H. A. and Hilbert, G. E. (1946). *J. Amer. Chem. Soc.*, **68,** p. 1377.
29. Bedford, G. R. and Gardiner, D. (1965). *Chem. Commun.*, p. 287.
30. Halpern, Y., Riffer, R. and Broido, A. (1973). *J. Org. Chem.*, **38,** p. 204.
31. Madorsky, S. L., Hart, V. E. and Straus, S. (1956). *J. Res. Nat. Bur. Stand.*, **56,** p. 343.
32. Wollwage, P. C. and Seib, P. A. (1969). *Carbohyd. Res.*, **10,** p. 589.
33. Knauf, A. E., Hann, R. M. and Hudson, C. S. (1941). *J. Amer. Chem. Soc.*, **63,** p. 1447.
34. Michael, F. and Kreutzer, Y. (1969). *Annalen*, **722,** p. 228.
35. Peat, S., Whelan, W. J., Edwards, T. E. and Owen, O. (1958). *J. Chem. Soc.*, p. 586.
36. Patai, S. and Houminer, Y., unpublished results.
37. Houminer, Y. and Patai, S. (1969). *J. Polymer Sci.* A, **7,** p. 3005.
38. Angyal, S. J. and Pickles, V. A. (1967). *Carbohyd. Res.*, **4,** p. 296.
39. Mora, P. T. and Wood, J. W. (1958). *J. Amer. Chem. Soc.*, **80,** p. 685.
40. Stoddart, J. F. (1971). *Stereochemistry of Carbohydrates*, Wiley–Interscience, New York, pp. 158–71.
41. Greenwood, C. T., Knox, J. H. and Milne, E. (1961). *Chem. and Ind.* (*London*), p. 1878; Bryce, D. J. and Greenwood, C. T. (1963). *Starke*, **15,** p. 359; Glassner, S. and Pierce, A. R. (1965). *Anal. Chem.*, **37,** p. 525; Schwenker, R. F. and Beck, L. R. (1963). *J. Polymer Sci.*, C, **2,** p. 331; Kato, K., Doihara, T. and Sakai, F. (1966). *J. Agr. Chem. Soc.* (Japan), **40,** p. 443; Byrne, G. A., Gardiner, D. and Holmes, F. H. (1966). *J. Appl. Chem.* (*London*), **16,** p. 81.
42. Walter, R. H. (1967). *Diss. Abs.*, (B), **28,** p. 228; Walter, R. H. and Fagerson, I. S. (1968). *J. Food Sci.*, **33,** p. 294.
43. Houminer, Y., Hoz, S. and Patai, S. (1969). *Israel J. Chem.*, **7,** p. 821.
44. Houminer, Y. and Hoz, S. (1970). *Israel J. Chem.*, **8,** p. 97.

DISCUSSION

Bathgate: Are any of the many products of carbohydrate pyrolysis toxic or carcinogenic?

Houminer: I know that some of the products are toxic but I don't know whether they are carcinogenic; I can tell you that some of the related products are.
Parker: In your proposed preferred mechanism for the formation of laevoglucosan in the thermal degradation of starch, via the 1,4-anhydroglucose, does this imply that (OR) ether elimination is favoured relative to hydroxyl (OH)?
Houminer: We haven't got enough data about this but I think the formation of laevoglucosan is faster than from any glycoside, but you cannot compare starch because then you are coming into the field of polymers. In starch any anhydro linkage in a glucose residue must be bonded to something else.
Parker: This is what I meant, that molecules other than glucose like the rest of the starch chain, undergo rearrangements of substituents and then elimination. I was wondering whether this was the basis you are suggesting.
Houminer: No, in starch you can form a 1,6-linkage without any problem. If you want to form a glucosan you have first to get 1,6-glucosan and then every adjacent group has to go through the same reaction. Have you asked whether reaction on the adjacent glucose residue would be faster?
Parker: I am sorry I am not clear in my question. I merely was wondering whether your proposed mechanism was based upon the fact that OR rather than OH is preferentially liberated or displaced.
Houminer: No, it is just based on the configuration but, if you are asking about 1,4-intermediates we could not find them, but recently they were prepared chemically. I think it would be very interesting to prepare them. They were prepared but I am not convinced about the structure—there is not enough evidence about it. But it would be very interesting to take the 1,4-anhydride and see if it was converted into laevoglucosan.
Fisher: It should be emphasised in a food symposium that the temperatures at which polysaccharides are converted to polycyclic aromatic hydrocarbons are far in excess of those used in food processing.

10

Lactose and Reverse Osmosis

R. A. M. DELANEY, J. K. DONNELLY and A. C. O'SULLIVAN

*Moorepark Research Centre, Agricultural Institute,
Fermoy, Ireland*

ABSTRACT

Reverse osmosis (RO) and Ultrafiltration (UF) are hydraulic pressure operated membrane separation processes. Both processes utilise specially structured and constituted polymeric films as molecular screens which discriminate between solute and solvent molecules on a basis of size, shape or chemical structure.

Reverse osmosis is the term applied to the separation of low-molecular-weight solutes (e.g. *salts, sugars, simple acids, etc.*). *In such cases, the driving pressure for efficient separation must exceed the osmotic pressure of the solute in the solution. Ultrafiltration is the term applied to the separation of relatively high-molecular-weight solutes* (e.g. *proteins, natural gums, polymers) and colloidal dispersed substances, such as clays, pigments, micro-organisms, etc., from their solvents. In these systems, the osmotic pressure of the solute is usually negligible and plays no part in the separation process.*

Basic differences in the two processes are considered. The properties and behavioural characteristics of some reverse osmosis membranes are compared and contrasted.

Mass transfer mechanisms across membranes are discussed. Data are presented on the main factors affecting separation and concentration of carbohydrate solutions (lactose, sucrose, dextrans) with special reference to molecular structure.

Applications of reverse osmosis in the food processing industry are reviewed.

INTRODUCTION

During the past 10 years reverse osmosis (RO) and ultrafiltration (UF) have been advanced from laboratory curiosities to important industrial unit operations. Practical applications have gone beyond the production of potable water and sea water desalination and include a broad spectrum of solution concentrations and/or fractionations.

Reverse osmosis and ultrafiltration are similar and related processes, since both use a semi-permeable membrane as the separation medium and applied hydraulic pressure as the driving force to achieve separation. There are important differences, however, which lead to different applications, process conditions and equipment for each of the two processes. These differences are summarised in Table 1.

TABLE 1

Differences between reverse osmosis and ultrafiltration

	Reverse osmosis	Ultrafiltration
Size of solute retained	Molecular weights generally less than 500 to 1 000	Molecular weights generally over 1000
Osmotic pressures of feed solutions	Important, can range to over 1 000 lb/in^2	Generally negligible
Operating pressures	Greater than 100 lb/in^2 up to 2 000 lb/in^2	10 to 100 lb/in^2
Nature of membrane retention	Diffusive transport barrier; possibly molecular screening	Molecular screening
Chemical nature of membrane	Important in affecting transport properties	Unimportant in affecting transport properties so long as proper pore size and pore size distribution are obtained

PRINCIPLE OF REVERSE OSMOSIS

The name 'reverse osmosis' is derived from *osmosis*, the term used to describe the spontaneous flow of pure water into an aqueous solution, or from a less to a more concentrated aqueous solution, when separated by a suitable membrane. Normal osmosis is illustrated in Fig. 1A. A certain quantity of potential energy exists between the two solutions on either side of the semi-permeable

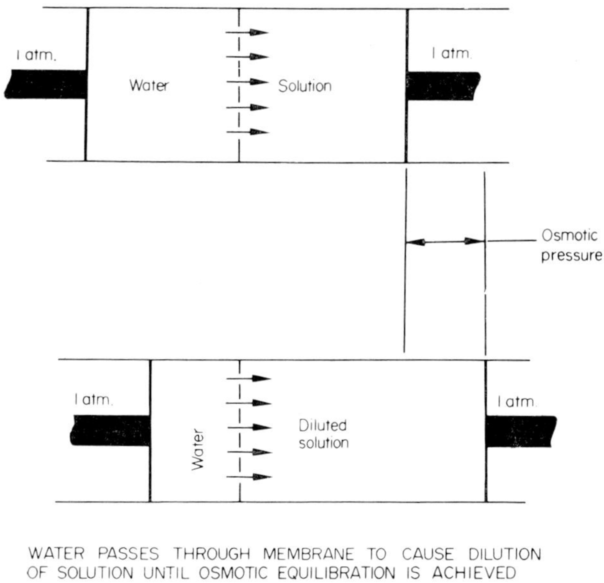

FIG. 1(A). Osmosis.

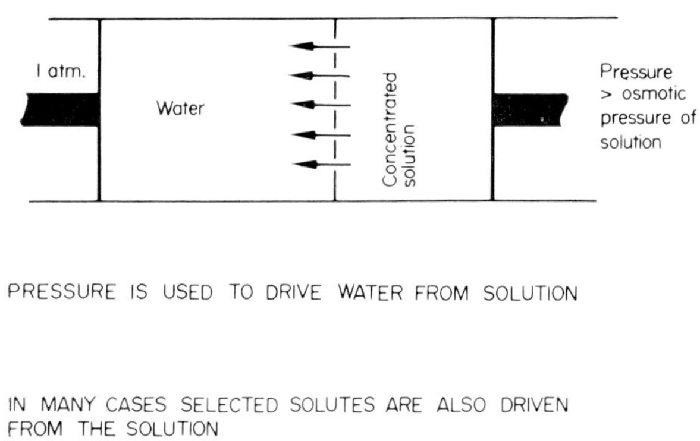

FIG. 1(B). Reverse osmosis, or ultrafiltration.

membrane. Because of this energy difference, water will flow from the less concentrated to the more concentrated solution until the system is in osmotic equilibrium. The addition of pressure energy to the concentrated solution will stop the transport of water across the membrane when the applied pressure equals the *apparent osmotic pressure* between the two solutions. The *apparent osmotic pressure* is a measure of the potential energy difference between the two solutions.

As further pressure is applied to the more concentrated solutions, as shown in Fig. 1B, the water will begin to flow from the more concentrated to the less concentrated solution. The rate of water transport is a function of pressure applied to the concentrated solution, the *apparent* osmotic pressure (*i.e.* the difference in the *absolute* osmotic pressure of each solution), and the membrane area being pressurised. The *absolute* osmotic pressure of a solution is the potential energy difference between it and pure water.

PROCESS FEATURES

Operationally, RO and UF are simple processes. As shown in Fig. 2, the solution under pressure flows over the surface of a suitably supported membrane. As a result of the applied pressure gradient across the membrane, solvent and certain solute species pass through

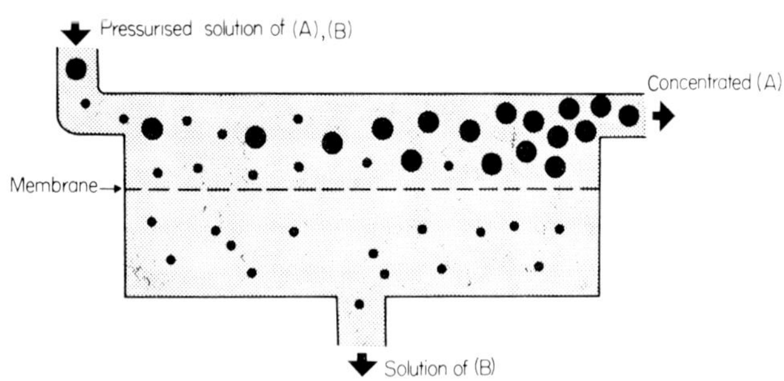

FIG. 2. Schematic diagram of membrane ultrafiltration process.

the membrane and are collected as *permeate* or *ultrafiltrate*. Depending on molecular size, other solute species are retained by the membrane and a concentrated solution of these species in the *concentrate* or *retentate* is recovered from the upstream chamber. By proper membrane selection it is thus possible to concentrate, purify and/or fractionate virtually any solution, the sole energy requirement being the compression energy of the feed solution. Thus in RO, virtually all substances except water are rejected or retained by the membrane and are concentrated. In UF, the membrane is permeable to both solvent and low-molecular-weight solutes, but is impermeable to higher-molecular-weight solutes.

PROPERTIES AND CHARACTERISTICS OF REVERSE OSMOSIS AND ULTRAFILTRATION MEMBRANES

Semi-permeable membranes are thin, fragile, plastics films. The earliest RO membranes were developed by Loeb and Sourirajan[1] and Majikian[2] at the University of California, Los Angeles, some 15 years ago. They were prepared from cellulose diacetate and served as very efficient RO desalination membranes, and this structure is still in widespread use today.

The membranes are asymmetric in structure, consisting of a very dense, thin layer of cellulose acetate on top of a fine-pore matrix. This dense layer is *ca.* 0·25 μ thick, with an overall membrane thickness of *ca.* 100 μ. The porous substructure is estimated to have a pore size of *ca.* 0·1 μ. It is this dense layer (or *active layer* as it is usually called) which is responsible for the membrane's ability to discriminate between different substances. The porous substructure plays no part in the rejection of solutes, but acts as a mechnical support for the active layer.

By suitably adjusting the polymer casting solution and proper control of post-casting treatment, asymmetric cellulose acetate membranes can be prepared with skin layers of varying pore texture. Thus a variety of membranes displaying widely different water permabilities and solute retentivities can be produced from this polymer. Cellulosic membranes, however, suffer from a number of limitations, most of which are attributable to the polymer properties. They can, as a rule, only be used with aqueous solutions since organic solvents either dissolve the membrane or plasticise it sufficiently to cause it to collapse. Most of them must be kept wet, because they irreversibly consolidate and lose their permeability if they are allowed to dry out. Because of the low glass transition temperature of cellulose acetate, these membranes cannot be operated at temperatures much above 50°C, as otherwise they collapse, consolidate and become impermeable. Because the polymer is both a polysaccharide and an ester, it is sensitive to hydrolysis at high and low pH's and, additionally, is susceptible to enzymic and microbial attack.

Over the past few years, however, techniques have been developed for producing asymmetric membranes from a range of synthetic polymers whose thermal, chemical and physical properties make them far more durable and versatile in general chemical and process applications, *e.g.* polyacrylamide nitrile.

MASS TRANSFER MECHANISMS

Studies of the filtration variation rate and solute rejection efficiency of various RO/UF membranes as functions of pressure, temperature and solute type and concentration indicate that there are two basic classes of mass transport mechanism which take place in such membranes. Tight membranes, which are those capable of retaining solutes whose molecular diameters are about 10 Å or less, function as diffusive transport barriers. In these membranes, both solute and solvent species migrate by molecular (Fickian) diffusion within the polymer, driven by concentration gradients established in the membrane by the applied pressure difference. Loose membranes, or those retaining particles larger than 10 Å, appear to function as molecular screens. Solvent moves through the membrane micropores in essentially viscous flow, while solute molecules are carried convectively with solvent, but only in those pores whose dimensions are large enough to accommodate them.

For diffusive-type membranes, the steady state relationships governing solvents and solute transport are as follows:

$$J_1 = \frac{K_1}{t}(\Delta P - \Delta\pi) = \frac{\bar{C}_1 D_1 \bar{V}_1}{tRT}(\Delta P - \Delta\pi) \qquad (1)$$

where:

- J_1 solvent flux (cm^3/cm^2-sec);
- t membrane thickness (cm);
- K_1 membrane permeability constant;
- ΔP hydrostatic pressure difference ($dynes/cm^2$);

$\Delta\pi$ solute osmotic pressure difference between upstream and downstream solutions (dynes/cm^2);
$\bar{C}_1$ mean concentration of solvent in membrane (cm^3/cm^3);
D_1 diffusivity of solvent in membrane (cm^2/sec);
$\bar{V}_1$ partial molar volume of water in solution (cm^3/mole);
R gas constant;
T absolute temperature.

For solute

$$J_2 = \frac{k_2 D_2}{t}(C_1 - C_0) \tag{2}$$

where:

J_2 solute flux (g/cm^2-sec);
k_2 solute distribution coefficient between membrane and solution;
D_2 solute diffusivity in membrane;
C_1 upstream solute concentration (g/cm^3);
C_0 downstream solute concentration (g/cm^3).

Mass conservation requires, however, that

$$J_2 = J_1 C_0 \tag{3}$$

For a highly retentive membrane (*i.e.* $C_0 \ll C_1$), Eqns. (1) and (3) can be solved simultaneously to find the membrane rejection efficiency, defined as the fraction of solute present in the feed solution which is retained by the membrane:

$$R = \frac{C_1 - C_0}{C_1} = \frac{B(\Delta P - \Delta\pi)}{1 + B(\Delta P - \Delta\pi)} \tag{4}$$

where

$$B = \frac{K_1}{k_2 D_2}$$

REJECTION EFFICIENCY

It is thus seen that, for diffusive membranes, the solvent flux is directly proportional to the effective pressure difference across the membrane, while the solute flux is not directly pressure dependent. This leads to the anomalous result that the rejection efficiency for a membrane, as in Eqn. (4), increases with increasing pressure, approaching unity in the theoretical limit as the applied pressure increases to infinity. In practice, no real diffusive membrane behaves in this way. Usually, there is some coupling of solute and solvent flow, indicating that as the pressure difference is increased, the solute permeability also increases somewhat. As a result, the membrane rejection efficiency does not tend to unity at high pressures, but rather approaches an asymptotic value less than unity. A good membrane will reach this asymptote at a reasonably low operating pressure.

For diffusive membranes, the rejection efficiency for a series of solutes of similar chemical structure will generally increase with increasing size of solute molecules. With electrolytes, rejection usually improves as ion-valency increases (*e.g.* $NaCl < CaCl_2$; $NaCl < Na_2SO_4$).

With solutes of dissimilar chemical structure, rejection efficiency cannot reliably be predicted on the basis of molecular size alone, since the affinity of the solute for the membrane substance is an equally important factor. For example, cellulose acetate membranes show no retention for phenol in water solution under conditions where they retain 98% of NaCl despite the fact that the phenol molecule is larger than sodium and chloride ions.

SIEVE-TYPE MEMBRANES

For microporous sieve-type membranes, the simplified transport relations are:

for solvent:

$$J_1 = \frac{K_1 \Delta P}{\eta t} \tag{5}$$

where η = the solvent viscosity;

for solute:

$$J_2 = \sigma_2 J_1 C_1 = \frac{\sigma_2 C_1 K_1 P}{nt} \tag{6}$$

where σ_2 = a dimensionless constant

$$(0 < \sigma_2 < 1)$$

since

$$J_2 = J_1 C_0 \quad (3)$$

and

$$\sigma_2 = \frac{C_0}{C_1} = 1 - R \quad (7)$$

The quantity (σ_2) represents, physically, the fraction of the total liquid flowing through the membrane passing through pores large enough to accommodate to solute molecules. Since this parameter is determined solely by the solute molecular dimensions and the pore size distribution in the membrane, the membrane rejection efficiency is independent of applied pressure. This is the most obvious and most easily determined functional difference between a sieve-type and a diffusive membrane. Whilst most sieve-type membranes display this general behaviour, many do show anomalies. In contrast to diffusive-type membranes (whose separative properties are largely governed by the chemical constitution of the polymer from which they are synthesised), sieve-type membranes owe their permeability almost entirely to microstructure, *i.e.* pore size and pore size distribution of the skin layer. Consequently, it is possible to produce sieve-type membranes of specified permeability and retentivity from a number of different polymer materials.

CONCENTRATION OF MEMBRANE POLARISATION

As solvent water passes through a reverse osmosis/ultrafiltration membrane, there will be a rapid increase in solute concentration on the original solution side of the membrane, with consequent local increase in osmotic pressure and a reduction in flux across the membrane. This phenomenon has been termed *concentration* or *membrane polarisation*. This is shown schematically in Fig. 3. The influence of polarisation upon membrane performance characteristics is always adverse and frequently severe. The membrane solvent and solute transport rates are governed solely by the composition of, and the hydrostatic pressure upon, the fluid in immediate contact with the upstream surface. If the membrane is not completely retentive for solute, the permeate will contain a substantially higher concentration of solute than would be predicted from the bulk solute concentration upstream. Hence the membrane's apparent

TABLE 2

Membrane configurations for ultrafiltration

System	Advantages	Disadvantages	Commercial status
TURBULENT FLOW			
A. Tubular	1. Easily cleaned for food applications; accepted for dairy and food processing 2. Well-developed equipment 3. Individual tubes can be replaced	1. High holding volume per unit membrane area 2. Presently moderately expensive (~10–20 $/ft^2) 3. Moderately parasitic pressure drop in tube connections (turnarounds)	Commercially available
B. Flat leaf[a]	1. Low holding volume per unit membrane area 2. Well-developed equipment	1. Susceptible to plugging at flow stagnation points; possibly difficult to clean for food, dairy and pharmaceutical applications 2. Presently expensive (~100 $/ft^2) 3. Moderate parasitic pressure drop losses 4. Entire membrane module must be replaced in case of failure	Commercially available
C. Spiral wound	1. Inexpensive (~3 $/ft^2) 2. Very compact with low holding volume per unit membrane area 3. Well-developed equipment 4. Low parasitic pressure drop losses	1. Very susceptible to plugging 2. Very difficult to clean and probably not acceptable for food, dairy and pharmaceutical applications	Currently available for RO only, but potentially adaptable to UF

LAMINAR FLOW			
A. Flat channels; annuli, etc.	1. Potentially more economical for highly viscous solutions 2. Very low holding volume per unit membrane area 3. High conversion obtainable; eliminates need for recycle operation 4. Low parasitic pressure drop losses	1. Equipment not well-developed 2. Susceptible to plugging 3. Potentially difficult to clean 4. Presently expensive 5. Membrane replacement difficult (depends on exact design)	Large-scale equipment under development
B. Hollow fibres (tubeside feed)	1. Same as above, plus potentially inexpensive	1. Not developed 2. Susceptible to plugging 3. Potentially difficult to clean 4. Entire fibre cartridge must be replaced upon single fibre failure	Not available
C. Hollow Fibres (shellside feed)	1. Same as above, plus potentially inexpensive	1. Excessive plugging excludes use for most UF applications 2. Non-cleanability excludes use for food, dairy and pharmaceutical applications	Commercially available for RO only

[a] Parallel flat leaves attached to a central permeate collection header.

efficiency will be substantially reduced. If the solution is sufficiently concentrated and the solute of relatively low molecular weight, the high solute osmotic pressure in the boundary layer will reduce the effective pressure for ultrafiltration, thus reducing UF flux. If the solution contains a high-molecular-weight solute or colloid, solute accumulation at the membrane surface produces a layer of finite, and frequently large, hydraulic flow resistance. This, of course, decreases the overall hydraulic permeability of the membrane and leads to a substantial decrease in ultrafiltration performance.

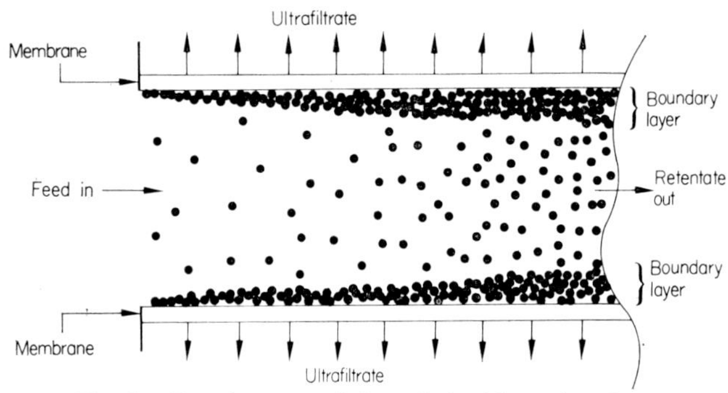

FIG. 3. Development of the polarised boundary layer.

MEMBRANE SYSTEM CONFIGURATIONS

Membrane systems are commercially available, or potentially available, in several configurations. Most of these have been developed for water desalination (RO) and some have been adapted to ultrafiltration. While mechanical strength is an important consideration for high-pressure RO systems, it assumes less importance for low-pressure ultrafiltration. Instead, mass transfer becomes exceptionally important and, correspondingly, system design and geometry.

Listed in Table 2 are different membrane configurations, divided into turbulent flow and laminar flow. Advantages and disadvantages of each for RO/UF applications are identified.

APPLICATIONS: LACTOSE SYSTEMS

Cheese and Casein Wheys

The disposal and/or utilisation of whey is a worldwide problem. With the programmed expansion in cheese and casein manufacture it is expected that current whey supplies in the Republic of Ireland (73 million gallons in 1971) may increase to about 230 million gallons by 1975. About 2200 million gallons of cheese whey are produced annually in the United States, of which somewhat less than half is treated to recover by-products and/or to abate water pollution. The remainder is discharged by various means and constitutes a major source of water pollution. New pollution control laws are forcing cheese manufacturers to process their whey. Disposal by land spreading as fertiliser is being discouraged because of run off into streams, especially during Spring thawing after build up from Winter application. In the rest of the world, producing several times more whey than the United States, land area and usage may be even more restrictive, or arid conditions may make water supplies even more sensitive.

An active research programme on the application of pressure-driven membrane concentration/separation processes in the dairy industry has been pursued at the Moorepark Research centre since 1971. The purpose of this work has been to examine the feasibility of using these processes to concentrate and fractionate whey and skim milk.

It is appropriate at this point to describe briefly the composition of skim milk and cheese whey. Skim milk contains *ca.* 2·5–3·5% by weight of casein, 0·5–0·7% of whey proteins (both the casein and whey protein fractions are in turn complicated mixtures of different proteins), 0·1–0·2% of lower-molecular-weight polypeptides, amino acids and urea (the so-called non-protein nitrogen fraction), 4·5% of lactose, 0·6–0·8% of mineral salts and varying quantities of citric acid, lactic acid and vitamins. Whey is that liquid portion of whole or skim milk which is left over when the casein has been coagulated and removed as curd for further processing into cheese (or casein). Whey therefore contains all the components of skim milk except the casein. In fact, it generally retains a small equilibrium amount of casein, either in its native form, or as fines retained in the curd during whey separation. For every pound of cheese produced, approximately 8–10 lb of whey are produced.

Figure 4 shows a simplified flow sheet for a two step Cheddar cheese whey treatment process based on the application of ultrafiltration and reverse osmosis. In Step 1, whey is pumped through a low pressure UF module for whey protein recovery and concentration. The permeate from the ultrafiltration step is concentrated by reverse osmosis for lactose recovery (*e.g.* by crystallisation). The bulk of the water contained in the whey is passed through the RO membranes and recovered as a low BOD water.

In Step 2, whey is concentrated 10 to 30 fold by volume. Membranes are used which preferentially retain whey proteins. Thus it is possible to obtain protein concentrates with a higher proportion of proteins in the dissolved solids, since lactose, non-protein nitrogen, lactic acid and minerals pass through the membranes. Operation is typically in the pressure range 3·5–12·0 kg/cm^2 and at temperatures of 15–30°C.

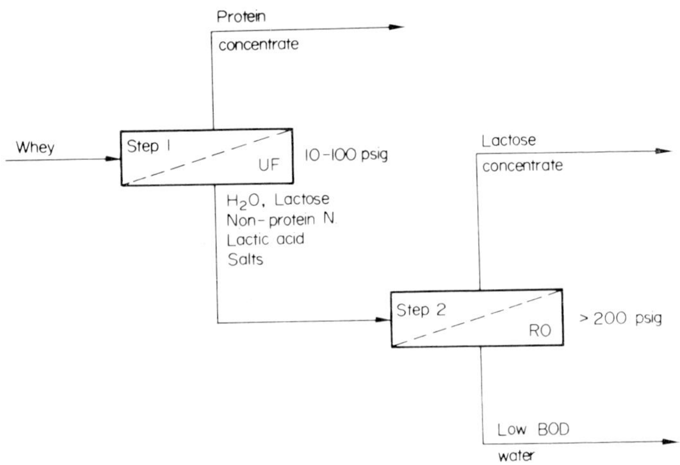

FIG. 4. Membrane process for whey treatment—flow schematic.

Table 3 contains data on a range of whey protein concentrates produced on pilot plant equipment at Moorepark. Two types of ultrafiltration plant, a tubular reverse osmosis/ultrafiltration (RO/UF) plant manufactured by Patterson Candy International (PCI) and a plate-and-frame plant manufactured by De Danske Sukkerfabrikker (DDS), were used for these trials. Flux rates averaged from 200 to 400 litres/m^2 of membrane surface/day (20 hr). Flux rate is a critical design parameter because it determines the membrane area requirement, or plant size, and thus capital cost. Major factors affecting flux are flow rate through the membrane unit, operating temperature and feed concentration level.

Figures 5, 6 and 7 show the effects of operating temperature, pressure and feed concentration on flux rate. Flux typically decreases

TABLE 3

Protein powder: Lactic casein whey—% composition

	Raw whey	Concentrate	Powder
Total solids	6·3	24·0	—
pH	4·75	4·85	4·76
Protein (N × 6·38)	0·68	14·5	50·6
NPN	0·25	1·05	—
Lactose	4·6	8·4	32·0
Fat	0·03	0·46	1·4
Acidity	0·45	1·5	5·6
Ash	0·61	0·83	3·23
Moisture	—	—	5·5

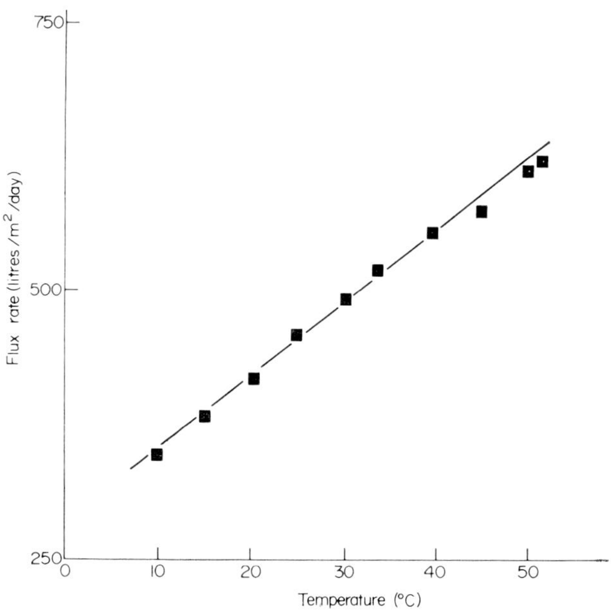

FIG. 5. Flux rate and temperature.

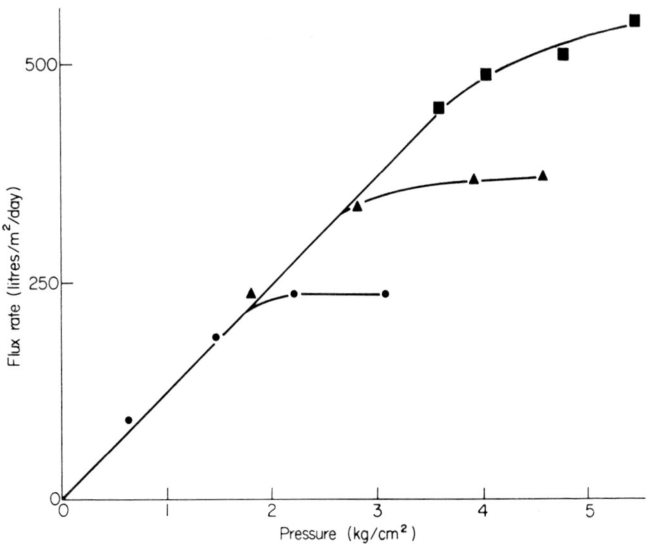

FIG. 6. Flux rate and pressure.

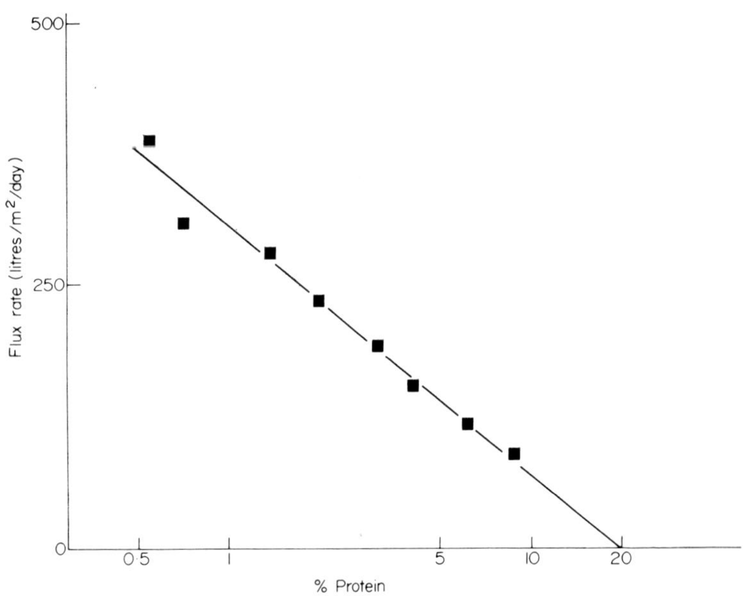

FIG. 7. Flux rate and feed protein concentration.

with increasing feed protein concentration, as well as decreasing temperature. In addition to causing a flux decline, the increasing protein level in the feed also increases feed viscosity and therefore the resultant pressure drop across the system. The exact magnitude of this increase in viscosity does not seem to be a function of the protein concentration alone, but also of certain other, as yet unidentified, substances present in whey, Also, flux is essentially independent of operating pressure above a certain value and increases almost in proportion with the linear velocity of the whey in the membrane system.

Ultrafiltration is applicable to all types of whey. One limitation of the process, however, requires that the fat content of the whey be such that no free fat is present. A separate fat phase can coat the membrane, greatly reducing flux. Emulsified fat, however, does not appear to constitute a processing problem. Similarly, the presence of residual casein fines presents no obstacle.

PROTEIN-PRODUCT FINAL RECOVERY, COMPOSITION AND PROPERTIES

Dried protein products can be recovered from the concentrate by spray drying.[3,4] Detailed laboratory evaluation has indicated that the products may be prepared with no evident loss of functionality. The composition of the protein product depends primarily on the

TABLE 4

Protein powder: cheddar whey—% composition

	Raw whey	Concentrate	Powder
Total solids	6·1	20·5	—
pH	6·4	6·5	6·1
Protein (N × 6·38)	0·62	13·32	64·6
NPN	0·19	1·34	—
Lactose	4·6	4·6	23·0
Fat	0·04	0·45	1·6
Acidity	0·12	0·62	2·0
Ash	0·56	0·88	3·3
Moisture	—	—	2·1

degree of water and impurities removal; the more water removed, the higher the protein content. This is illustrated in Fig. 8. Even higher protein content products can be prepared by rediluting with water and reconcentrating by ultrafiltration.

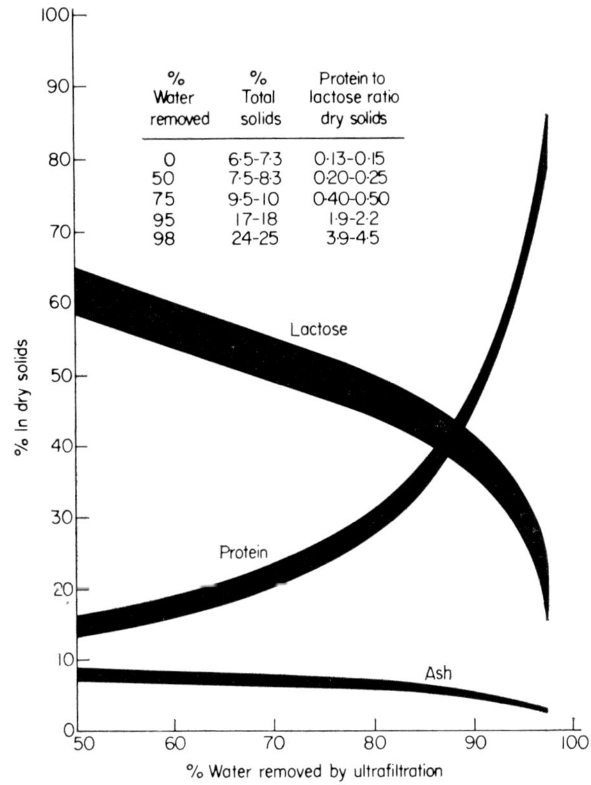

FIG. 8. Composition of whey protein concentrate.

High protein concentrates have been prepared from both Cheddar cheese and casein wheys. Typical compositional data for these products are given in Tables 3 and 4. The products have excellent nutritional and functional properties and have a wide range of food applications.[5]

REVERSE OSMOSIS CONCENTRATION OF ULTRAFILTRATION PERMEATE (LACTOSE) OR WHOLE WHEY

In contrast to the UF step, reverse osmosis requires high pressure operation (pressure in excess of 50 kg/cm^2) and the use of a 'tight' or retentive membrane. Figure 9 shows representative data obtained for the concentration of lactose permeates from the ultrafiltration

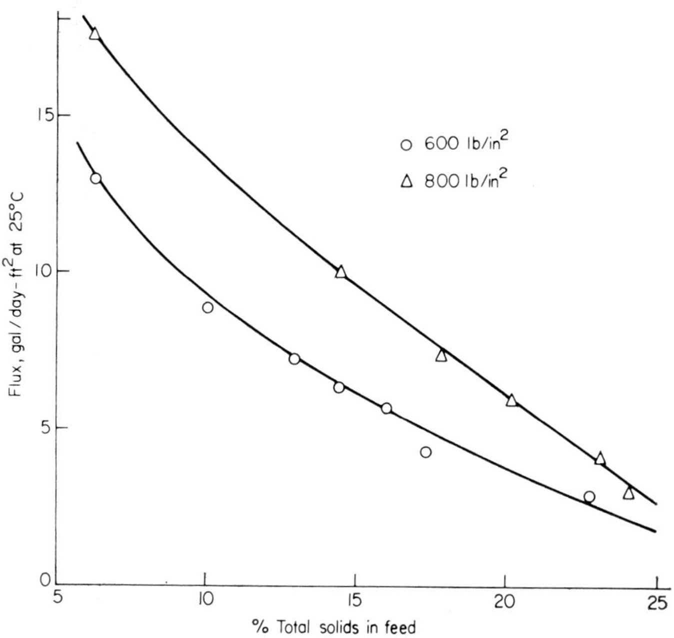

FIG. 9. Reverse osmosis flux as function of pressure and concentration.

step. Data for whole whey would be similar. Flux decreases with concentration due to the increasing osmotic pressure of the lactose or whole whey solution. It is possible to achieve a five-fold concentration of the ultrafiltration permeate (or whole whey), giving an effective total solids level of 25–30% in the concentrate.

The reverse osmosis concentration of ultrafiltration permeate (lactose) or whole whey is important because it determines the BOD level of the treated whey effluent. A reduction in BOD of the order of 98% can be achieved.

The concentrated permeate may be used for the recovery of lactose as a pharmaceutical or food grade product, as a microbial growth substrate or as an energy feedstuff for pigs or calves.

ULTRAFILTRATION AND REVERSE OSMOSIS OF SKIM MILK SYSTEMS

In a similar manner to whey, ultrafiltration may be applied to fractionate skim milk into a colloid-rich protein fraction and a lactose-cum-salts fraction.[6] Operation is typically at low pressures of about 5 kg/cm^2. During the process, no phase changes take place and as the operation is effected at temperatures below 10°C, there is no denaturation or chemical change in the thermolabile milk proteins. A six-fold volumetric reduction is possible, but this requires a high temperature (45–50°C) operation for the latter part of the ultrafiltration cycle in order to counteract the viscosity increase in the feed. For this duty, flux rates of 180 litres/m^2/membrane surface/ 20 hr are possible using the DDS plate-and-frame system fitted with membranes type 600.[7]

A milk concentrate containing up to 70% protein (with correspondingly low lactose content) is possible, having a wide range of special diabetic and health food applications.

Reverse osmosis of skim milk is an additional possibility. This may be of value as a preliminary step before evaporation or spray drying, or in order to economise on transport or other costs. The concentration ratio is 1:3 maximum corresponding to 30% dry matter in the concentrate.[8] For concentration duties up to 30%, processing costs for RO are lower than for conventional thermal evaporation.

REFERENCES

1. Loeb, S. and Sourirajan, S. (1963). *Advan. Chem. Ser.*, **38**, p. 117.
2. Manjikian, S. (1967). *Indus. Engin. Chem. Prod. Res. Div.*, **6**, p. 23.
3. Delaney, R. A. M., Donnelly, J. K. and O'Sullivan, A. C. (1972). *Ir. J. agric. Res.*, **11**, p. 181.
4. Delaney, R. A. M., Donnelly, J. K. and O'Sullivan, A. C. (1973). *Ir. J. agric. Res.*, in press.
5. Delaney, R. A. M. and Donnelly, J. K. (1972). Paper presented at Symposium on 'Processing of Whey and Milk by Membrane Separation Techniques and Related Processes', Organised by the International Circle of Dairy Research Leaders, Cork, Dec. 11–12.
6. Delaney, R. A. M. and Donnelly, J. K. (1973). *Tech. Ireland*, **4**(13).
7. Neilsen, I. K., Bundgaard, A. G., Olsen, O. J. and Madsen, R. F. (1972). *Proc. Biochem.*, **7**(9), p. 27.
8. Bundgaard, A. G., Olsen, O. J. and Madsen, R. F. (1972). *Dairy Ind.*, **37**(10), p. 539.

DISCUSSION

Wiggall: I wonder whether Dr Delaney could comment upon the expected life of the membrane systems available. Presumably this is a very important consideration from the commercial standpoint.

Delaney: A very important factor. This has been one of the reasons why commercialisation did not come sooner. In our lab we have used membranes for periods in excess of one year without a significant loss. At the end of each working day you may have to clean the membranes. We have one year now as a conservative estimate for using most membranes. We have operated a 20-hr day continuously for about a 200-day period at about 10 000 litres of whey a day.

Until recently there has not been sufficient experience with large-scale pilot plant equipment to reliably predict membrane life. Our results indicate that one year may be regarded as a reasonably conservative working life for the best commercially available membranes working continuously on whey.

Nicol: Would it be possible to separate lactose and ash by ultrafiltration or reverse osmosis?

Delaney: Yes, that is possible. In the transcript we have submitted data on this. We have in fact used membranes which will give you retention of lactose with a 90% reduction in the ash content.

Parker: Have you looked into the economic viability of the process?

Delaney: Yes, but it is very difficult to give you blanket costs because they depend on the individual operation.

For example, any pretreatment which is necessary may dramatically increase costs. Also the membrane life will affect cost and the membrane life will be determined by the duty required. It is possible to make general cost assessment based on costs for treatment of brackish water (this is a reverse osmosis process). Experience here would suggest costs of 20–25p per 1000 gal of water treated. As a general guide I would suggest that the cost of buying and operating an RO plant at £1/1000 gal of water removed is reasonable and this compares favourably with current dairy costs of £2–£2.50/1000 gal removed by conventional thermal evaporation. With RO you do of course have a concentration ceiling of about 25–30% solids.

Brennan: How does it stand up from the sanitary point of view? Are there any microbiological problems arising from the long term use of UF or RO plants?

Delaney: Well designed sanitary plants are commercially available—a laminar flow system of plate-and-frame design manufactured by De Danske Sukkerfabrikker (DDS), Copenhagen and turbulent flow tubular design plant from Abcor Inc. (USA).

Our cleaning and sanitising procedure is something as follows:

1. water-wash flushing for 15 min;
2. 0·2% of biological detergent circulated for 2 hr at 40°C. For marked protein film deposition, treatment with 0·5% trypsin solution may be required to remove the film;
3. finally, sanitisation is achieved by recirculating 50 ppm hypochlorite.

11

The Structure of Starch

W. BANKS, C. T. GREENWOOD and D. D. MUIR

Flour Milling and Baking Research Association,
Chorleywood, Herts., England

ABSTRACT

The structure of starch must be considered at two quite distinct levels.

First, at the molecular level, we are concerned with the fine-structures of the two macromolecular components of starch, amylose and amylopectin. Current models for these two polysaccharides, and the evidence on which these models are based, will be reviewed.

Second, the morphology of the granule must be considered—in many industrial applications it is the physical and mechanical properties of granular *starch that assume dominant importance. Starch granules have been the subject of repeated investigations dating back to the development of the optical microscope. The type of information that can be obtained by means of optical microscopy will be discussed, as will the more recent use of X-ray diffraction, scanning electron microscopy and laser beams for determining the structure of the granule. The structure of the granule will be compared with the spherulitic structures exhibited by many synthetic, crystalline polymers.*

INTRODUCTION

Starch occurs in all higher plants as semi-crystalline granules of polymeric material. The starches of major economic importance are reserve starches, laid down by the plant as an energy store, for example, in the seeds of cereal grains or in the tubers of potato plants. As starches are polymers of glucose with a high nutritive value, cultivation of plant sources rich in starch is widespread, and a high proportion of the world's food energy intake is as starch.

The role of starch in some foods is well known—large quantities of starch, or derivatives of starch, are used as thickening agents, as

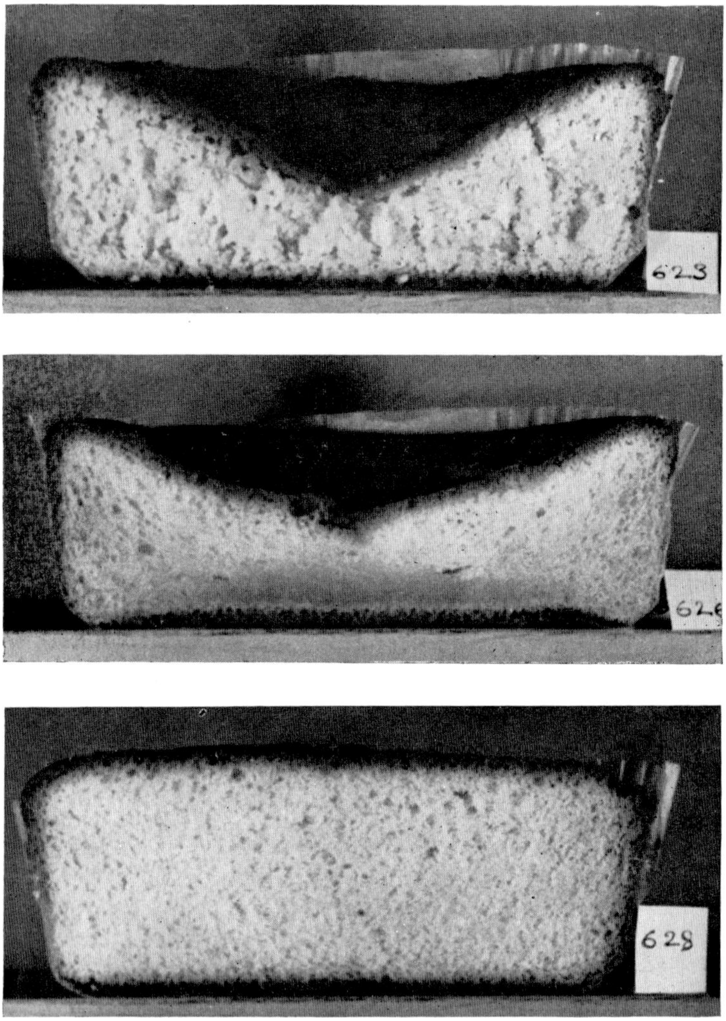

FIG. 1. High-ratio yellow cakes baked from mixtures of various types of maize starch and wheat gluten as a replacement for wheat flour. 623 Cake baked using maize starch of apparently 55% amylose content. 626 Cake baked using waxy maize starch (waxy maize starch contains <1% amylose). 628 Cake baked using normal maize starch (with ~28% amylose, corresponding to wheat starch).

edible films and for modification of food textures. However, in an important class of food, namely baked goods, the part played by starch in the overall structure is often less widely appreciated. Wheat flour contains about 80% of its weight as starch, but the contribution of this material in baking processes often tends to be overshadowed by the presence of 8–14% proteinaceous material. Whilst protein undoubtedly plays a significant role in the quality of bread, it by no means determines the form of the product. If bread is prepared from wheat flour, from wheat gluten and from wheat starch, although obviously lacking in qualities such as loaf volume and lightness of crumb, the loaf made from starch is comparable to that made from flour, but no such similarity is observed when using gluten. Not only is the presence of starch important in the structure of baked goods, but the starch type is also critical, a point well demonstrated in Fig. 1. In this case, high-ratio yellow cakes were baked using different types of maize starch (waxy maize, normal maize and amylomaize) in place of the wheat starch in flour. Major differences are shown in the resulting cakes—only that from normal maize starch gave a cake without collapse. These results demonstrate the profound relation that exists between the properties of the starch granules and those of the ultimate baked product. If, therefore, we are to understand and control the baking process, one of our major aims must be to determine the structure and properties of granular starch.

Starch may be considered at two distinct levels:

(*a*) on a molecular level, the structure, shape and size of the component molecules must be known; and,

(*b*) the organisation of these polymeric molecules on a macromolecular level should be determined.

Only then can the complex interactions resulting in the ultimate granular structure be elucidated, and improvements in the manufactured end-product in the cases outlined—baked goods—be achieved.

THE STARCH COMPONENTS

Fractionation of Starch

Fractionation of starch may be achieved by a variety of different procedures. The most efficient technique involves dispersion of the starch granule in water, after a pre-treatment with either liquid ammonia[1] or dimethyl sulphoxide[2] to shatter the granular structure. The components are then separated by differential complex formation with either thymol or butan-1-ol.[3] The amylose component forms an insoluble complex and is readily removed by centrifugation, then purified by dissolution in boiling water and recrystallisation with butanol, on cooling. The amylopectin component is isolated from the initial supernatant, after removal of the amylose complex. The supernatant is freed from alcohol by repeated solvent extraction with diethylether, reduced in volume, and freeze-dried. Fractions of starch prepared in this way are readily dispersed in hot water to yield true solutions.

Amylose

Amylose, isolated by the above technique, has been shown to be an essentially linear polymer of glucose units linked by α-1:4- bonds.[4] However, when the enzyme beta-amylase is allowed to hydrolyse amyloses derived from cereal or potato starches, conversion to maltose is incomplete. Beta-amylase hydrolyses alternate bonds in chains of α-1:4-linked glucose residues, from the non-reducing end of the chain, to yield maltose. The partial inaccessibility of amylose molecules to the action of beta-amylase has been shown to be due to the presence of small amounts of branching through α-1:6- bonds.[5] Although the extent of branching is slight (of the order of one branch-point per 500 residues), these points effectively block the action of beta-amylase. Small amounts of Z-enzyme, a weak alpha-amylase[6]—conveniently found as an impurity in crude cereal beta-amylase preparations—effectively bypass these points, and allow complete conversion to maltose by concurrent hydrolysis with beta-amylase and Z-enzyme. The properties of some typical amyloses are shown in Table 1.

The behaviour of amylose in foods is dominated by two features: (a) the ease with which the polymer forms inclusion complexes; and (b) the ability of the molecules to form crystalline bodies with strong molecular interactions. Disregarding the slight extent of long-chain branching, both these properties of amylose may be attributed to the stereoregularity of the polymer backbone. In dilute solution, amylose adopts a randomly coiled form, despite earlier published models to the contrary,[7] and on the addition of one of a wide variety of complexing agents, such as lipid, iodine or most primary aliphatic alcohols, a helical structure, of 6 or 7 glucose residues per turn, is formed with the complexed molecules occupying the central cavity of the helix.[8] As will be seen later, the ability of amylose to interact with iodine, forming a characteristic deep-blue complex, has been developed into a powerful diagnostic tool invaluable in the characterisation of starch.

TABLE 1
Properties of amyloses

Starch	$[\beta]^a$	$[\beta + Z]^b$	$[\eta]^c$	Reference
Potato	81	99	530	
Barley	83	101	391	
Wheat	72	101	330	2
Rye	72	98	335	2
Smooth-seeded pea	81	100	—	21
Wrinkle-seeded pea	82	100	—	21

[a] Percentage conversion into maltose under the action of crystalline beta-amylase.
[b] Percentage conversion into maltose under the concurrent action of beta-amylase and Z-enzyme.
[c] Limiting viscosity number (ml/g) in 0·15 M KOH.

If concentrated solutions of amylose are cooled slowly, crystallisation occurs with the formation, in some cases, of spherulites, similar in appearance to starch granules.[9] Crystallisation phenomena are, however, more widely observed as retrogradation, a process in which the starch molecules become irreversibly insoluble in water due to the formation of very powerful intermolecular bonds. Retrograded amylose possesses a crystalline structure,[10] but the exact nature of the bonding within the insolubilised material is not yet known.

Amylopectin

The highly branched fraction of starch, amylopectin, is as yet relatively poorly characterised. As in amylose, the predominant linkage between monomer residues is by α-1:4- bonds, but the extent of branching, through α-1:6- branch-points, is greater than in amylose, ranging from one in sixteen to one in twenty-five residues, depending on the source of the amylopectin. As shown in Fig. 2, the generally accepted model for the arrangement of chains in amylopectin is that of a randomly branched structure.[11] Doubts have recently been cast on the adequacy of this type of amylopectin structure,[12] but conclusive evidence on this point is not yet available. Beta-amylase hydrolyses approximately 55% of the amylopectin molecule to maltose, leaving a high-molecular-weight beta-limit dextrin. Because of the presence of short-chain branching, the addition of small quantities of Z-enzyme effects little or no change in the extent of conversion to maltose. However, if a debranching

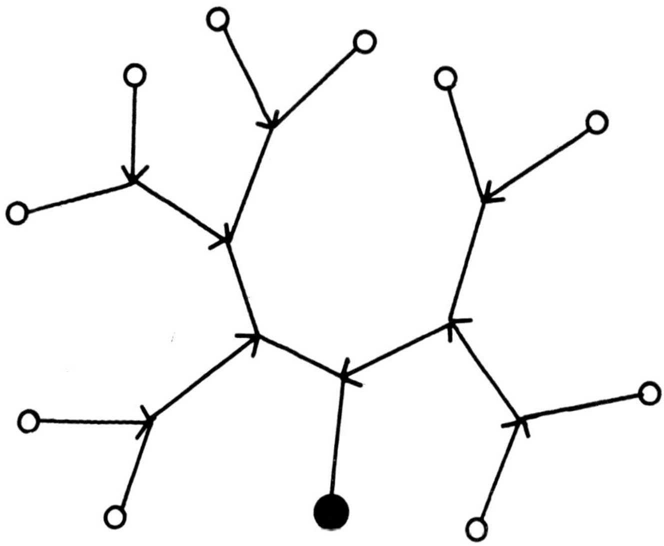

FIG. 2. The randomly branched structure of amylopectin. ○ non-reducing end, ● reducing end, → α-1:6- bond.

enzyme, for example pullulanase, is added to the beta-amylase digest, the molecule once more becomes totally accessible to the action of beta-amylase and conversion is complete. Table 2 shows the properties of some typical amylopectins.

The structure of amylopectin is generally thought to be analogous to that of glycogen, the mammalian reserve polysaccharide, but major differences in behaviour exist which may be attributed to the shape of the amylopectin molecule. Whilst glycogen exists in solution in a compact spherical shape, experiments have shown that amylopectin has a significantly higher volume in solution than would be expected on the basis of a similar, though less highly-branched, molecule.[13] In addition, amylopectin is reputed to form crystalline retrograded material,[14] and also inclusion complexes. The ability to form these complexes is, however, more limited than in the case of amylose. At pH 12 in the presence of salt, amylose is thought to exist in a helical conformation,[15] and since this is a most favourable conformation for the formation of complexes, addition of butan-1-ol causes immediate precipitation of the amylose as the butanol complex.

TABLE 2

Properties of amylopectins

Starch	$[\beta]^a$	$[\beta + Z]^b$	$[\beta + Pu]^c$	$\overline{CL}^d$	$\overline{MW} \times 10^{-6e}$	Ref.
Potato	54	55	100	21	~250	
Barley	57	58	101	21	~250	
Wheat	54	55	n.d.[f]	20	n.d.	2
Rye	58	57	n.d.	20	n.d.	2
Smooth-seeded pea	58	n.d.	n.d.	26	n.d.	21
Wrinkle-seeded pea	65	n.d.	n.d.	35	n.d.	21

[a] Percentage conversion into maltose under the action of crystalline beta-amylase.

[b] Percentage conversion into maltose under the concurrent action of beta-amylase and Z-enzyme.

[c] Percentage conversion into maltose under the concurrent action of beta-amylase and pullulanase.

[d] Average length of unit-chain.

[e] Molecular weight by light scattering.

[f] n.d. = not determined.

When amylopectin is dissolved in a similar solvent system, the hydrodynamic volume of the polymer decreases with respect to that in water, indicating that a similar coil–helix transition occurs, but the addition of butanol does not yield a complex unless the solution is cooled to 4°C and held at this temperature. Amylopectin in concentrated solution may also be induced to form aggregates, if the molecule is subjected to alternate cycles of freezing and thawing. It seems, therefore, that the crystallisation behaviour of amylopectin may differ only in degree from that of amylose. As stressed earlier, the ability of a polymer to crystallise is directly related to the stereoregularity of the polymer chain, and, though the basic units in both amylose and amylopectin are the same, in a 3-dimensional structure such as that of glycogen, crystallisation would be entirely prevented by the branching of the polymer chains. The concept of amylopectin existing in a 2-dimensional, *i.e.* planar, form, however, does not preclude crystallisation,[16] and could explain observations of chain folding in the case of complexes of amylopectin.[17] Further work is required before the structure and shape of amylopectin can be put on a sound theoretical basis.

The Amylose–Amylopectin Ratio in Starches

We have described how two quite distinct polymer types may be fractionated from starch, and shall now discuss the relative proportions of these polymer types found within native starch granules.

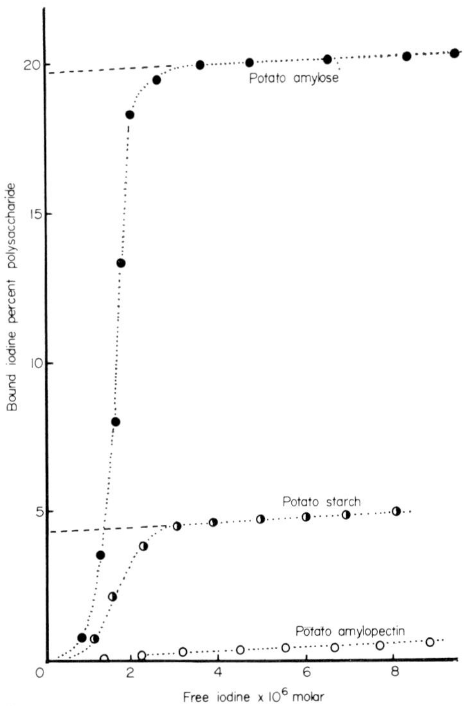

FIG. 3. The iodine-binding curves of potato starch, potato amylose and potato amylopectin measured at 20°C by the technique of Banks *et al.*[18]

The differing abilities of amylose and amylopectin to complex with iodine have already been mentioned and provide a useful means of analysis.[18] Potentiometric titration of the polymers with iodine readily differentiates between the two types as shown in Fig. 3;

amylose binds 19–20 mg iodine percent polysaccharide at 20°C and, under identical conditions, amylopectin binds none. The amount of amylose within any starch may thus be measured by:

$$\% \text{ amylose} = \frac{\text{iodine-binding capacity of the starch}}{\text{iodine-binding capacity of amylose}} \times 100\%$$

provided both iodine-binding capacities are measured at the same temperature. Most normal varieties of starch contain between 20–30% amylose, and in Table 3 the amylose contents of starches isolated from various cultivars are shown. It should be noted that

TABLE 3

Apparent amylose contents of various starches

Starch	IBC[a]	Amylose content (%)
Potato	4·5	23
Barley (normal)	5·7	29
Barley (high-amylose)	8·2	42
Wheat	5·4	28
Rye	5·5	28
Maize	5·3	27
Amylomaize	~10·5	~54
Smooth-seeded pea	7·0	36
Wrinkle-seeded pea	14·1	72

[a] Iodine-binding capacity (mg/100 mg starch), measured at 20°C.

mutant varieties of plants do exist, in which starches, composed entirely of amylopectin—the waxy starches—or starches, with amylose contents greatly in excess of 30%, do occur. Caution must be exercised in interpretation of the iodine-binding curves of some of the starches of high, apparent amylose content. Certain varieties of maize starch contain material which binds considerable quantities of iodine, but which is not adequately described as either amylose or amylopectin.[19,20] No fixed value of amylose content can be given for starch from any particular variety as the amylose content of all starches examined to date changes during growth.[21–23] Bearing this in mind, the way in which the polymers are arranged within the granule will now be discussed.

STARCH IN THE GRANULAR FORM

Starch granules have a diversity of shapes and sizes, often uniquely characteristic of the cultivar from which the starch is isolated. The microscopic examination of starch, isolated from the plant by techniques devised to minimise experimental artifacts,[24] reveals several characteristic features of which two are of special significance:

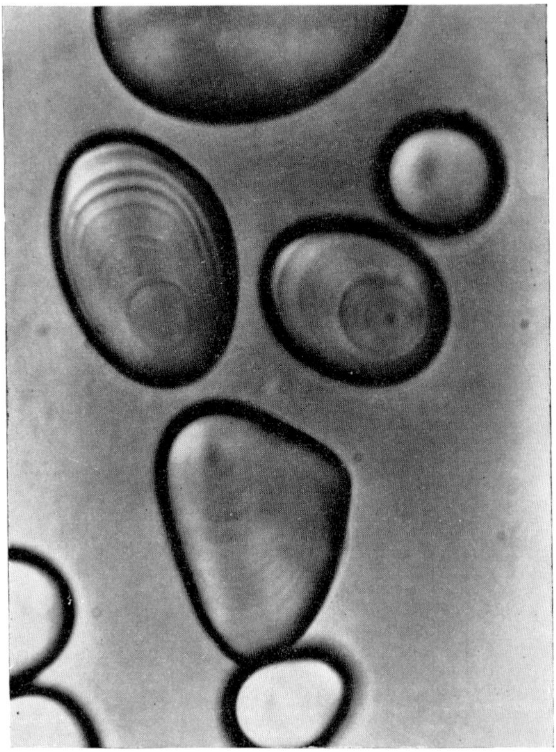

FIG. 4. Potato starch granules, between 20 and 60 μ in size, which exhibit distinct rings.

(1) starch granules tend to possess radial symmetry and often exhibit well-defined rings or lamellae; and (2) when viewed between crossed polarisers the granules are optically anisotropic and have a well-defined birefringence pattern. These features are exemplified in Figs. 4 and 5 for potato starch.

The appearance of rings is widely interpreted as indicating a layering of the structure of the granule, though starch from many plants (*e.g.* maize, wheat and barley) seldom exhibits rings unless pretreated by acid or by amylolytic enzymes. A strong argument has been advanced for the correlation between rings in wheat starch and growth layers, for starch from wheat grown in continuous daylight

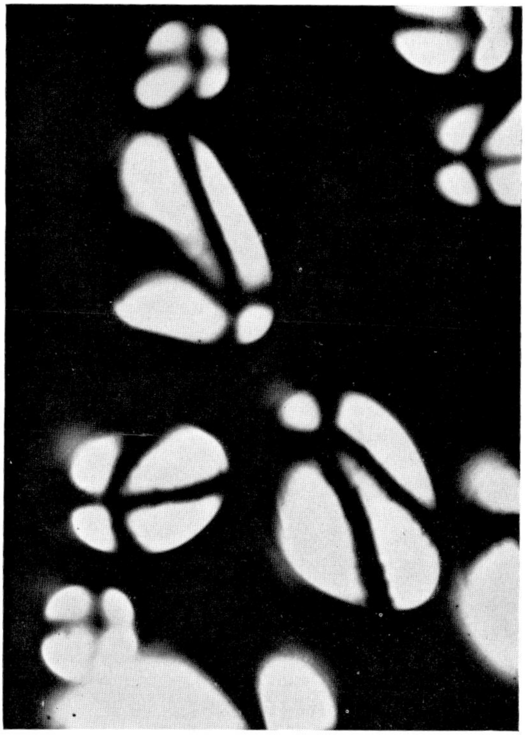

FIG. 5. The potato starch granules of Fig. 4 viewed between crossed polarisers, with marked birefringence patterns.

showed no rings after hydrolytic treatment, whilst starch from wheat grown in an alternating light–dark regime had a definite ring structure after similar treatment.[25] However, parallel experiments with potato starch showed no correlation between the light–dark environment used during growth and ring structure,[26] and cast some doubt upon the interpretation of rings on starch granules.

The well-defined birefringence pattern of starch is due to the alignment of light-scattering bodies, thought to be crystalline in nature. The sign of birefringence is positive,[27] and this is interpreted as being due to starch molecules lying with their molecular axes in a radial direction.[28] This conclusion is based on the premise that the highest index of refraction lies along the molecular axis. Whilst this fact undoubtedly is true for amylose in an extended chain conformation, caution must be exercised if the molecule is in a helical or folded form, and, in view of the lack of detailed knowledge of the crystalline structure of starch, the alignment of the starch molecules is open to question. The intensity of birefringence of starch varies widely between cultivars, and between mutant varieties of the same plant, but, in general, waxy starches are as birefringent as their normal counterparts,[29] whilst starches of high apparent amylose content are usually less birefringent. These observations imply that amylopectin is the structure-ordering component of starch—a concept supported by later evidence.

When starch granules are examined by X-ray diffraction techniques, complex spectra result,[30] and these have been classified into a number of types depending on certain spectral characteristics. Interpretation of the data is limited, and no simple model has yet emerged for the crystalline patterns of starch granules. In a recent review of the available data, French[27] advanced a structure based on parallel or anti-parallel chains of starch molecules in a double helix. No evidence at present exists to vitiate this hypothesis. The differences in degree of crystallinity of starches, as measured by X-ray diffraction, are similar to those differences for birefringence measurements. Waxy starches exhibit diffraction patterns of similar intensity to their normal counterparts,[29] so that once again amylopectin alone is shown capable of forming the granule structure.

Recent work has applied light-scattering techniques to single starch granules by the use of lasers,[31] but the data are exceedingly complex, and, as in X-ray diffraction measurements, interpretation of the results is inconclusive.

Despite the lack of precise knowledge of the granular structure of starch, the granule has many similarities to a polymer spherulite,[32] but although much information is available concerning the nature of polymer spherulites, little attempt has been made to relate these data to those on starch granules. Consideration of extensive review articles[33–35] provides a concensus of opinion for the appearance of spherulites—when the polymer crystallises it does so from primary nuclei; as the process of crystallisation continues, progressive layers of material are deposited on these nuclei, imperfections or defects being excluded and pushed outwards into the melt or solution. Often defects or dislocations change the orientation of the crystal and cause branching or twinning. When such defects occur frequently, the mode of crystallite extension is dominated by branching, and a radially orientated skeleton quickly develops with large amounts of imperfect material, rejected from the crystalline fibrils, incorporated in the overall structure.

It is at once apparent that analogies to this form of structure exist in the starch granule. Amylopectin has been suggested to be the basic structural component, and the branch-points may provide the defects necessary for spherulitic growth. Radiating fibrils of material have been observed (*e.g.* in potato starch[36]) using scanning electron microscopy, though little information on the nature or orientation of the molecules within the fibrils was given. A model for starch granules of radiating, para-crystalline fibrils of amylopectin, the interstices of which contain predominantly amylose, is consistent with many of the experimental observations on starch, and conforms to the typical spherulite structure. Such a model is substantiated by gentle leaching experiments[37] where amylose is preferentially leached from potato starch at its gelatinisation temperature, and by other experiments, at elevated temperatures, where extensive leaching of granular starch leaves a residual starch structure rich in the branched component.[20,38]

In polymer spherulites, ringed structures are commonplace, and have been explained in theories *not* involving successive layers of material.[33,39] Both theories interpret ring phenomena as due to twisting of crystalline fibrils during the growth of the spherulite.

GRANULAR STRUCTURE AND USEFUL PROPERTIES

In the foregoing discussions, the nature of starch components and their relation within the starch granule have been considered. So far no attempt has been made in this review to relate the useful properties of starch to what is known about the granule. However, as shown in Fig. 1, starch type plays a very important part in determining the appearance of the final product in baked goods. In this particular context, the swelling behaviour of the starch is of paramount importance.

When starch granules are progressively heated in water, at a certain temperature, the granules swell irreversibly and the birefringent properties of the granule are lost. The process, known as gelatinisation, is due to an irreversible breakdown in the order and crystallinity of the molecules within the granule, and the bonding forces may conveniently be measured by differential scanning calorimetry.[40] Further heating of the granule in water above the gelatinisation temperature causes greater swelling in a pattern characteristic of each type of starch. The swelling process is followed in Fig. 6 for three types of maize starch (with apparent amylose

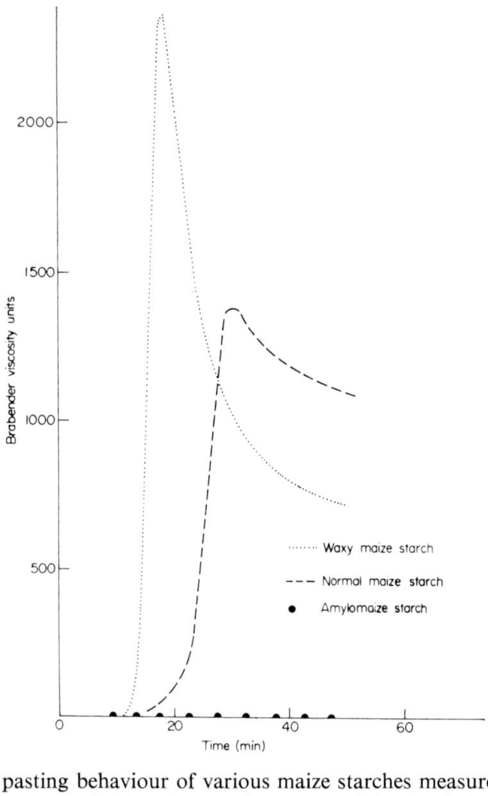

FIG. 6. The pasting behaviour of various maize starches measured in a 'Brabender' visco-amylograph. Starch concentration was 40 g starch in 460 ml water. The heating programme was (*a*) started at 50°C; (*b*) heated at a rate of 1·5°C/min to 95°C; (*c*) held at 95°C for 30 min.

contents of 0 %, 28 % and 55 % respectively) by measurement of the pure viscosity as a slurry of starch is heated in water over a programmed temperature rise. As the granules swell, they impinge upon each other and increase the viscosity of the starch paste; the swelling continues as the temperature rises until the cohesive forces in the original granular structure become excessively weakened, and the structure of the paste—and in consequence the observed viscosity—collapses as the integrity of the granules is lost. Reference to Fig. 6 shows quite different swelling behaviour for the starches from the maize genotypes. As the apparent amylose content increases, the forces holding the molecules within the granule tend to increase, for whilst waxy maize starch swells greatly under the observed conditions, the starch of apparently high amylose content registers no swelling at all. As the intermolecular forces are weaker in waxy maize starch, the granules break down more readily during cooking to give a resulting weak paste structure.

The behaviour of the three starch types on baking may now be rationalised. In normal maize, the starch is similar in swelling behaviour to that from wheat, and a normal type of cake is produced; in waxy maize starch, structural bonding is weak, so that, although the starch granules swell upon baking, the cake structure cannot stand the stresses involved during baking or subsequent cooling, and collapse of the structure occurs. Although producing a cake similarly sunken in appearance, the starch of high amylose content is a different case, for here the granules never swell sufficiently to provide a true structure during baking and the resulting cake is a failure. Although these explanations are a gross oversimplification of the interactions which occur during the baking process, they do stress the importance of the behaviour of starch granules and their relation to baking performance.

CONCLUSIONS

We have attempted to underline the areas of starch chemistry where further research is required, and summarise our conclusions thus:

(*a*) the structure of the linear component of starch, amylose, is now well established, but its role within the granular structure is somewhat obscure;

(*b*) amylopectin, the branched component of starch, is relatively poorly characterised, but many aspects of its behaviour may be rationalised by considering the molecule as a planar structure;

(*c*) the structure of the starch granule may be usefully regarded as that of a typical polymer spherulite, and the formation of granules may be similar to the crystallisation processes involved in the formation of spherulites;

(*d*) the nature of the intermolecular forces within the starch granule is a predominant factor in determining the subsequent behaviour of starch on cooking.

It is surmised that the strength of the non-valence bonding within the starch granule, and the ratio of amylose to amylopectin, control many of the properties in which the technologist is interested. Only by a more thorough understanding of the nature of the starch granule will control of baking phenomena and product improvement be achieved, to the mutual advantage of manufacturer and consumer.

REFERENCES

1. Hodge, J. E., Montgomery, E. M. and Hilbert, G. E. (1948). *Cereal Chem.,* **25,** p. 19.
2. Banks, W. and Greenwood, C. T. (1967). *Stärke,* **19,** p. 394.
3. Greenwood, C. T. and Robertson, J. S. M. (1954). *J. Chem. Soc.,* p. 3769.
4. Banks, W. and Greenwood, C. T. (1959). *Stärke,* **10,** p. 294.
5. Banks, W. and Greenwood, C. T. (1967). *Stärke,* **19,** p. 197.
6. Banks, W., Greenwood, C. T. and Jones, I. G. (1960). *J. Chem. Soc.,* p. 150.
7. Szejtli, J. and Augustat, S. (1966). *Stärke,* **18,** p. 38.
8. Rundle, R. E. and French, D. (1943). *J. Amer. Chem. Soc.,* **65,** p. 1707.
9. Schoch, T. J. (1969). *Journal of Japanese Soc. of Starch Science,* **17,** p. 5.
10. Whistler, R. L. and Johnson, C. (1948). *Cereal Chem.,* **25,** p. 418.
11. Meyer, K. H., Bernfeld, P. and Hohenemser, W. (1941). *Helv. Chim. Acta,* **23,** p. 885.
12. Gunja-Smith, Z., Marshall, J. J., Mercier, C., Smith, E. E. and Whelan, W. J. (1970). *Febs. Lett.,* **12,** p. 101.
13. Banks, W., Geddes, R., Greenwood, C. T. and Jones, I. G. (1972). *Stärke,* **24,** p. 245.
14. Doi, K. and Nikuni, Z. (1962). *Stärke,* **14,** p. 461.
15. Banks, W. and Greenwood, C. T. (1971). *Stärke,* **23,** p. 300.
16. Greenwood, C. T. (1956). *Advances in Carbohydrate Chem.,* **11,** p. 335.

17. Vasko, P. D. and Koenig, J. L. (1972). *J. Macromol. Sci. Phys.*, **B6**(1), p. 117.
18. Banks, W., Greenwood, C. T. and Muir, D. D. (1971). *Stärke,* **23,** p. 118.
19. Adkins, G. K. and Greenwood, C. T. (1969). *Carbohydrate Res.,* **11,** p. 217.
20. Banks, W., Greenwood, C. T. and Muir, D. D. (1971). *Stärke,* **23,** p. 199.
21. Greenwood, C. T. and Thomson, J. (1962). *Biochem. J.,* **82,** p. 156.
22. Harris, G. and MacWilliam, I. C. (1958). *Cereal Chem.,* **35,** p. 82.
23. Geddes, R., Greenwood, C. T. and MacKenzie, S. (1965). *Carbohydrate Res.,* **1,** p. 71
24. Banks, W., Greenwood, C. T. and Muir, D. D. (1971). *Stärke,* **23,** p. 380.
25. May, L. H. and Buttrose, M. S. (1959). *Australian J. Biol. Sci.,* **12**(2), p. 146.
26. Buttrose, M. S. (1963). *Stärke,* **15,** p. 213.
27. French, D. (1972). *Journal of Japanese Soc. of Starch Science,* **19,** p. 8.
28. Frey-Wyssling, A. (1953). *Submicroscopic Morphology of Protoplasm,* Elsevier, Amsterdam.
29. Baker, F. and Whelan, W. J. (1950). *Nature,* **166,** p. 34.
30. Bear, R. S. and French, D. (1941). *J. Amer. Chem. Soc.,* **63,** p. 2298.
31. Finkelstein, R. S. and Sarko, A. (1972). *Carbohydrate Res.,* **23,** p. 31.
32. Geddes, R. and Greenwood, C. T. (1969). *Stärke,* **21,** p. 148.
33. Price, F. P. (1959). *J. Polymer Sci.,* **37,** p. 71.
34. Lindenmeyer, P. H. (1963). *J. Polymer Sci.,* C, **1,** p. 5.
35. Mandelkern, L. (1964). *Crystallization of Polymers,* McGraw-Hill, London.
36. Sterling, C. (1971). *Stärke,* **23,** p. 193.
37. Banks, W. (1960). Ph.D. Thesis, University of Edinburgh.
38. Cowie, J. M. G. and Greenwood, C. T. (1957). *J. Chem. Soc.,* p. 2862.
39. Keller, A. (1959). *J. Polymer Sci.,* **39,** p. 151.
40. Stevens, D. J. and Elton, G. A. (1971). *Stärke,* **23,** p. 8.

DISCUSSION

Chairman: To open the discussion, we at Detmold have tried to make bread with different sorts of starch and even tried very different qualities from the best down to the worst. This confirmation means the molecules in the starch are the dominant factors.
Shallenberger: I am troubled by your statement that the starch molecule is two-dimensional. I am having a problem. What do you mean by the structure of a starch molecule?
Greenwood: No, I did not say starch molecule, I said amylopectin. The chemist put forward the branched structure mentioning it was a three-dimensional branched structure. I suggest that for a variety of reasons

amylopectin is synthesised off against the energy from synthesised polymer starch—I think it is synthesis, not stereochemistry. I think that amylopectin is laid down in the granule; it is laid down in two directions, but I think the enzymes are constrained in the plant in a way in which to me it doesn't seem improbable that synthesis takes place in two directions. When you put the granule into dispersal, because this no longer holds, the molecule is capable of undergoing different forms, but inherently it is laid down in two dimensions and that is why the behaviour of amylopectin is so different from that of glycogen. Glycogen is branched with a chain length about half that of amylopectin but the molecular weights are the same and when you put them in water you find the viscosity of glycogen is 7 and that of amylopectin is 170. You tell me why. It behaves as a spherical molecule. I think this is a result of the fact that amylopectin is not three-dimensional and this comes into everything from solution behaviour to the fact that in granule synthesis it is possible for things to go together. To amplify that a little, as Dr Norris well knows I don't believe that in the polysaccharides helices come from nowhere to form gels, but in starch I think it is there in the form of a helix. I believe that in the granule, amylose is there in helical form; that is why it is soluble.

Hood: Do you think that the ratio of amylose to amylopectin is constant throughout the granule?

Greenwood: I would not put it that way round. We haven't evidence to suggest the opposite. What I feel is important in this context is that this amylose/amylopectin ratio is a changing quantity. If you take the simplest example, potato starch, and measure the content, it can be as low as 5%, but in mature potato it is up to 20 or more. This applies to any other starch material. What one has to take into account is the fact that this ratio amylose/amylopectin is changing as the plant matures and somehow we have to reconcile that and the question how is it laid down in the granule.

McMichael: Can you comment on the effects of cooking starches and the rate of their hydrolysis by alpha- and beta-amylases?

Greenwood: I think this is a very difficult question leading into hours of discussion. We automatically differentiate into three areas—we deal with bread, confectionery and biscuits, and when we come to try to define in these three areas the role of the starch granule, there is a different answer to your question in each area. I don't think we have the time to deal adequately with your question.

Spencer: One of the slides showed the effects of the action of beta-amylase and a combination of alpha- and beta-amylases on various types of amylopectin. Surprisingly, the results showed very little difference. Why should this be the case?

Greenwood: This is one of the difficulties of nomenclature. When we treat it with alpha- and beta-amylases we are treating it with what you will find is Z-enzyme and that, as far as we are able to show, lets in the other amylase, but it so happens that there is a critical amount of alpha-amylase at a level below which you can detect no effect. This simply means that there is no action.

12

The Molecular Basis of Starch Technology in New Food Products

G. G. BIRCH, J. G. BRENNAN, R. J. PRIESTLEY and G. SODAH-AYERNOR

National College of Food Technology, University of Reading, Weybridge, Surrey, England

ABSTRACT

The preparation, processing and storage of starch-based products involves changes which have been somewhat loosely described as gelatinisation and retrogradation but which have not been properly described on a molecular basis.

This paper investigates the possibility of defining these changes in terms of the macromolecules which exist in the starch granules of rice and yam, with a view to achieving a more fundamental understanding of how food processing operations can affect the texture, appearance and quality of new starch-based products.

INTRODUCTION

Processing and storage of starch-based products involve changes of texture in which polymers may be shown to coalesce, crystallise, hydrate or dissolve. These changes may be accompanied by changes in the chemistry and morphology of the food particles involved resulting in clear differences of texture, flavour and appearance. These changes may be collectively described as 'retrogradation', 'hydration' and 'gelatinisation', but since none of these terms has been described as a discreet molecular event it is impossible to quantify any of them on an absolute molecular basis. For example, although previous workers have referred to hydration and gelatinisation of starch as a network formation of hydrogen bonds,[1] a recent review[2] makes no direct mention of hydrogen bonding, van der Waals' forces or London dispersion forces in the gelatinisation of macromolecules. It follows that methods reported for the quantification of gelatinisation based on the chemical determination of released amylose or the physical binding of water are empirical and in no way serve to explain the molecular changes which take place during the cooking and storage of starch. Rather they describe some of the effects of these changes, and the results of measurements depend largely on the method selected.

In investigating optimum quality changes in the cooking of rice products a chemical method for measuring degree of gelatinisation has been developed and tested. It is also tentatively suggested that gelatinisation may indeed be a hydrogen bonding phenomenon as evidenced by a related change which can be observed in the infrared spectrum.

We are also concerned with the phenomenon of retrogradation in starch-based foods with particular reference to reconstituted, dehydrated yam flour. Retrogradation in the wider sense is a term used to describe the changes which occur in starch pastes or gels on ageing.[3] More precisely, it is a crystallisation process[4] during which a system moves towards a more thermodynamically stable condition. Such a process has a profound effect on the rheological characteristics of the system in which it occurs and it is in this context that it concerns the work reported here.

THE MEASUREMENT OF MOLECULAR CHANGES DURING THE GELATINISATION OF RICE

Rice grains contain a number of small starch granules ranging in diameter from 6 μ to 9 μ and which, on the bulk of modern evidence, are not considered to have a surrounding membrane. Probably the characteristic shape of the starch granule is maintained by some form of organisation at the surface of the granule, due to its chemical composition. As the rice is heated the granules swell and burst above gelatinisation temperature releasing amylose and amylopectin, the former giving a blue-coloured complex with iodine. Although it is clear from this description that blue-value methods for measuring degree of gelatinisation are in reality measuring disruption of the starch granule, the popularity of the method attests to its convenience as a technique. For this reason, and because the rate at which gelatinisation proceeds may affect the texture and eating quality of starch, it was decided to investigate a recently published method[5] for measuring degree of gelatinisation in Australian biscuits. This method consisted essentially of the determination of amylose–iodine blue value before and after the cooking process, the initial determination being done on a water extract of starch and the final determination on a dilute alkali (0·5N) extract. This technique was not suitable for use with rice because the released amylose was not quantitatively dissolved by water.

The method for determination of degree of gelatinisation which has been developed at this College is based on the amylose–iodine complex, but depends on the solubilisation of the gelatinised starch by 0·2N potassium hydroxide and all of the starch by 0·5N potassium

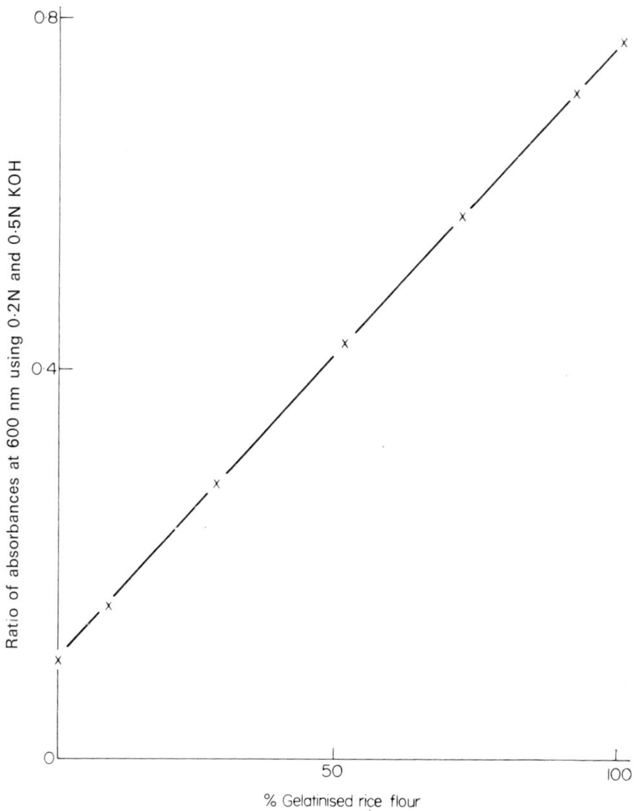

FIG. 1. Ratios of absorbances at 600 nm using 0·2N and 0·5N KOH against % gelatinisation of rice flour.

hydroxide. These conditions appear to be optimum for distinguishing between raw and gelatinised rice starch. The method was tested by preparing a range of standard mixtures of raw, water-washed rice starch (defined as ungelatinised) and rice starch autoclaved for 1 hr at 15 lb/in^2 (defined as 100% gelatinised). When these mixtures were separately dissolved in 0·2N potassium hydroxide solution and 0·5N potassium hydroxide solution and the iodine blue value of each solution was determined by colorimetry, the ratio of the two blue values for each mixture was found to be proportional to the defined degree of gelatinisation (Fig. 1). This method therefore gives a useful measure of a series of changes which we have previously defined as proceeding from an ungelatinised to a completely gelatinised state, but offers no explanation of the molecular events which are taking place.

This technique has also been extended to the indirect determination of gelatinisation temperature of milled rice and the results correlate well with those obtained from the well-known alkali test.

Kerr describes starch gelatinisation first as a process of hydrogen bond rupture within the starch granule, followed by a process of

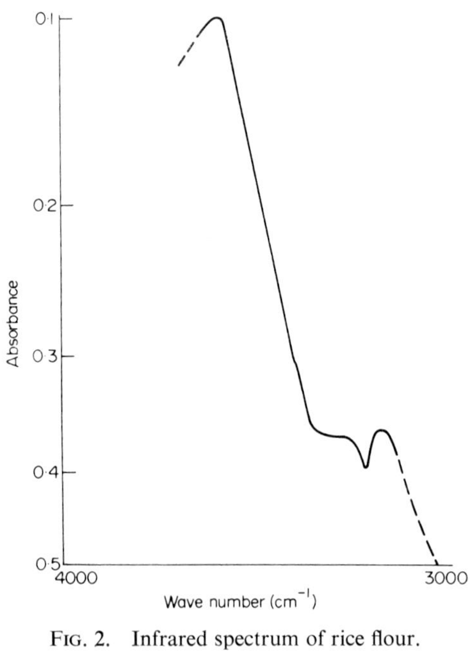

FIG. 2. Infrared spectrum of rice flour.

water penetration into the loosened disorganised structure. It is a consequence of this plausible explanation that on cooling gelatinised starch the total hydrogen bonding energy should become considerably greater than in the native starch granule. Indeed, increase in hydrogen bond energy may be the best means available for defining the process of gelatinisation. This hypothesis was tested by examining the infrared spectra of the same mixtures which were used for the

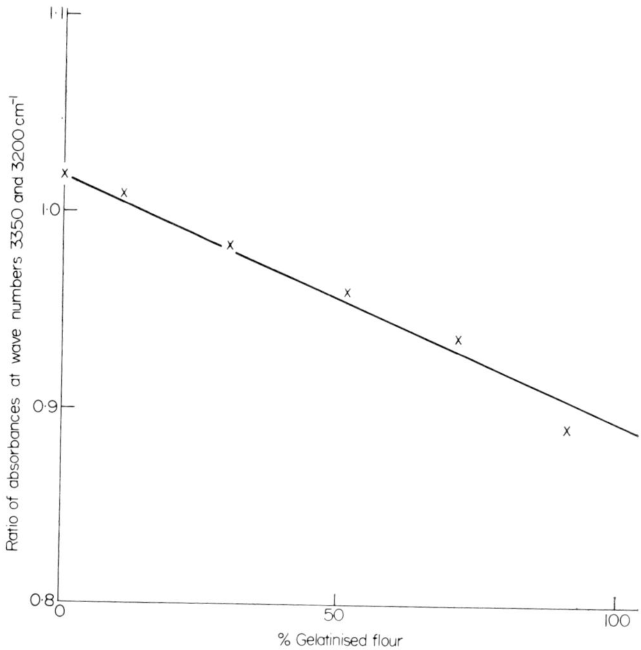

FIG. 3. Ratios of absorbances at wave numbers 3350 and 3200 cm^{-1} against % gelatinisation of flour.

chemical determination of the degree of gelatinisation with particular reference to the peaks at wave numbers of 3200 and 3350 cm^{-1} (Fig. 2) attributed by Shallenberger[6] and other workers[7,8] to free and hydrogen-bonded hydroxyl groups. Since both the gelatinised and ungelatinised starches used in our mixtures were dried to the same carbohydrate content, the ratio of the peak heights at 3200 and 3350 cm^{-1} should give a measure of increase in bonded hydroxyls and hence degree of gelatinisation. Plotting of this ratio against degree of gelatinisation gives a straight line as shown in Fig. 3 and this is interpreted as evidence in favour of the hydrogen-bonded character of gelatinised starch. This may prove to be a rapid and convenient method of following the gelatinisation process in cooking rice.

MOLECULAR CHANGES RESULTING IN CHANGES IN THE RHEOLOGICAL CHARACTERISTICS OF YAM DOUGH

Yam dough may be prepared from a flour obtained from the yam (*Discorea rotundata* (Poir L.)), which is an important tuber crop in the tropics and sub-tropics. It is a highly perishable material and the broad aim of this work is to study factors influencing the production of a dried yam product.

D. rotundata has the typical composition shown in Table 1, the amylose content being of the order of 20% (similar to that of potato, cassava and other root crop starches). Rasper and Coursey[9] have noted that the yam starches have less swelling capacity than potato or cassava starches but exhibit greater viscosities on gelling. These facts may be indicative of greater intermolecular forces in yam starches as compared with potato or cassava starches.

PEELING	—	tuber
↓ DICING	—	$\frac{1}{2} \times 1 \times 1$ in
WASHING	—	0·2% $Na_2S_2O_5$ water
PREHEATING	—	steam; atm. 10 min
COMMINUTION	—	slurry 15% solids
DEHYDRATION	—	drum—80 lb/in^2—dt 20–30 sec
FLAKES		
MILLING	—	hammermill
FLOUR	—	
SCREENING	—	BS 100 mesh
RECONSTITUTION	—	RT 2 min 30 g:50 ml water
↓ DOUGH		

FIG. 4. Processing of yam flour and dough.

TABLE 1

Approximate composition (%) of Yam tuber compared with potato and sweet potato

Tuber	Water	Carb.	Fat	Crd. prot.	Fibre	Ash
Yam D.r.	58–73	23	0·12	1·09–1·99	0·35–0·79	0·68–2·56
Potato	68–82	14–27	0·02–0·18	1·14–2·28	0·28–0·55	0·78–1·16
Sweet potato	58–81	17–43	0·18–0·68	0·45–4·37	0·60–4·54	0·66–1·98

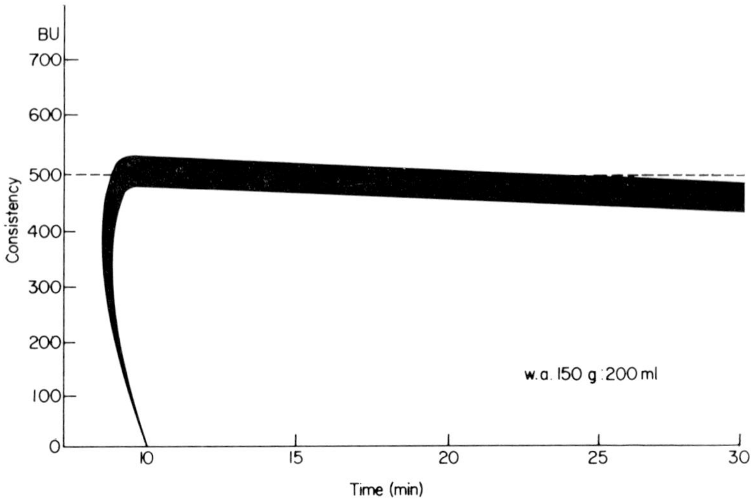

FIG. 5(*a*). Brabender Farinogram of pregelatinised yam flour.

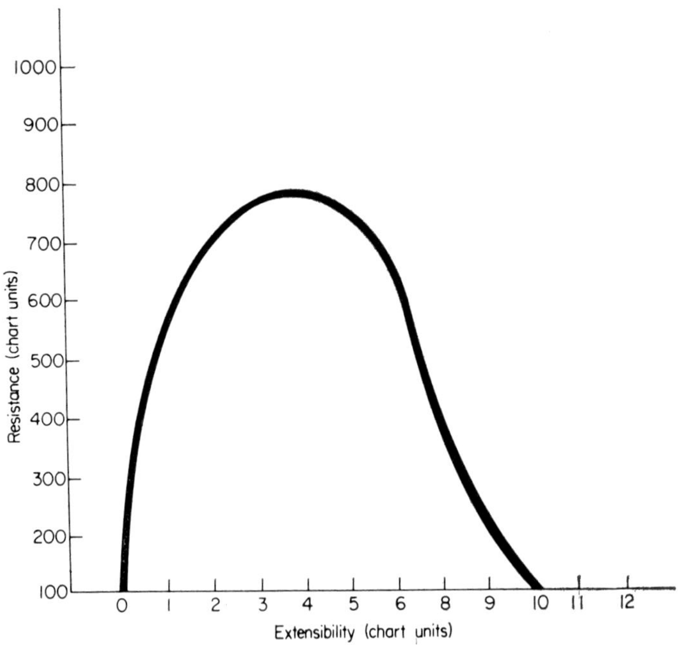

FIG. 5(*b*). Extensometry of yam dough.

The stages in the production of dried yam flour and its reconstitution into a dough are shown in Fig. 4, conditions being typical of those used. The dough characteristics during and immediately after reconstitution are illustrated by typical Brabender Farinograph (Fig. 5*a*) and Simon Extensometer (Fig. 5*b*) curves. The rheological characteristics of the dough were determined experimentally by compressing cylindrical samples using an Instron Universal Test

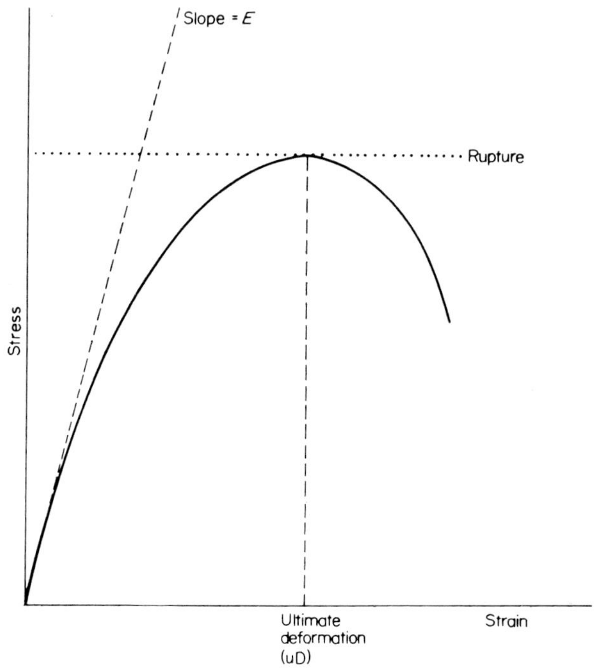

FIG. 6. Typical stress–strain curve of yam dough.

Instrument.[10] Typical stress–strain curves constructed from the results of such tests are shown in Fig. 6. From these curves, moduli of elasticity and 'ultimate deformations' were calculated.

As a result of the preheating, comminution, drum-drying and dry milling stages in the preparation of the flour, a considerable amount of damage was incurred by the starch granules. This was confirmed by blue-value measurements. A high degree of starch damage is desirable in order that the physical characteristics of the reconstituted dough resemble those of the traditional 'fufu' produced by cooking and pounding the fresh tubers.[11]

Early attempts to characterise the dough rheologically as a pre-requisite to studying the effects of processing variables revealed that these rheological characteristics changed markedly on standing after reconstitution. These changes in dough characteristics are the subject of this part of the paper.

Typical patterns of dough behaviour after reconstitution are shown in Figs. 7*a*, 7*b*. There is an initial lag phase after which the physical characteristics, quantified in terms of modulus of elasticity and 'ultimate deformation', change rapidly and the material loses its dough-like character, stiffens and hardens.

The most plausible explanation of these rheological changes is in terms of starch retrogradation. Ceh[12] has concluded that retrogradation results when starch hydroxyl–water bonds are replaced by intra- or intermicellar hydroxyl–hydroxyl hydrogen bonds. Hollo and

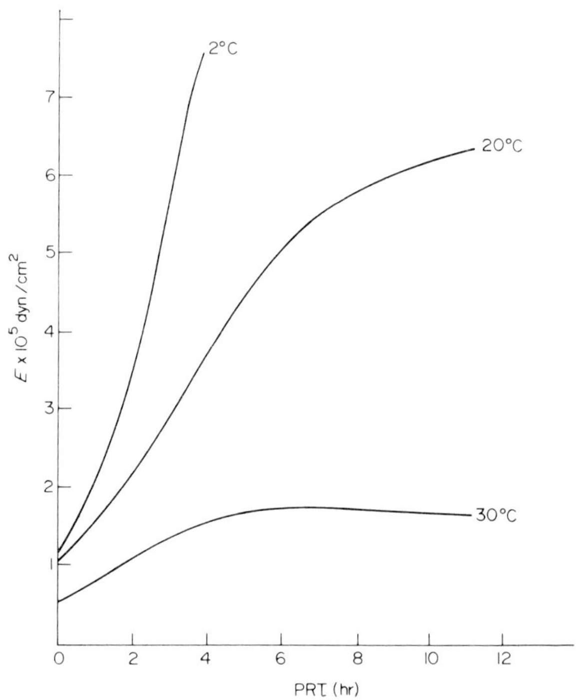

FIG. 7(*a*). Elasticity of yam dough *vs* time (after reconstitution).

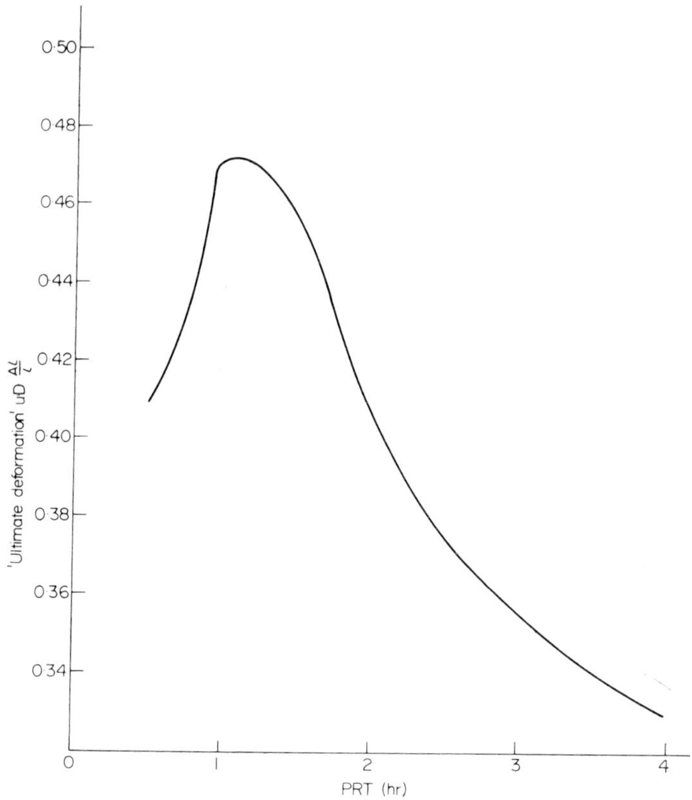

FIG. 7(*b*). Typical uD *vs*. PRT.

co-workers[13] conclude that retrogradation takes place in three stages:

(i) chain stretching due to the breaking of intermolecular bonds which maintain the helical configurations;

(ii) loss of bound water, followed by a suitable reorientation of the molecules;

(iii) hydrogen bond formation between adjacent molecules.

The first two stages of the above sequence are endothermic and the last exothermic.

The temperature changes in the centre of a ball of the dough placed in an environment of constant ambient temperature were recorded

(Fig. 8). These indicate that in the period immediately after reconstitution an endothermic reaction is occurring and that after about 1 hr this situation changes to one in which energy may be released.

When the results of the compression tests were presented in the form of an Avrami plot, as used by McIver *et al.*[14] for wheat starch gels, reasonably straight line patterns were obtained. The constants obtained from these plots indicate a high rate of crystallisation. The effects of ageing temperature on the physical characteristics of

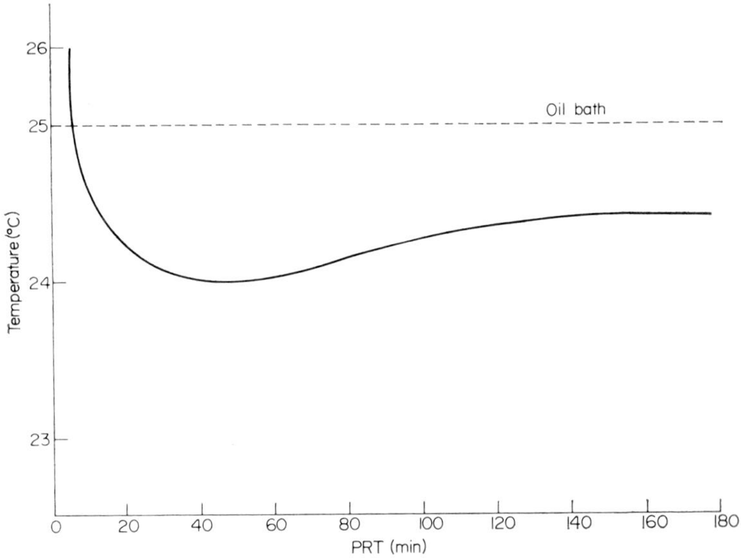

FIG. 8. Thermal change in dough.

the dough also follow those of wheat starch gels, the rate of change of dough characteristics increasing as the temperature is lowered (Fig. 7). The main difference in the behaviour of the yam dough and starch gel is in the rapidity with which the changes occur in the former. This may be accounted for by the high degree of processing to which the material has been subjected or it may be due to some particular characteristic of yam starch itself. The progressive increase in the ordered arrangement in the yam dough during ageing after reconstitution was confirmed by X-ray studies.

It would appear, therefore, that the physical changes in the yam dough which occur after reconstitution might be explained in terms of a change in the nature of the bonding, in particular an increase in water–starch and starch–starch hydrogen bonds, *i.e.* a form of retrogradation.

The importance of this phenomenon in the context of the wider objective of the work is that in order to specify the physical characteristics of the dough the time that has elapsed after constitution must also be specified. Work is in progress to study the factors influencing the rate of retrogradation.

CONCLUSIONS

The technological observations reported in this paper for two different foodstuffs have in common that they may be explained in terms of the known bonding properties of a common polymer, starch. Such a fundamental approach is an essential prior step to understanding the technological changes which may result from partial or total substitution of one starch foodstuff for another.

REFERENCES

1. Kerr, R. W. (1944). *Chemistry and Industry of Starch,* Academic Press, New York.
2. Rees, D. A. (1972). *Chem. and Ind.,* **16,** p. 630.
3. Collison, R. (1968). In *Starch and its Derivatives,* 4th Ed., Ed. by J. A. Radley, p. 194, Chapman and Hall, London.
4. Katz, J. R. (1930). *Z. Phys. Chem.,* A, **150,** p. 37.
5. Wooton, M., Weedon, D. and Munk, N. (1971). *Fd. Tech. Austral.,* **23,** p. 612.
6. Shallenberger, R. S. (1963). *J. Fd. Sci.,* **28,** p. 584.
7. Barker, S. A., Brimacombe, J. S., Foster, A. B., Whiffen, D. H. and Zweifel, G. (1959). *Tetrahedron,* **7,** p. 10.
8. Brimacombe, J. S., Foster, A. B., Stacey, M. and Whiffen, D. H. (1958). *Tetrahedron,* **4,** p. 351.
9. Rasper, V. and Coursey, D. G. (1967). *J. Sci. Fd. Agric.,* **18,** p. 240.
10. Brennan, J. G., Jowitt, R. and Mughsi, O. A. (1970). *J. Texture Studies,* **1,** p. 167.
11. Sodah-Ayernor, G. (1970). Unpublished report (No. 1) on 'The Utilization of the Yam as a Food in West Africa', National College of Food Technology.
12. Ceh, Von M. (1958). *Die Starke,* **10,** p. 103.
13. Hollo, J., Szektli, J. and Gantner, G. S. (1960). *Die Starke,* **12,** p. 106.
14. McIver, R. G., Axford, D. W. E., Colwell, K. H. and Elton, G. A. H. (1968). *J. Sci. Fd. Agric.,* **19,** p. 560.

13

The Starch $\rightleftharpoons$ Sugar Transformation in Potato Tubers During Drying and Cooling

G. LISINSKA

Department of Food Technology and Storage of the Agricultural University in Wroclaw, Poland

ABSTRACT

The changes in total dry matter, starch, saccharose and reducing sugar which occur during the drying and cooling of potato tubers are presented under different conditions of sub-division and through the agency of different drying gases. Changes of either temperature or gas will alter the extent of carbohydrate transformation by several hundred per cent, and certain selected conditions will reduce the extent of the transformation to a negligible level.

The potato is of great importance in a number of countries for feeding people or cattle. It is also used as a raw material in the distillation industries, and for starch and dehydrated potato manufacture. The growing requirements for its industrial use have resulted in continual and comprehensive study of its properties and biochemical transformations in tubers. One of the more important biochemical processes which occurs in potato tubers is the transformation of carbohydrate compounds. In a tuber, being in a state of repose, the process of starch $\rightleftharpoons$ sugar transformation is slow. Its intensity increases either with germination or under the influence of such factors as: cold storage,[1] drying,[1-13] mechanical damage[3] and ionising radiation.[10]

The aim of the work reported here was to study the effect of such factors as cold storage and drying on the content of carbohydrate compounds in potato tubers. Moreover, the optimum conditions for the various carbohydrate transformations in potato tubers according to the drying temperatures, the kind of gas and the degree of tuber crushing have been investigated.

EXPERIMENTAL DETAILS

Potatoes of the variety 'Lenino' were used for experiments. The tubers were cut into slices 3–4 mm thick and then they were dried or cooled in an atmosphere of air, oxygen, nitrogen and carbon dioxide. The slices were dried at the temperatures: 20°, 40°, 60°, 80°C, and cooled at +1·5°C. Moreover, tubers having different crushing as pulp or slices, 1–2 mm and 3–4 mm thick, were dried in air at a temperature of 20°C. As well as crushing, the tubers were cut into quarters and cooled in the same gases at a temperature of +1·5°C.

In the fresh, dried and cooled potato tubers the contents of dry matter, starch, reducing sugars and saccharose were determined.

RESULTS AND DISCUSSION

Figure 1 presents the decrease or increase of starch content in potatoes dried in an atmosphere of oxygen, air, nitrogen or carbon dioxide at 20°, 40°, 60° and 80°C, expressed in percent in relation to the starch content in fresh material.

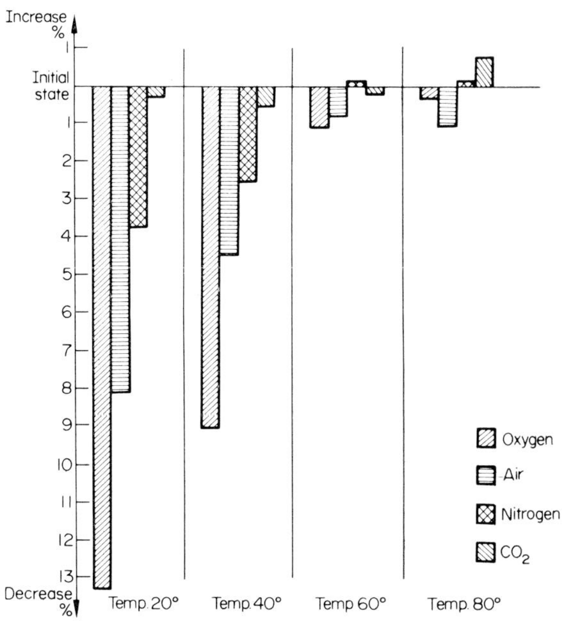

FIG. 1. Changes in the content of starch in potatoes dried under various conditions, expressed in % in relation to the starch content in fresh material.

The greatest decrease of starch amounting to 13·56%—in relation to the initial state taken as 100%—was achieved when drying the potato slices in an atmosphere of oxygen at 20°C. The decrease of starch content in potatoes dried at the same temperature in air was 8·17%, and in nitrogen it was 3·71%. Compared with fresh potato tubers, the slices dried in carbon dioxide did not show any important changes in starch content.

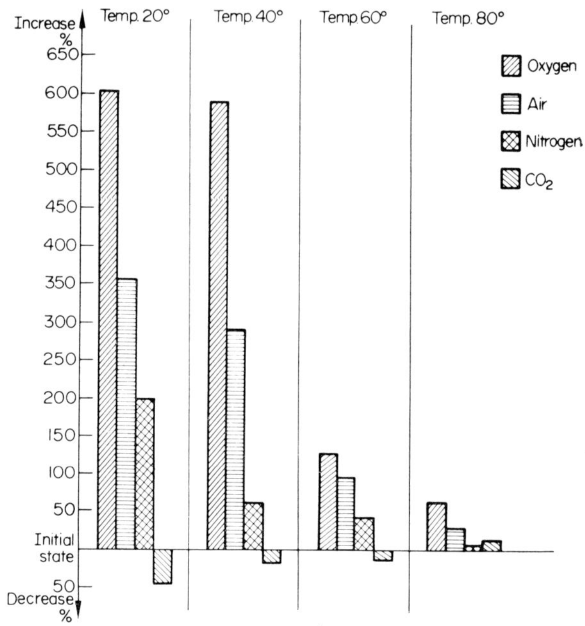

FIG. 2. Changes in the content of saccharose in potatoes dried under various conditions, expressed in % in relation to the saccharose content in fresh material.

At temperatures of 60° and 80°C the changes of starch content in potatoes dried in the above-mentioned gases are not large, compared with the content of fresh potato tubers.

In these conditions the inactivation of enzymes decomposing the starch is likely to have occurred, and a slight decrease in content of polysaccharide should result from the action of enzymes in the initial phase of drying when the temperature is rising to the fixed level.

Figure 2 presents the changes in the content of saccharose in potatoes dried under various conditions. The largest increase was found when drying at 20° and 40°C in oxygen. The content of saccharose in these potatoes was about 600% larger than it was in the initial state. In potato tubers dried in air at 20°C the increase of saccharose content was about 350%, and about 280% at a temperature of 40°C. When dried in nitrogen it was only 200%. Carbon dioxide completely stopped the formation of saccharose during potato drying, and compared with the content of saccharose in fresh tubers, it even decreased its content slightly.

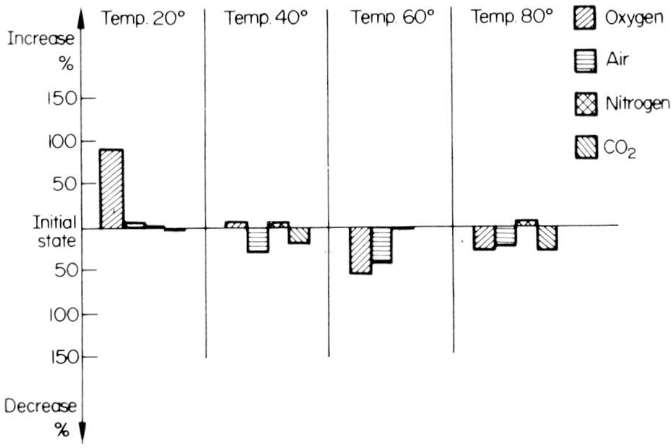

FIG. 3. Changes in the content of reducing sugars in potatoes dried under various conditions, expression in % in relation to the contents of these sugars in fresh material.

At the drying temperatures of 60° and 80°C the changes of saccharose content in potato slices were slight.

Figure 3 shows some changes in the content of reducing sugars in potatoes dried in various gases and at different temperatures. It can be seen that the changes were slight as compared with the initial state.

Some changes in the content of carbohydrate compounds in potatoes kept for 7 days at a temperature of +1·5°C in oxygen, air, nitrogen and carbon dioxide are shown in Fig. 4.

Compared with fresh potatoes, the decreases of starch in tubers kept at a temperature of + 1·5°C in oxygen, air and nitrogen were respectively about 9%, 8% and 5%. The content of starch in tubers did not, however, change whilst kept in carbon dioxide.

In tubers cooled in oxygen and air the content of reducing sugars underwent a big change—it increased 100% and 126% respectively. A large increase of reducing sugars was also noted in tubers cooled

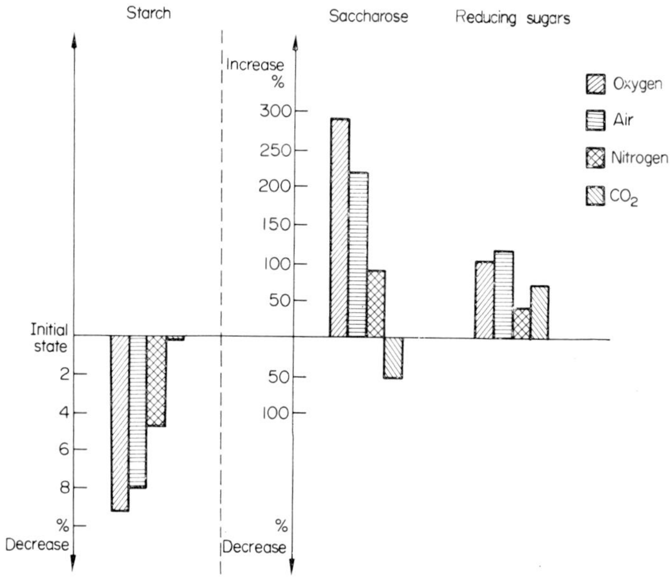

FIG. 4. Changes in the content of starch, saccharose and reducing sugars in potatoes during cold storage under various conditions, expressed in % in relation to the contents of these compounds in fresh material.

in carbon dioxide, amounting to 70% of their initial content. In all probability, these sugars originated at the expense of saccharose as the content of the latter, in relation to its content in fresh tubers, decreased 60%. The content of saccharose increased in those tubers which were cooled in gases other than carbon dioxide—about 280% in oxygen, 225% in air, and least in nitrogen (only 80%).

Figure 5 shows the changing content of starch, saccharose and reducing sugars in potato tubers in the form of pulp, and thin and thick slices, dried in air at 20°C. As shown in the figure, the content of several carbohydrate compounds in dried potato pulp is the same as in fresh tubers, whereas in dried potato slices a large decrease of starch content and increase of saccharose content, compared with their contents in fresh potatoes, can be seen. At the same time, these changes are larger in slices 3–4 mm thick than in slices 1–2 mm thick.

Figure 6 shows the changes in the content of carbohydrate compounds in potato pulp, in thin and thick tubers and in quarters of tubers cooled at +1·5°C, as compared with their content in fresh

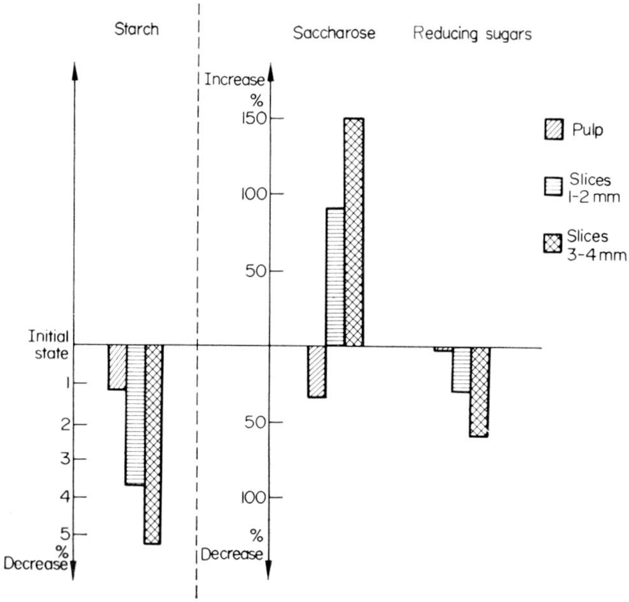

FIG. 5. Changes in the content of starch, saccharose and reducing sugars in pulp and potato slices dried at 20°C in air, expressed in % in relation to the contents of these compounds in fresh material.

tubers. As shown in the figure, the content of starch, saccharose and reducing sugars in these potatoes depends on the degree of potato crushing. The greater the crushing of tubers the smaller the changes in the contents of the above-mentioned compounds, as compared with the normal chemical composition of fresh potatoes.

CONCLUSIONS

The results of this investigation of the changes of carbohydrate components in potato tubers dried or cooled under various conditions suggest that:

1. Drying of the tubers in an atmosphere of oxygen, as well as cooling them in the same atmosphere, creates the best conditions for carbohydrate transformations. On the other hand, nitrogen, as a potato drying gas, decreases the process of starch decomposition and sugar accumulation in tubers more than oxygen, while carbon dioxide stops the process completely.

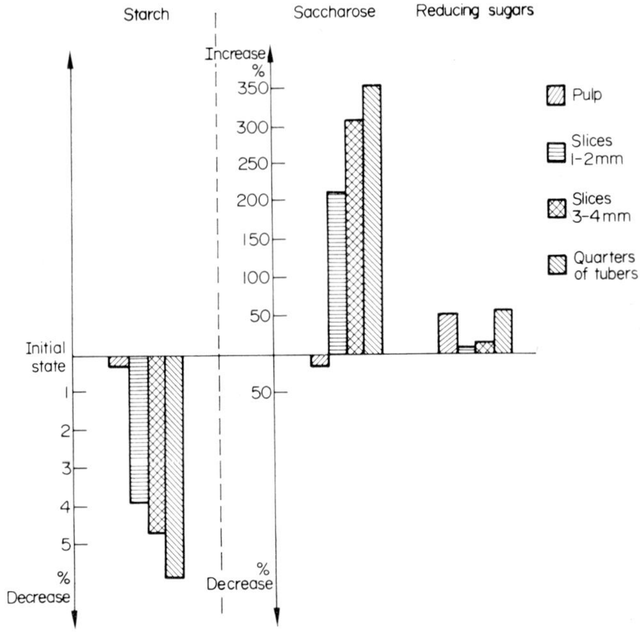

FIG. 6. Changes in the content of starch, saccharose and reducing sugars in pulp, slices and quarters of potato tubers during cold storage in air, expressed in % in relation to the contents of these compounds in fresh material.

2. Increase of drying temperature above 40°, 60° and 80°C inhibits carbohydrate transformations in dried tubers, independently of the type of drying gas used.
3. In cooled potatoes, carbon dioxide stops the process of starch decomposition. It does not, however, inhibit the decomposition of saccharose into monosaccharides.
4. In potato tubers dried at 20°C or cooled in air, the transformation of starch into sugars increases as the degree of tuber crushing decreases.

REFERENCES

1. Burton, W. G. (1965). *Eur. Potato J.*, **8,** p. 2.
2. Craft, C. C., (1956). *American Potato J.*, **33,** p. 259.
3. Hopkins, E. F. (1927). *Botanical Gazette,* **84,** p. 75.
4. Kamienobrodzki, W. and Lisinska, G. (1967). *Scientific Papers of the Agricultural University in Wroclaw,* XXI, **66,** p. 83.

5. Kamienobrodzki, W. and Lisinska, G. (1968). *Scientific Papers of the Agricultural University in Wroclaw,* XXV, **77,** p. 45.
6. Kamienobrodzki, W. and Lisinska, G. (1968). *Scientific Papers of the Agricultural University in Wroclaw,* XXV, **77,** p. 53.
7. Lisinska, G. (1971). *Ann. Food Techn. and Chem.* **XXI,** p. 101.
8. Müller-Thurgau, H. (1882). *Landw. Jahrb.,* **11,** p. 751.
9. Nowotny, F. and Samotus, B. (1965). *Die Stärke,* **17**(10), p. 313.
10. Nowotny, F., editor. (1969). *Starch,* Warsaw.
11. Prokoszew, S. M. (1947). *Biochimija kartofiela,* Moscow–Leningrad.
12. Samotus, B. and Schwimmer, S. (1963). *J. Food Sci.,* **28**(2), p. 163.
13. Wolff, C. J. (1926). *Biochemische Zeitschrift,* **176,** p. 22.

N.B. Due to difficulties with the language, discussion did not take place.

14

The Structural Basis of Carbohydrate Digestion and Absorption

J. E. G. BARNETT

Department of Physiology and Biochemistry, University of Southampton, Southampton, England

ABSTRACT

The utilisation of the carbohydrate part of the diet is governed by three main factors; its breakdown by digestive enzymes in the intestinal tract, the transport of monosaccharides across the mucosal membrane of the small intestine and finally intracellular phosphorylation allowing entry into the metabolic processes. Only carbohydrates which have structures compatible with the structural requirements of each of these systems will be of nutritional value. It is important, therefore, to understand the scientific basis for this structural specificity.

After a brief review of the specificity and location of the human digestive enzymes, the specificity of intestinal absorption is discussed. Two major transport systems can be distinguished—a sodium ion-dependent active transport system for glucose and galactose, and a separate system for fructose.

The structural requirements of the active transport system are defined and explained in terms of hydrogen bonds and a covalent bond at C-2 between sugar and carrier. Glucose and galactose, actively concentrated in the mucosal epithelial cells, enter the blood and lymph systems directly by diffusion, but fructose is partially phosphorylated in the intestinal tissue and metabolised to glucose and lactate. The rapid metabolism of fructose maintains the 'downhill' gradient of the free sugar into the epithelial cells, ensuring rapid absorption.

The utilisation of the carbohydrate part of the human diet is governed by three main factors: its breakdown by digestive enzymes in the intestinal tract, the transport of monosaccharides across the mucosal membrane of the small intestine and finally intracellular phosphorylation allowing entry into the metabolic processes. A further factor is present in some mammals, namely the ruminants (cows, sheep, etc.), and other herbivores (*e.g.* rabbits), where digestion of carbohydrate by symbiotic bacteria in the ruminant stomach, or in the caecum, plays a dominant role, allowing, in particular, the digestion of celluloses. In contrast, the influence of the normal human intestinal flora on digestion may be disregarded. Only carbohydrates which have structures compatible with the structural requirements of digestion, absorption and metabolism will be of nutritional value. It is important, therefore, to understand the scientific basis of this structural specificity.

HUMAN CARBOHYDRATE DIGESTIVE ENZYMES

In relation to the wide variety of carbohydrate polymers found in nature, and in contrast to some other animals, notably some molluscs such as the snail *Helix pomatia*, the ability of the human digestive system to hydrolyse polysaccharides is extremely limited. Polysaccharide activity is mainly limited to one enzyme, the α-amylase secreted from the salivary glands or pancreas into the mouth or duodenum respectively. The enzymes from both sources have been crystallised, and their properties appear to be identical.[1,2] Their specificity is absolute for the α(1 → 4) linkage between glucopyranosyl residues, which are cleaved randomly, although not close to α(1 → 6) linkages on amylopectin or glycogen. Oligosaccharides are only very poor substrates, so that maltotetraose is only slowly attacked. Maltotriose and maltose do not appear to be substrates, although α-D-glucopyranosyl fluoride, first shown to replace maltose as a general substrate for α-glucosidases and glucoamylase,[3,4] has recently been shown to be a substrate for human salivary amylase.[5]

The remaining human digestive enzymes are found in the mucosal lining of the small intestine, where they are an integral part of the brush-border of the epithelial cells responsible for the active absorption of monosaccharides. There is a multiplicity of these enzymes, all basically oligosaccharidases, but the range of activities that they display is fairly limited. The enzymes, which are particulate, but which can be distinguished by selective heat denaturation,[6] or solubilised and separated by the action of proteolytic enzymes followed by Sephadex chromatography,[7] may be classified either

TABLE 1

Classification of the oligosaccharidases of the human intestine

Classification			Relative rates of hydrolysis of specified sugars					
As glycoside	Zurich[a]	By sugar hydrolysed (trivial) name[b]	Amylose	Maltose	Sucrose	Isomaltose	Maltotriose	Trehalose
α-Glucosidase 1 α-Glucosidase 2	Maltase 1 Maltase 2	Maltase 1 Maltase 2	40	40	0	Trace	24	0
α-Glucosidase 3	Maltase 3	Sucrase 1	0	10	20	—	—	—
α-Glucosidase 4	Maltase 4	Sucrase 2	0	50	80	—	28	—
α-Glucosidase 5	Maltase 5	Isomaltase	0		—	100[c]	48	—
α-Glucosidase 6	Trehalase	Trehalase	0	0	0	0	0	100
			Lactose	Cellobiose				
β-Galactosidase 1	Lactase 1	Lactase 1	100[c]	20				
β-Galactosidase 2	Lactase 2	Lactase 2	100[c]	50				

[a] Zurich classification.

[b] Lund classification.[6]

[c] Arbitrarily set at 100.

by their specificity for the glycosyl residue hydrolysed, as is usual for glycosidases, or by their ability to hydrolyse sugars commonly found in the diet. Both classifications are complicated and unsatisfactory, because of the marked specificity for the aglycone which is not indicated by the former classification, and the considerable overlap of activities not indicated by the latter (*see* Table 1). Classified as glycosidases, there appear to be 5 α-glucopyranosidases and a β-galactosidase. There is a second, soluble β-galactosidase which is probably lysosomal in origin, and a brush-border β-glucosidase which hydrolyses phloretin β-glucopyranoside (phlorizin), but not cellobiose.[8] The same enzymes contain maltase, sucrase, isomaltase, trehalase, amylase, lactase and cellobiase activities (Table 1). Hydrolase activities are not confined to those listed in Table 1. For instance, α-glucosidase 5 (maltase 5, isomaltase) hydrolyses, in addition to maltose (4-*O*-α-D-glucopyranosyl-D-glucose) and isomaltose (6-*O*-α-D-glucopyranosyl-D-glucose), maltitol, panose (*O*-α-D-glucopyranosyl (1 → 6)-*O*-α-glucopyranosyl (1 → 4)-D-glucose), palatinose (6-*O*-α-glucopyranosyl-D-fructose) and other dextrins produced by the action of α-amylase on glycogen or amylopectin.

There are minor species differences, but generally the same pattern of activities is found in other mammals. Some human genetic variants occur which lack one or more of the enzymes; while low adult β-galactosidase activities could be regarded as 'normal' because high levels of this enzyme predominated only in Northern European and Puerto Rican stocks out of several tested, including oriental (all deficient) and negro.[9] These genetic disorders are discussed in the next paper.

INTESTINAL ABSORPTION

Figure 1 shows a diagrammatic representation of a section of small intestine.[10] Sugars and other foods are absorbed by the epithelial cells which are formed in the crypts and move towards the tips of the villi where they are shed. The process takes about 3–6 days in man and active absorption is highest at the tips of the villi. Actively absorbed molecules diffuse from the epithelial cells (Fig. 2) into the blood and lymphatic systems.

Mammalian intestine does not absorb sugar phosphates, oligo- or polysaccharides, except perhaps in traces. The oligosaccharidases and alkaline phosphatase of the epithelial cell brush-border release monosaccharides, and it is these that are transported. Several workers have shown that the enzymes are not only physically part of the brush-border, using cell-fractionation methods[11] or fluorescent antibody techniques,[12] but they are so closely associated with the

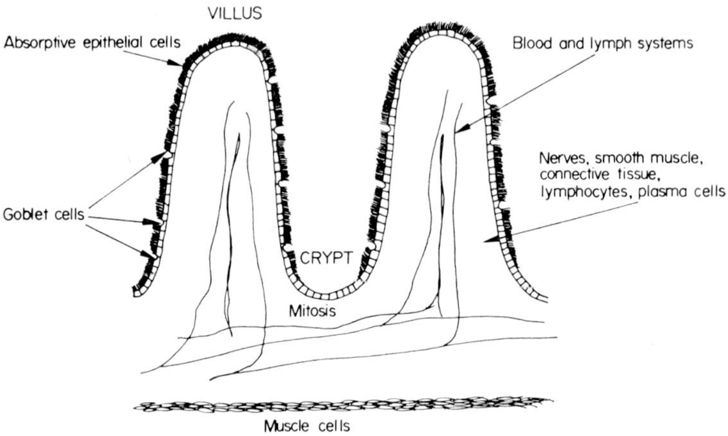

FIG. 1. Cross section of the small intestine.

transport sites that the monosaccharides released are immediately transported. Thus Miller and Crane[13] have shown that the glucose units of sucrose or maltose accumulate inside the epithelial cells even if a large excess of glucose oxidase is added to the outer, mucosal

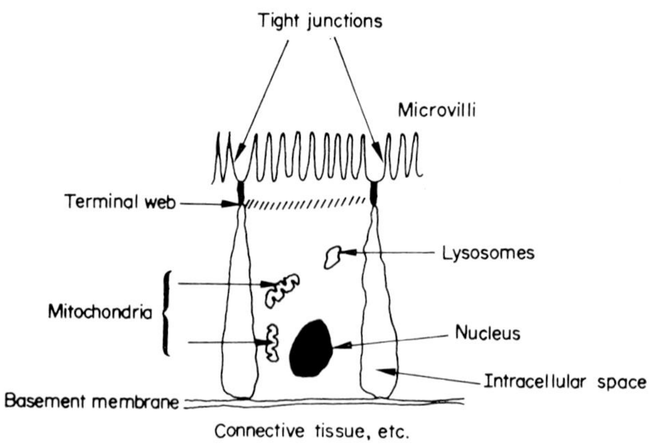

FIG. 2. Typical intestinal epithelial cell.

solution. However, by using the transport inhibitor, phlorizin, they proved that the release was outside the transport system. The extracellular location was confirmed in a different way by Barnett *et al.*[3]

Monosaccharides are absorbed in the mammalian small intestine by two independent transport systems, an active, sodium-dependent system which actively accumulates glucose and galactose, and a second, facilitated system for fructose. The distinction between the systems is nicely shown by a human genetic defect[14] in which the glucose/galactose system is entirely absent. Patients with the disease have a perfectly normal, or enhanced, absorption of fructose.

Although fructose entry in most mammals may not be active, fructose is rapidly removed from the intestine, either by metabolism or by diffusion into the blood and lymph systems. Particularly *in vitro,* a high rate of conversion into lactate and glucose is observed.[15,16] The rate at which this occurs is species-dependent, and is high in the hamster and guinea-pig, but low in the rat and man.[16–18] This high rate of metabolism makes it very difficult to study the transport process in isolation, and for this reason almost nothing is known about its specificity. Such evidence as exists suggests that it is high.

Recently Gracey *et al.*[19] have shown that the fructose accumulation in rat intestine is both sodium-dependent and active, and these findings warrant re-investigation of earlier work in other species.

SPECIFICITY OF THE SODIUM-DEPENDENT GLUCOSE/GALACTOSE TRANSPORT SYSTEM

The main transport system for monosaccharides is the sodium-dependent active transport system which transports glucose, galactose and many other monosaccharides. The specificity requirements of this system are well known. In three papers, Barnett *et al.*[20–22] have described the transport of a series of D-glucose or D-galactose analogues which differ from the parent sugars by substitution for a particular hydroxyl group of either the hydrogen or fluorine atoms, or other atoms or groups of known size and binding properties. They considered that two major factors would influence the binding of sugar to the carrier. These were the positive binding, either covalent or hydrogen bonding between specific hydroxyl groups of the sugar and the carrier protein, and the possibility of steric hindrance caused by substituting a large atom or group into the D-glucose structure.

If a hydrogen bond normally occurs between any particular hydroxyl group and the carrier (Fig. 3*a* or *b*), replacement of the hydroxyl

```
                     H
                     |
(a) Sugar————O- - - -H————X————Protein
(b) Sugar————O————H- - - -X————Protein
(c) Sugar————H    H————X————Protein
(d) Sugar————F- - - -H————X————Protein
```

FIG. 3. Possibilities for hydrogen bonds between substituted or parent sugar and the carrier protein.

group by the smaller hydrogen atom, either as the deoxy sugar or by inversion to the epimer, would abolish the bond (Fig. 3*c*) and lead to a reduction in affinity for the carrier. Replacement of the hydroxyl group by the fluorine atom, also smaller, which can form hydrogen bonds in a similar way to oxygen (Fig. 3*d*), will be expected to restore the affinity if the original bond is of the type shown in Fig. 3*a*, but not if the original bond required the hydrogen of the hydroxyl group for binding (Fig. 3*b*). A covalent bond (such as an ester) would be formed only by this hydroxyl group.

Direct measurement of transport is not necessarily a good method of measuring affinity for the carrier, so in addition to a simple test for transport, the Michaelis constant (K_m) for the analogue and its competitive inhibition constant for transport of another sugar (K_i) were measured for each of the sugars transported. K_m was originally conceived as the dissociation constant (K_s or k_{-1}/k_{+1}) of an enzyme–substrate, or in this case carrier–sugar, complex (Fig. 4).

$$S_{out} + C_{out} \underset{k_{-1}}{\overset{k_{+1}}{\rightleftharpoons}} SC_{out} \underset{k_{-2}}{\overset{k_{+2}}{\rightleftharpoons}} SC_{in} \underset{k_{-3}}{\overset{k_{+3}}{\rightleftharpoons}} C_{in} + S_{in}$$

FIG. 4. Sugar–carrier transport process.

However, it has a component due to the rate of transport, and for the simplified system shown, $K_m = (k_{-1} + k_{+2})/k_{+1}$. For this reason K_i, the dissociation constant of the sugar–carrier complex when the analogue was used as the inhibitor of transport of another sugar, was considered to be a better measure of binding, although if the competing sugar is transported, K_i itself is not a true dissociation constant. The values obtained for this constant should not be regarded as absolute for such a complex process, and care was taken to measure inhibition of the same sugar under identical conditions wherever possible, so that the measurement of affinity would be accurate in a relative sense.

All sugars were first tested for accumulation into everted hamster intestinal tissue rings over 30 min at 37°C. The tissue water/medium concentration ratios (t/m ratios) were then measured. For weakly transported sugars this was measured in the presence and absence of sodium ions, previously shown[24] to be obligatory for active transport. Any sodium ion-stimulated transport was considered to

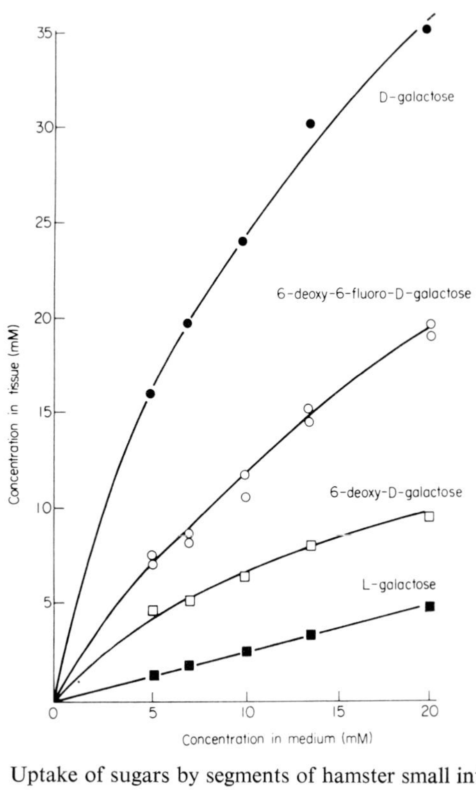

FIG. 5. Uptake of sugars by segments of hamster small intestine.

be due to the glucose/galactose carrier. For some sugars K_m was measured. Sugars which were actively transported were then tested as competitive inhibitors of one of two transported sugars, methyl α-D-glucopyranoside or D-galactose, neither of which are metabolised by the intestine.

Figure 5 shows the rate of transport as a function of concentration for several D-galactose analogues modified at C-6. The saturation at high concentrations can clearly be seen. Substitution of the hydroxyl group at C-6 by the hydrogen atom leads to a marked diminution in transport; replacement of the hydrogen atom by the fluorine atom partially restores it.

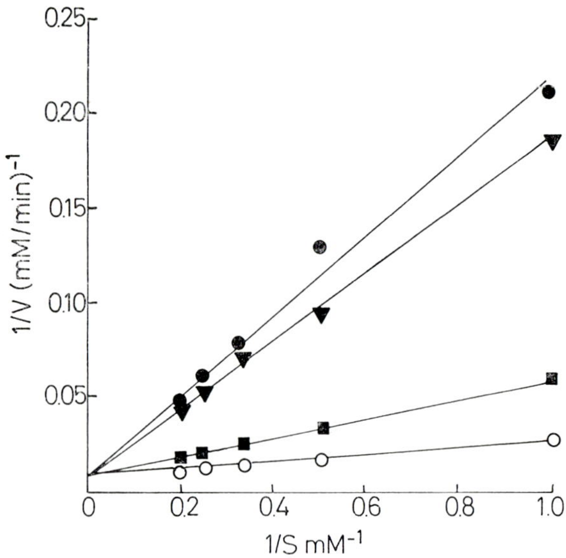

FIG. 6. Lineweaver–Burk plot showing competitive inhibition of D-galactose accumulation by 3-substituted D-glucoses. ○: No addition; ■: 20 mM-3-deoxy-D-glucose; ▼: 17·5 mM-3-deoxy-3-fluoro-D-glucose; ●: 20 mM-D-glucose.

Figure 6 shows a Lineweaver–Burk plot for the inhibition of D-galactose transport by D-glucose analogues modified at C-3. Substitution by the hydrogen atom (3-deoxy-glucose) markedly reduces the competitive inhibition, but substitution by the fluorine atom gives a sugar with the same affinity as D-glucose.

Both at C-6 and at C-3, there appears to be a hydrogen bond between the hydroxyl group and the carrier protein.

Table 2 shows the *t/m* ratios and inhibition constants (K_i) for some selected D-glucose and D-galactose analogues modified at C-1, C-2, C-3, C-4, C-5 and C-6. It can be seen that replacement of the hydroxyl groups at C-1, C-2, C-3, C-4 or C-6 leads to a reduced affinity for the carrier. Substitution of the C-5 (ring) oxygen by sulphur which cannot hydrogen bond does not alter the affinity, but substitution of the C-1 oxygen of methyl β-D-galactopyranoside to

TABLE 2

Tissue water/medium concentration ratios and K_m *values for selected analogues of* D-*glucose and* D-*galactose*

t/m ratios were measured after incubating the sugar (1 mM) with everted hamster intestinal tissue rings. Inhibition constants were measured by finding the apparent K_m of galactose using the concentration range 1–10 mM in the presence and absence of 20 mM sugar

Alteration to D-glucose	Sugar	Tissue/medium ratio (initial conc. 1 mM)	K_i (mM)
	D-glucose	16·4	2·3
C-2	2-deoxy-D-glucose	0·17[a]	
C-2	2-deoxy-2-fluoro-D-glucose	0·3[a]	
C-2	D-mannose	0·18[a]	
C-3	3-deoxy-D-glucose	2·1	24
C-3	3-deoxy-3-fluoro-D-glucose	26·6	2·5
C-3	D-allose	1·7	40
C-3, C-6	3,6-dideoxy-D-glucose	0·5	—
C-3, C-4	3-deoxy-D-galactose	1·0	—
C-4	D-galactose	8·3	2·5[b]
C-5	5-thio-D-glucose	12·5	2·9
(C-1)[c] C-4	methyl α-D-galactopyranoside	10·0	—
(C-1)[c] C-4	methyl β-D-galactopyranoside	5·6	—
C-1, C-4	methyl β-D-thiogalactopyranoside	0·5	—
C-1, C-4	1-deoxy-D-galactose	0·4	—
C-1, C-4	α-D-galactopyranosyl fluoride	1·2	—
C-4, C-6	6-deoxy-D-galactose	1·45	16[b]
C-4, C-6	6-deoxy-6-fluoro-D-galactose	4·3	7[b]

[a] Unchanged if sodium ion omitted (cf. D-galactose, 0·39).

[b] K_i for methyl α-D-glucopyranoside transport.

[c] The oxygen of the methoxyl group can still hydrogen bond.

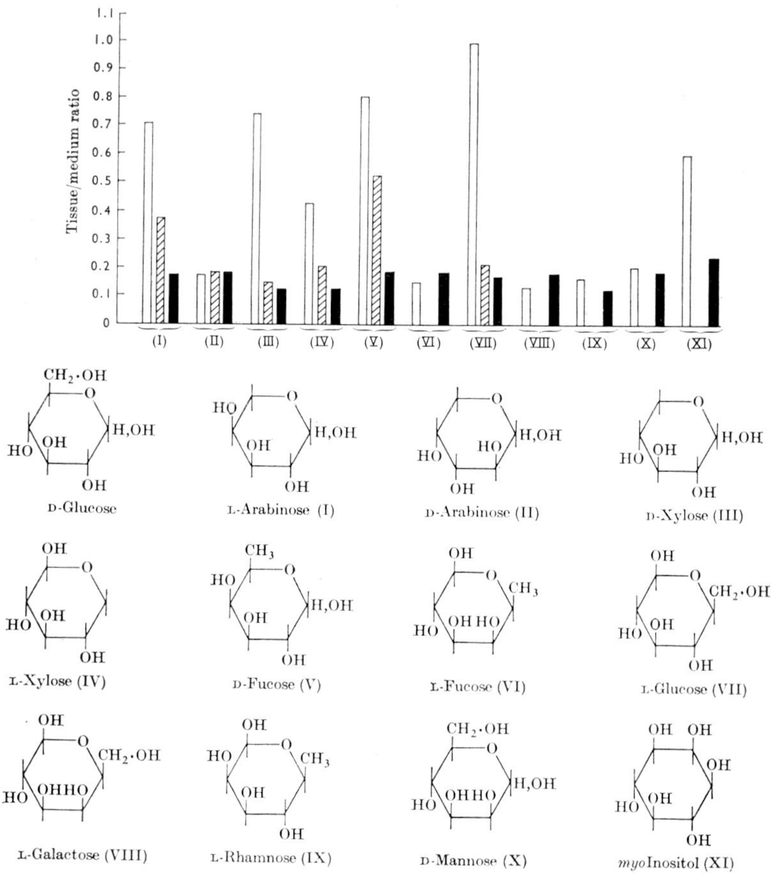

FIG. 7. Comparison of the structures of weakly transported sugars with their accumulation into hamster intestinal slices under various conditions. The sugars (initial concentration 1mM) were incubated for 1 hr in the presence of Na^+ (145 mequiv.) (□), in the presence of Na^+ and 1,5-anhydro-D-glucitol (▨) and in the absence of Na^+ (■). Sugars are drawn so that the oxygen falls in the position usually occupied by the oxygen in D-glucose, so that the hydroxymethyl group falls either at the position normally occupied by C-6 of D-glucose or in the aglycone position of a β-D-glucopyranoside. If the reducing group is in the position occupied by C-1 of D-glucose, no preference is indicated for the α- or β-anomers, but if the reducing group falls at the position occupied by C-5 of D-glucose the β-anomer is drawn since this occupies the C-6 position of D-glucose. (Reproduced by courtesy of *Biochemical Journal*.)

give methyl β-D-thiogalactopyranoside does. It must be concluded that each hydroxyl group of D-glucose, with the exception of that involved in ring formation at C-5, contributes to the carrier–sugar binding. Furthermore, replacement of the hydrogen atom by the fluorine atom restores the affinity either partially (C-1, C-6) or completely (C-3) at every position tested but C-2. For C-1, C-3 and C-6, a hydrogen bond using a hydrogen from the carrier to the oxygen of the hydroxyl group can be envisaged (Fig. 3*a*). Because 4-deoxy-4-fluoro-D-glucose has not been tested, the direction of the hydrogen bond at C-4 is unknown.

The complete lack of transport caused by modification at C-2 is unique. It might be due to the loss of a hydrogen bond of the type *b,* Fig. 3, where the hydroxyl group donates the hydrogen atom, or to covalent bonding of the hydroxyl group. Comparison with the data for other weakly transported sugars favours the latter.

By inspection of the data in Table 2, Fig. 7, and the original papers, it can be shown that one deviation from the D-glucose structure as in allose or galactose, does not lead to abolition of active transport. Similarly both 1-deoxy-glucose and 6-deoxy-glucose are actively transported.[23] Two deviations from the D-glucose structure: 1-deoxy-galactose, 1,3-dideoxy-D-glucose (Table 2), L-arabinose (Fig. 7), 1,6-dideoxy-glucose,[23] give a sugar which is not always actively transported, but is stimulated by sodium ions. In contrast, any modification at C-2 of D-glucose leads to complete loss of sodium-dependent transport, suggesting that the bond at this position

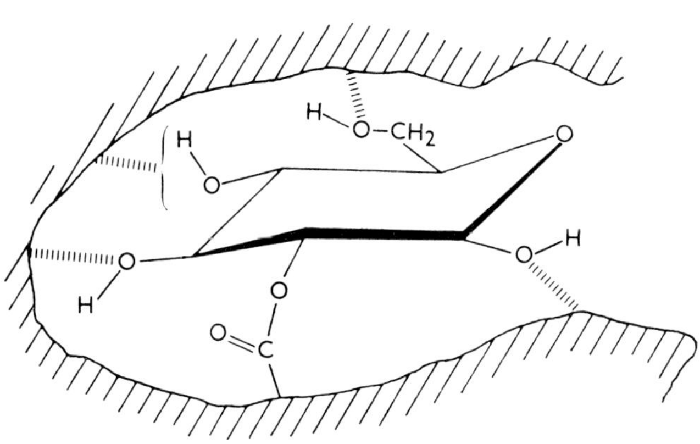

FIG. 8. Diagram of the possible binding of D-glucose to the hamster intestinal sugar carrier. Broken lines represent hydrogen bonds.

is of a different type to that at the other positions, and is probably covalent.

A model for the carrier–sugar binding is shown in Fig. 8. Sugars must bind in the pyranose ring form, but it is possible to fit the steric requirements by binding with the hydroxymethyl group at the position normally occupied by a hydroxyl group at C-1. In this way L-glucose can bind to the carrier (Fig. 7). The steric constraints on binding have been explored by the use of analogues specifically substituted with halogen atoms or alkyl groups of increasing size and may be summarised briefly. The carrier protein approaches the sugar closely at C-6 and in the *allo*-configuration at C-3, but there is some space in the *gluco*-configuration at C-3 and a large space in both α- and β-configurations at C-1.

A MECHANISM FOR ACTIVE TRANSPORT IN THE INTESTINE

Crane[24] has shown that the binding of sugars to the membrane is strong in the presence of sodium ions and weak in their absence. He has suggested that the sugar binds to the membrane strongly in the high sodium concentration outside the cell, and that the membrane rearranges so that the sodium ion and sugar are transferred to the inside of the cell where the sodium ion diffuses off in the low intracellular sodium ion concentration. This in turn leads to release of sugar even when the intracellular concentration of the sugar is higher than that of the extracellular fluid. The sodium ion gradient is maintained by the sodium pump.

Since this hypothesis for active transport demands that the sugar should bind reversibly to the membrane carrier, and without net

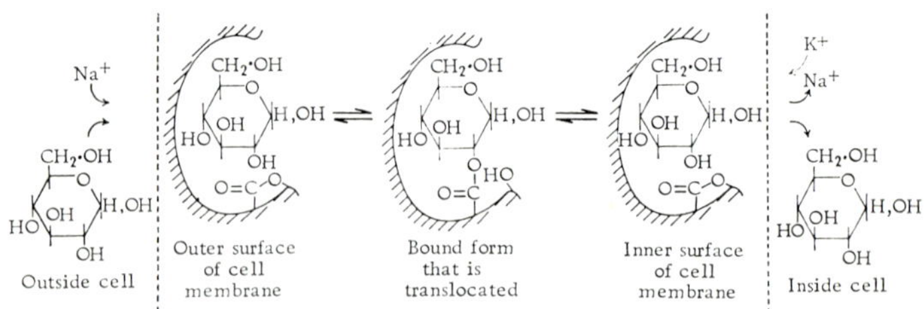

FIG. 9. Possible mechanism for the active transport of D-glucose into the hamster intestine.

utilisation of energy, it is envisaged that the proposed covalent bond at C-2 may be an ester formed by cleavage of an intramolecular ester on the membrane after initial absorption as shown in Fig. 9. On release of the sugar, the intramolecular bond on the membrane would be regenerated.

NON-SPECIFIC ABSORPTION

Some sugars, particularly those lacking a hydroxyl group at C-2, are not transported by either sugar carrier, but if introduced into the intestine, or incubated with everted intestinal rings, are slowly, passively absorbed and converted into the corresponding 6-phosphate by hexokinase.

Examples of this behaviour are found with 2-deoxy-D-glucose[25] and possibly mannose,[26] neither of which have a structure accepted by the two sugar carriers. Two possibilities exist to explain the

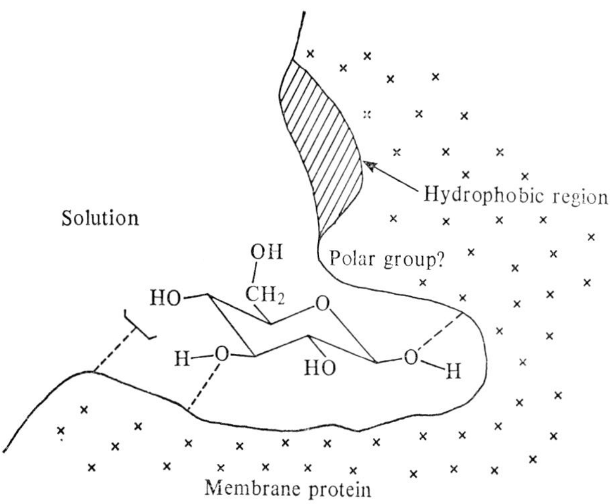

FIG. 10. Model for the glucose–carrier complex in the human erythrocyte. (Reproduced by courtesy of *Biochemical Journal*.)

penetration. The first, that entry is by simple diffusion, is unlikely in view of the large size and poor lipid solubility of the sugars. A possible alternative is that a third carrier exists in the epithelial cell, capable of slowly equilibrating these and other sugars. The latter appears more probable, and a good candidate for the carrier is the normal glucose entry mechanism found in all cells of the body. If the human red blood cell can be regarded as a typical cell with respect to this carrier, the structural requirements are known[27] and are shown in Fig. 10. They would favour entry of 2-deoxy-D-glucose and D-mannose.

THE METABOLISM OF TRANSPORTED SUGARS

It can be seen from the foregoing considerations of specificity that only D-glucose, D-galactose and D-fructose are likely to be absorbed in any quantity. Before these sugars can be metabolised they must be phosphorylated. This occurs either in the intestine, where, under some conditions and in some species, fructose is extensively converted into glucose and lactate, or in the liver to which the absorbed sugars are transported in the portal vein.

The major enzymes capable of phosphorylating sugars in mammals are hexokinase and fructokinase in the intestine and liver, and glucokinase and galactokinase found only in the liver.

The specificity of hexokinase has been widely studied,[28] but the results have been complicated by the subsequent discovery of three isoenzymes, hexokinase I–III, which have different abundances in different tissues.[29] The enzyme occurring in rat intestine is 90% type II,[30] whereas the most complete specificity studies have been on brain hexokinase, predominantly type I. However, the specificities of all the hexokinases appear to be qualitatively similar, with D-glucose as the best substrate, together with sugars modified only at C-2 (2-deoxy-glucose, mannose, 2-amino-2-deoxy-glucose). Modification of the D-glucose structure at other carbon atoms causes at least a 100-fold, and in the case of C-4 (galactose) a 10 000-fold, increase in K_m. Fructose is also a substrate, but with a K_m about 100 times that of glucose. Table 3 shows the effect of using 90 mM sugars as inhibitors of the phosphorylation of 0·6 mM D-glucose using purified type II hexokinase from rat.[29]

Intestinal fructokinase, which converts fructose into its 1-phosphate ester, will also accept L-sorbose as a substrate.[31] Galactokinase, which also converts the sugar into the 1-phosphate ester is found in mammalian liver and appears to be very specific,[32] as is glucokinase, an enzyme which, like hexokinase, converts glucose into its 6-phosphate. It differs from hexokinase in its high specificity and high K_m for glucose.[33]

TABLE 3

Inhibition of the phosphorylation of 0·6 mM glucose using hexokinase type II

Sugar (90 mM)	% Inhibition
D-mannose	100
2-deoxy-D-glucose	90
D-fructose	58
D-glucosamine	100
N-acetyl-D-glucosamine	100
D-xylose	37
D-galactose	0
D-sorbitol	0

CONCLUSION

For a sugar to be digested, absorbed and metabolised, it must pass the specificity requirements of each of the processes. It can be seen from the foregoing discussion that the most stringent of these is digestion, if any contribution of the intestinal flora is regarded as negligible. In normal circumstances, this assumption appears to be reasonable, but continual feeding of an abnormal carbohydrate may be expected to attract a flora which can utilise it. Thus, it has been shown that the ability to convert cyclamates to cyclohexylamine is a property of the intestinal flora which is acquired by feeding cyclamate.[34,35]

REFERENCES

1. Bernfeld, P., Duckart, P. and Fischer, E. H. (1950). *Helv. Chim. Acta,* **33,** p. 1024.
2. Semenza, G. (1968). In *Handbook of Physiology*, Section 6, Alimentary Canal, Vol. V, ed. by C. F. Code, American Physiological Society, Washington, D.C., p. 2637.
3. Barnett, J. E. G., Jarvis, W. T. S. and Munday, K. A. (1967). *Biochem. J.,* **103,** p. 699.
4. Barnett, J. E. G., Jarvis, W. T. S. and Munday, K. A. (1967). *Biochem. J.,* **105,** p. 699.
5. Hehre, E. J., Genghof, D. S. and Okada, G. (1971). *Arch. Biochem. Biophys.,* **142,** p. 382.

6. Dahlquist, A. (1962). *J. Clin. Invest.,* **41,** p. 463.
7. Semenza, G. and Auricchio, S. (1962). *Biochim. Biophys. Acta,* **65,** p. 173.
8. Malahi, P. and Crane, R. K. (1968). *Fed. Proc. Fed. Am. Soc. Exp. Biol.,* **27,** p. 385.
9. Gray, G. M. (1972). In *The Metabolic Basis of Inherited Disease,* 3rd edn, ed. by J. B. Stanbury, J. B. Wyngaarden, and D. S. Frederickson, McGraw-Hill, New York, p. 1455.
10. Trier, J. R. (1968). In *Handbook of Physiology,* Section 6, Alimentary Canal, Vol. III, ed by C. F. Code, American Physiological Society, Washington, D.C., p. 1125.
11. Miller, D. and Crane, R. K. (1961). *Biochim. Biophys. Acta,* **52,** p. 293.
12. Duell, R. G., Rosen, G. and Kritchener, W. (1965). *Proc. Nat. Acad. Sci., U.S.,* **54,** p. 1268.
13. Miller, D. and Crane, R. K. (1961). *Biochim. Biophys. Acta,* **52,** p. 281.
14. Lindquist, B., Meeuwisse, G. and Melin, K. (1962). *Lancet,* **2,** p. 666.
15. Wilson, T. H. and Vincent, T. N. (1955). *J. Biol. Chem.,* **216,** p. 841.
16. Kiyasu, J. V. and Chaikoff, I. R. (1957). *J. Biol. Chem.,* **224,** p. 935.
17. Holdsworth, G. D. and Dawson, A. M. (1965). *Proc. Soc. Exp. Biol. Med.,* **118,** p. 142.
18. Cook, G. C. (1969). *Clin. Sci.,* **37,** p. 675.
19. Gracey, M., Burke, V. and Oshin, A. (1972). *Biochim. Biophys. Acta,* **266,** p. 397.
20. Barnett, J. E. G., Jarvis, W. T. S. and Munday, K. A. (1968). *Biochem. J.* **109,** p. 61.
21. Barnett, J. E. G., Ralph, A. and Munday, K. A. (1969). *Biochem. J.,* **114,** p. 569.
22. Barnett, J. E. G., Ralph, A. and Munday, K. A. (1970). *Biochem. J.,* **118,** p. 843.
23. Bihler, I., Hawkins, K. H. and Crane, R. K. (1962). *Biochim. Biophys. Acta,* **59,** p. 94.
24. Crane, R. K. (1965). *Fed. Proc. Fed. Am. Soc. Exp. Biol.,* **24,** p. 1000.
25. Elsas, J. L. and MacDonell, R. C. (1972). *Biochim. Biophys. Acta,* **255,** p. 948.
26. Csaky, T. A. and Ho, P. M. (1966). *Life Sci.,* **5,** p. 1025.
27. Barnett, J. E. G., Holman, G. D. and Munday, K. A. (1973). *Biochem. J.,* **131,** p. 211.
28. Crane, R. K. (1962). In *The Enzymes,* Vol. 6, 2nd edn, ed by P. D. Boyer, H. Lardy and K. Myerback, Academic Press, New York, p. 47.
29. Grossbard, L. and Schimke, R. J. (1966). *J. Biol. Chem.,* **241,** p. 3552.
30. Srivasta, L. M., Shakespeare, P. and Hubscher, G. (1968). *Biochem. J.,* **109,** p. 35.
31. Cadenas, E. and Sols, A. (1960). *Biochim. Biophys. Acta,* **42,** p. 490.
32. Cardini, C. E. and Leloir, L. F. (1953). *Arch. Biochem. Biophys.,* **45,** 55.
33. Katzen, H. M. and Schimke, R. T. (1965). *Proc. Nat. Acad. Sci. U.S.,* **54,** p. 1218.
34. Renwick, A. G. and Williams, R. T. (1972). *Biochem. J.,* **129,** p. 869.

35. Draser, B. S., Renwick, A. G. and Williams, R. T. (1972). *Biochem. J.*, **129**, p. 881.

DISCUSSION

Buss: Have you looked at how D-glucosamine is transported by your system? This could be interesting in the light of your theory that a covalent bond must be formed at C-2.

Barnett: D-glucosamine is not transported. In fact it is a non-competitive inhibitor at 20 mM concentration with transport down by about 25%. This property appears to be a general one of amines.

Parker: I would like to note that Professor A. Foster found 6-fluoroglucose to have, unexpectedly in his opinion, anti-carcinogenic activity implying transport across the gut, which is a corollary of your conclusions.

Barnett: One must be careful to distinguish between the specificity of the sodium-dependent intestinal system I have discussed and other sugar transport systems, for instance that of the red blood cell (Barnett, Holman and Munday (1973) *Biochem. J.*, **131**, p. 211) which is quite different. The transport of a sugar with a cancer cell will probably therefore have a very different specificity from that of the intestine. However, as you say, 6-deoxy-6-fluoroglucose is absorbed by the intestine.

Parker: Are you implying that sucrose is not actively transported as such, or is there in fact a concerted transport of glucose and fructose?

Barnett: Sucrose is not actively transported as such, but the glucose and fructose are released by the mucosal surface directly onto the carrier sites in high concentration and do not equilibrate with the mucosal solution. However, you may be interested in the paper by Semenza (*Febs Letters*, 1972) (Amsterdam meeting edition) in which he added intestinal sucrose to an artificial membrane and showed that, although sucrose was not actively transported, fructose and glucose appeared on the inside of the membrane.

Nicol: What about fructose itself? Can you tell me whether inulin is hydrolysed?

Barnett: I don't think inulin, as such, would be hydrolysed, but it may be by sucrose, to give fructose. Particularly in animals other than man, fructose is very rapidly metabolised to glucose and lactate.

Grenby: Could you tell us about the transport of fructose across the intestinal barrier? We heard yesterday about the possible nutritional value of fructose and its polymer, inulin. How are they absorbed?

Barnett: I believe that inulin is not absorbed since it is not hydrolysed by any of the intestinal enzymes (confirmed by the chairman). However, fructose is absorbed very rapidly by a separate carrier as detailed in this paper.

Birch: I'd like to ask about the odd occurrence of trehalase in the alimentary system, because trehalose is not part of the diet. What do you think of Gray's suggestion that trehalase is the carrier?

Barnett: It has the wrong specificity, but you may know how it differs from the other carbohydrases.
Birch: It differs in being resistant to papain and I think it must therefore be located differently.
Barnett: The carbohydrases are all associated with the brush-border region of the small intestine, but in answer to your first question although trehalose is not now part of the diet it may once have been.
Hood: Do substituent groups linked to the glucose through an ether linkage, such as a hydroxypropyl group, have any effect on the transport mechanism you have described?
Barnett: Yes. You mean putting ether groups around the ring? This is the other part I did not talk about today. We have explored steric effects of different size groups as well, starting generally with chlorine, bromine and iodine then right up to various alkyl groups. The methyl substitution at position 3 does go and ethyl doesn't go very well, so there is a cut-off about there. In this position bromide doesn't go.
Macdonald: So you find 2 and 3 to be quite simple in terms of specificity?
Barnett: 2-*O*-Methyl glucose is not transported. 6-*O*-Methyl glucose is not transported, nor 4-*O*, but 3-*O* is.
Parker: It is interesting that 3-*O*-methyl glucose is actively transported. I understand that it is not metabolised and is excreted unchanged. Would you please comment on this?
Barnett: Yes, many of these sugars I used are not metabolised, particularly 3-deoxy-3-fluoroglucose.

15

Carbohydrates and Human Performance

J. D. Brooke

Human Performance Laboratory, Salford University, Salford, Lancs., England

ABSTRACT

Food carbohydrates (CoH) provide fuel for skeletal muscle metabolism. Body CoH stores can limit performance of hard physical work maintained over hours. Provision is mainly endogenous to the active muscle through local glycogen storage. Muscle glycogen stores increase with high CoH diet. Preliminary repeated physical work exhaustion of the stores markedly boosts this increase and the time before exhaustion from work appears. Glucose syrup drink supplements during work extend performance time through exogenous provision and after exhaustion they result in faster recovery. Efficiency of performance increases with adequate glycogen and glucose available for muscle metabolism or with exogenous provision through simple CoH supplements. With exhaustion of CoH stores during work, fats seem incapable of completely supporting further skeletal muscle metabolism.

Food CoH also provides fuel for central nervous cells, with reserve support from ketone bodies. The grossness of studies to demonstrate the effect of transient (meal omission) or sustained inadequacy of supply of food CoH permits only limited interpretation. Within the normal range, starvation increases reaction time. Blood glucose in the range 50–70 *mg*/100 *ml evokes in some subjects changes in emotional response, reaction time, feelings of fatigue and response to 'stress'. This range is observed during normal performance. There is much inter- and intra- individual variation in blood glucose response to glucose loads: the causes are little investigated. In some states oral* vs. *intravenous loading provides different results. Circadian rhythm exists in the response. An undershoot occurs hours after loading: it has implications for the quality of normal performance at such times.*

Recent work on relationships between transient food CoH insufficiency, glucose syrup supplements and reduction in factory accidents is reviewed. Attention is drawn to present interest in vehicle driving accidents on motorways and transient CoH insufficiency. In study of food CoH, central nervous states and performance, there is need for rigorous research into the subtle changes that occur normally.

This review is concerned with the relationship between food carbohydrates (CoHs) and task performance by normal human beings; it is not concerned directly with the biochemistry of the functioning of these substances.

Such a brief eliminates also concern for clinical matters and animal experimentation other than human. The focus is normal human performance, the study perspective is wide and the attention to the detail of more micro levels accordingly less intense. Of the food CoHs reported, most information is available about glucose and glucose syrups,[1] sucrose and fructose specifically or by inference from glucose: sucrose comparisons, together with less precisely defined work using mixed diets estimated to contain a certain proportion of CoHs, fats and protein.

Two important roles appear for food CoHs in human performance, one as a major fuel in the metabolism providing for the activity of skeletal muscles and the other as a primary fuel for nerve cells. Neither provision involves an exclusive role so that we are concerned not with the existence of the functions, which is beyond debate, but with the effect of use or restriction of these roles upon normal human behaviour.

SKELETAL MUSCLE ACTIVITY

Energy from skeletal muscle is derived immediately from one of three metabolic sources as shown in Table 1. For the first source, phosphogen splitting at the onset of activity is a very short term matter and need not concern us. For the second source, during food combustion with adequate oxygen potentials, fats and CoHs fuel the muscle metabolism. There is no conclusive evidence that protein contributes normally as an additional energy source for physical work. This was clear from as early as 1866, von Pettenkofer and Voit[2] observing no increase in urinary nitrogen excretion with physical activity, and it has been confirmed repeatedly since by many investigations.[3,4]

In states of starvation, gluconeogenesis does occur with metabolism of glucogenic amino acids,[5] but this is the exception to the normal state. Free fatty acids, muscle triglycerides and glucose/glycogen stores are the combustible end products of foods utilised normally when adequate oxygen is available. In such conditions work can be sustained over hours.

The third immediate source of energy in muscular activity is by addition to the contribution from combusted fuel, the contribution from glycolysis when there is insufficient oxygen for only combustion to provide the energy. The normal process of break-down of muscle glycogen to pyruvic acid is continued a stage further under inadequate oxygen potential to the formation of lactic acid, with the

TABLE 1

Primary metabolic sources of energy for skeletal muscle activity

Type of activity	Metabolic source of energy	Time span
A. Initiation of performance	Phosphogen splitting (alactacid—Margaria 1933)	$\leq$15 sec
B. Tolerable load for O_2 homeostasis	Food combustion, measured by O_2 consumption	Many hours
C. Severe load beyond O_2 homeostasis	Food combustion and glycolysis with incomplete phosphogen resynthesis (lactacid—Margaria 1933)	$\geq$20 sec dependent upon severity of O_2 disequilibrium

latter's subsequent release and buffering in the blood. This process is self-limiting in that the feelings of distress associated with its development inhibit further performance. It is also wasteful of glycogen as an energy source. With glycolytic breakdown (anaerobic), 1 molecule of glycogen provides 2 molecules of adenosine triphosphate (together with phospho-creatine this is the higher energy source in muscle) whereas in food combustion (aerobic) the conversion of 1 molecule of glycogen provides 38 molecules of ATP. Glycolysis as a source of skeletal muscle energy is limited theoretically by the fast approach to complete breakdown of the phosphogens and extravagant use of glycogen: it is limited practically by the distress associated with the process: it does not concern us further in the present topic.

The significance of food CoHs to human performance involving primarily activity of skeletal musculature is in the oxidative aspects of muscle metabolism, for in normal conditions there are immense reserves of oxygen available in the atmosphere and with moderate work load these may be transported by respiration to maintain the metabolic process. Attention then turns to the gradual use of fuel, CoH and fats. The specific metabolism of fats as a source of muscular energy is established.[6] With low intensities of external power demand [requiring $\leq 50\%$ of the maximum oxygen uptake ($\dot{V}O_2$ max)] for subjects on normal diets, fat and CoH contribute almost equally as the fuel supply to the exercising muscle.[7] At very low loads fats may be the predominant fuel. As the external power demand is increased, so there is an increasing participation of CoH to the neglect of fats in the muscle metabolism; this statement applies up to the maximum ability to generate physical power, but in the upper part of the power range the CoH contribution is partly by glycolysis.

It is the intention to leave the issues of fat metabolism at this point, merely noting that where proportional contributions of CoH to energy release are reported below it is often possible merely to abstract the proportion remaining to identify the contribution from fats.

A methodological note is necessary. Prior to the advent of muscle biopsy techniques (referred to below) the standard method for estimation of the metabolic fuel was the non-protein metabolic respiratory quotient (RQ), the ratio of carbon dioxide eliminated to oxygen utilised.[8] In homeostasis for oxygen provision, respiratory quotients equal to one indicate that solely CoH is being combusted, that is,

$$C_6H_{12}O_6 + 6O_2 \rightarrow 6CO_2 + 6H_2O$$

In similar conditions an RQ of 0·7 is commonly taken to indicate solely fat metabolism. With glycerol tristearate,

$$\begin{array}{l} CH_2O \cdot CO \cdot C_{17}H_{35} \\ | \\ 2CHO \cdot CO \cdot C_{17}H_{35} + 163O_2 \rightarrow 114CO_2 + 110H_2O \\ | \\ CH_2O \cdot CO \cdot C_{17}H_{35} \end{array}$$

With RQ values intermediate in the range 1·0 to 0·7, differing proportions of carbohydrate and fat are taken to be metabolised. The various percentage contributions are tabulated.[9–11] The energy provided per litre of oxygen used also varies over this RQ range, being from 21·1 kJ/litre O_2 with complete CoH metabolism, RQ = 1·0, to 19·6 kJ/litre O_2 with complete fat metabolism. These data are similarly tabulated op. cit. From such information the mechanical efficiency of work performed can be calculated as

$$E\% = \frac{\text{external power generated}}{\text{internal energy expended}} \times 100$$

This is particularly facilitated if the external power output can be expressed in watts (*i.e.* J/sec) as on a cycle ergometer. The use of RQ analysis from respiratory gases is a sound way to estimate the overall metabolic mixture. The method does have limits that should be observed. One of the assumptions is to a non-protein calculation, that is, the experimental conditions are assumed not to alter the protein metabolism. A further assumption is a stable acid–base state. Disturbances of this balance by metabolic or respiratory dynamics will much complicate interpretation of the RQ as an index of the metabolic fuel.

In studies of human performance, attempts have been made to extend the limits of physical power expenditure by supplying additional CoHs to the body, sometimes orally, sometimes intravenously and more recently with additional benefits through initiation of physiological adaptation. For maximum short term physical work ($\leq$15 min) little or no effect is seen.[12] Haldi and Wynn[13] found no difference in 100 yd swim time $2\frac{1}{2}$ to 3 hours after heavy meals (4·399 MJ) or light meals (2·306 MJ), even when the latter were supplemented with 50 or 100 g of sucrose immediately before the swim. Taylor *et al.*[14] found no decrement in muscle glycogen stores following maximal short term cycle ergometer work, indicating no apparent limit from CoH stores. Clarke *et al.*[15] did find reduction in 100 yd and 600 yd run times for Indian schoolgirls during the Ramadam festival when no food is taken during the day. However, there was weak experimental control of the subjective expectation of being less able to work whilst under the scourge of fasting and this effect may be contained within these results.

In comparison, when the work load is moderately hard (demanding 60 to 75% $\dot{V}O_2$ max) yet such that physical work can be maintained for hours, the role of dietary CoH stands out. At the whole-body level of analysis, more work is possible for a given oxygen uptake with CoH than with fat metabolism[16] and the condition of marathon runners is related[17] to the level of the blood glucose. The effect of supplementing the provision to body CoH stores by manipulating the pre-work diet was investigated by Christensen and Hansen.[7] Subjects worked to incapacity over hours on cycle ergometers at moderate work loads. In comparison to performance on a normal diet, a week of low CoH/high fat diet reduced by up to half the work time to exhaustion. Conversely work times increased by approximately one third of the normal with a week of high CoH diet.

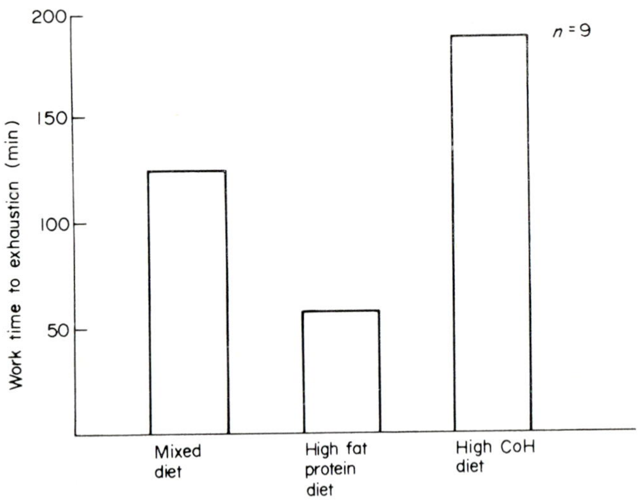

FIG. 1. Work abilities after various pre-work diets for three days (drawn from data of Saltin and Hermansen[18]).

Recent work has confirmed this effect of nutrition on performance,[18] as shown in Fig. 1. The work time to exhaustion of 9 subjects working on a cycle ergometer at 75% $\dot{V}O_2$ max was assessed. On the day of the experiment the subjects took no food. The second trial was preceded by the normal mixed diet. Between the first and second trials 6 subjects were given a 3-day diet high in fats and protein: the subsequent work time decreased as shown in Fig. 1. Between the second and third trials the 6 subjects took a 3-day diet high in CoH: the work time for the final trial increased by 50% over the second trial. The experimental work followed the treatment sequence on the figure, reading from left to right, and it has been proposed that the full sequence of diets is necessary to obtain this effect on the work performance. However, recent work[19] has demonstrated a similar effect with a replication of the physical work demands of that experiment, but with limited dietary manipulation. Subjects followed a regime of feed, 20-hr fast and work to exhaustion of available CoH over hours three times with 72 hours between trials. Feeding for the 50 hr was on their normal sportsman's diets high in CoH.

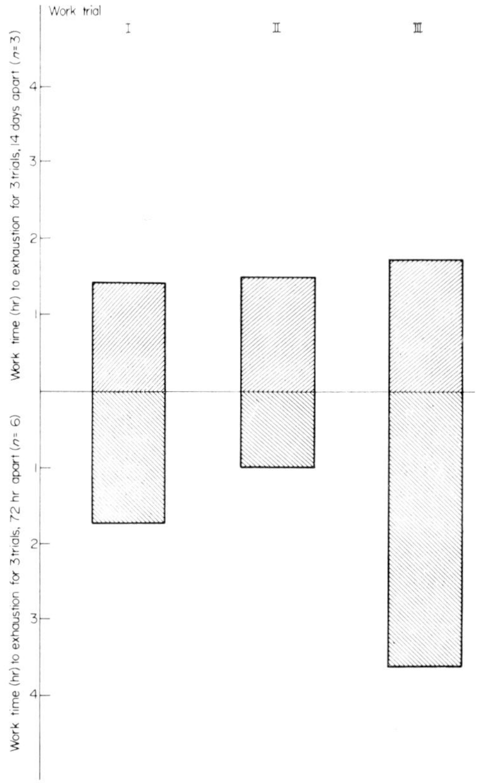

FIG. 2. Work times to exhaustion for three trials, close spaced (72 hr) and open spaced (14 days).

The effect upon performance of this repeated exhaustion of CoH available for work is shown in Fig. 2. A marked reduction occurred in the second trial performance with third trial times showing an increase over the first trial of more than 100%. The underlying state of the available carbohydrate stores is demonstrated by the respiratory quotients shown in Fig. 3. The full and subsequent extended rises in work performance were obtained merely by the experimental treatment, with dietary significance being reduced to the provision of a diet adequately high in CoHs.

It is clear from these two pieces of research that repeated depletion of CoH stores leads to adaptive responses so strong that an overshoot in restoration occurs. In the previous study[18] the fat and protein diet only aided this process, the exhaustion of the CoH stores again

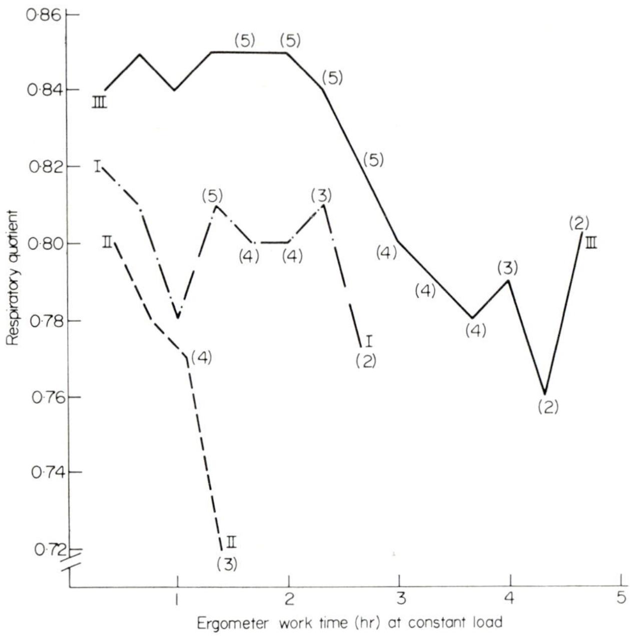

FIG. 3. Mean repiratory quotient during three work trials (I, II, III) 72 hr apart [6 subjects unless indicated: ( )].

in the second work trial probably being critical in obtaining the third trial response to high CoH feeding. This suggestion is supported by the Scandinavian data on three subjects who took the high CoH diet first, in place of the fat and protein. Both CoH available and work times to exhaustion were low when the second trial was used in this way to assess the effectiveness of the diet high in CoHs. Two additional factors contribute to the very marked adaptation seen in the recent work of Brooke and Green.[19] One was the effect of extended fasting before performance which would act as an additional and preliminary depletion of CoH stores that were low already. The other is that racing cyclists were used as subjects and the ergometer load was applied with a new device,[20] the Ergowheel,* that could be attached to the cyclists' own racing cycles to which they were habituated by daily training. Unlike the pilot attempts with this research, postural factors as a limit to the performance on the ergometer were then removed. With an adequately high CoH content in the diet, repeated work exhaustion elicits an adaptive response in body carbohydrate storage that overshoots and results in increased capacity to sustain performance.

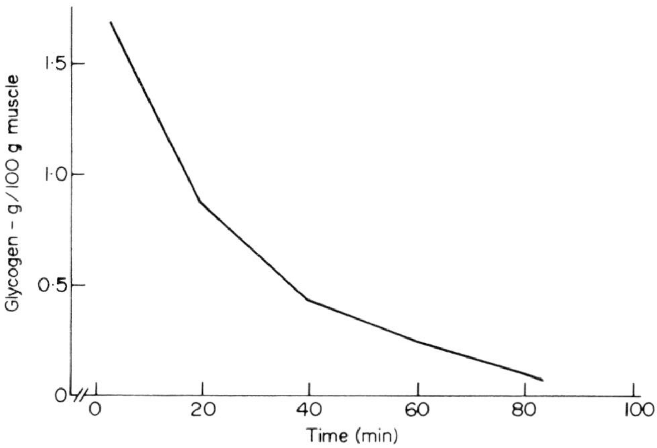

FIG. 4. Glycogen content of quadriceps femoris muscle during extended work to exhaustion (drawn from data of Saltin and Hermansen[18]).

Light has been cast recently on the specific CoH stores in the body that limit such performances and that are adapted by the exhaustion. The introduction[21] of muscle biopsy techniques allowed direct assays to be made of the glycogen content of exercising muscle by removing small samples from the muscle. Such information had not been obtained before for normal human performance. With physical work over hours, muscle glycogen values at exhaustion are very low;[22] at rest the values approximate 7 g glycogen per 100 g fat and glycogen-free solids and at exhaustion 1·7 g/100 g.

There is continuous reduction of this store as physical work is carried out.[23] After work on a high CoH diet there is very rapid restoration of these muscle glycogen levels and a marked rebound

* Worthwhile Designs Ltd, Grange Road, Eccles.

effect,[24] with exercised muscle glycogen levels then exceeding the normal range by as much as 100% after several days on the diet. Normal levels of 1·75 g/100 g of wet muscle might increase to 3·3 g/100 g after exercise and subsequent high dietary CoH levels. With the assumption of 30 kg of muscle in the body composition of the adult male, this indicates muscle glycogen stores of up to 1000 g with adaptation. This is in accordance with Saltin and Hermansen's[18] calculated use of up to 800 g during exhaustive cycle ergometer exercise. It has been suggested that, with the additional 3 to 4 g of water retained with each gramme of glycogen, increase in glycogen levels could cause performance deterioration because of the extra weight to be carried. However, this disadvantage appears to be over-ridden by the gains in energy resources, for performance gains, not decrements, are seen even in tasks where movement of the body weight predominates.

During these prolonged hard work tasks the respiratory functions, *e.g.* $\dot{V}O_2$ or Hf, are submaximal: they do not approach limits.[25] In addition, with many subjects, blood glucose levels at exhaustion do not fall much below 60 mg/100 ml blood and liver glycogen stores are not greatly depleted.[23] Rowell *et al.*[26] state that 10% of energy is contributed by splanchnic glucose production in young men fasting for 16 hr, after 1 hr moderate exercise. In addition, as shown in Fig. 4, it is possible to have rising blood sugar levels with adequate total body CoH and subjects still become exhausted. Costill *et al.*[27] make a similar note, and possible hormonal effects (catecholamine) on liver glycogen release close to exhaustion are discussed briefly by Bergström and Hultman.[23] It appears that endogenous supplies of glycogen are the main CoH energy substrate for exercising skeletal muscle and that the major role of dietary CoH is in making available adequate glucose for these local stores to be replete. Without exercise, muscle glycogen levels can be increased somewhat with a high CoH diet and by glucose or fructose infusion.[28] However, the effect is much more marked after exercise. With starvation and a low CoH diet, levels are reduced, as is work ability, and post-work restoration of muscle glycogen is very slow (> 1 week). There appears to be little transfer from one local body store to another, for in subjects exercising only one leg, glycogen values at exhaustion were very low for the exercised muscles and normal for the contralateral ones. A similar localisation is seen in the subsequent glycogen adaptation.

It is clear that the performance changes reported by Brooke and Green[19] and Saltin and Hermansen[18] are primarily the result of changes in the levels of glycogen in skeletal muscles used for the physical activity. The beneficial effects of a high CoH diet on running 30 km races,[29] and the detrimental effect of denying free sucrose intake to runners prior to marathon running[30] appear to have a similar basis.

The pre-work diets defined as high CoH have been a mixture of food CoHs, *e.g.* bread, spaghetti, potatoes, sugar, fruit and juices contributing at least 95% of the energy. Exploration is still required into the effects of specific food CoHs as pre-work diets. Also, while the source of the performance changes is clear, work still remains to be done on the specific biochemistry of the adaptive response in re-synthesis of muscle glycogen: it has been suggested that the force is upon the I-form of glycogen synthetase, but knowledge of glycogen storage in skeletal muscles is incomplete.[29,31] More information is also needed on the time course of the adaptation, for the work of Costill *et al.*[32] exercising subjects on three trials on successive days resulted in a continued depletion of muscle glycogen levels, in comparison to the third trial elevation of performance with 72 hr between trials.[18,19]

In addition to pre-work diets some information is available about the effects of diets during work. While endogenous muscle glycogen stores provide much of the CoH for moderately hard and extended physical work performance, when these stores are low use is also made of liver glycogen from glucogenic[23] and gluconeogenic sources,[33] and of blood glucose.[18] For loads a little lighter than those considered at present, up to one-third of the glucose oxidised might be provided exogenously.[34] The following hypothesis was therefore tested;[35] that a specific high CoH diet during work would be more effective in maintaining work performance than a low energy diet or a normal intake (for the sport of time trial cycle racing). As a full stomach is not recommended for vigorous physical activity,[36] 'let your stomach be free of excessive food and drink', the high CoH diet used was a glucose syrup[37] (GS) drink* with added salt, providing the high energy/volume ratio of 5·944 MJ/litre of fluid. The other merit of this CoH-rich fluid is its palatability in comparison with isocaloric amounts of sucrose,

* 'Dynamo'—Beecham Products.

for the latter tastes excessively sweet. Macdonald[38] states that glucose syrup has a sweetness value of 0·33 in comparison with an arbitrarily assigned value of 1·00 for sucrose. There is also suggestion of clinical benefits in the consumption of glucose rather than sucrose.[39]

With eight male cyclists working as described above at approximately 70% $\dot{V}O_2$ max, their internal energy expended was replaced every 20 min by the equivalent energy as GS supplements, by isocaloric normal dietary intake (rice pudding, fruit salad and added

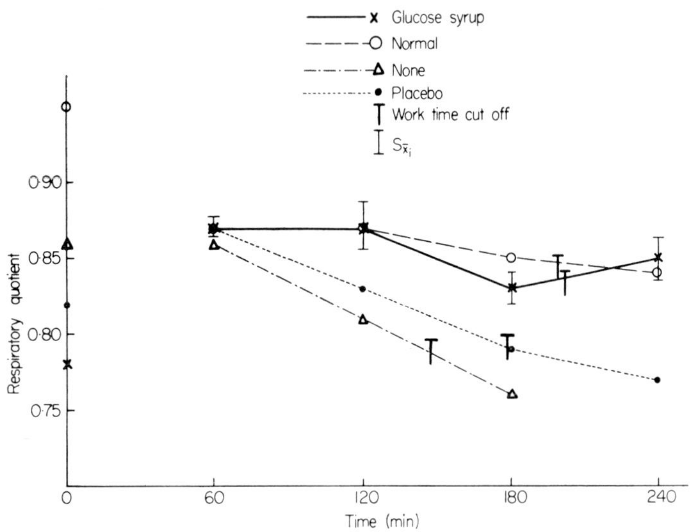

FIG. 5. Mean respiratory quotients during rides on different feeds ($n = 8$).

sucrose) or replacement was mimicked by the same volume of very low calorie fluid as the GS drink. In addition, one trial was made without food. The two fluids were presented to the subjects as two experimental treatments that were being assessed. 10% of the energy requirement was taken 3 hr before starting work. 150 ml of an electrolyte solution approximating the concentration of sweat was presented also every 20 min. The total work time per trial extended for 3 to 4 hr. As shown in Fig. 5, most work was done on the GS supplement, followed by the normal diet, the control fluid and, finally, no food (all differences statistically significant, $p < \cdot05$).

Significantly more work was done on the GS diet. There was decreasing availability of CoH with the low energy diets as shown by the course of the RQ. This work extends the early work of Dill *et al.*[40] who elicited more work from dogs maintained on glucose, and is in accord with Bergström and Hultman's work,[23] for with a continuous glucose infusion during a trial, muscle glycogen consumption was lowered and blood sugar remained high. The action of the dietary CoH was seen to occur after the first two hours, with elevated levels of blood sugar in comparison with the low energy treatments and also increased proportions of CoH combusted.

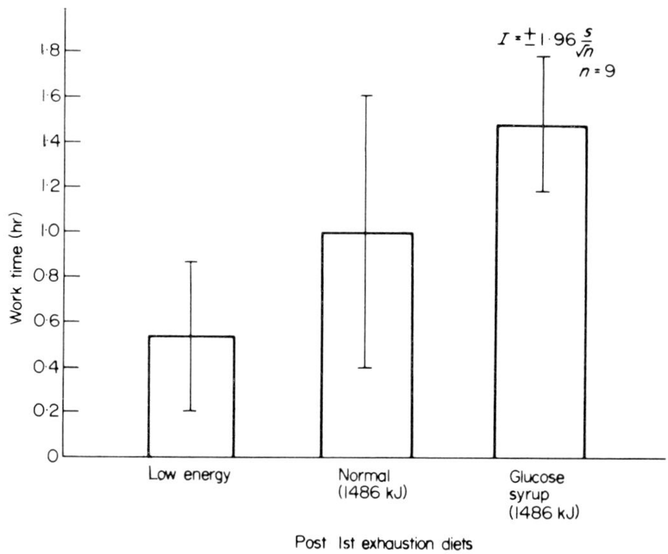

FIG. 6. Recovery work following work exhaustion and feeds ($n = 9$).

A high CoH dietary supplement during work normally increases the capacity for performance: the effect is much slighter than that achieved by prior adaptation of the glycogen resynthesis by exhausting work. It is improbable that inhibition of gastric emptying during cycling would restrict use of this work diet,[41] although such inhibition has been seen with a group of four marathon runners.[27]

The capacity of a dietary supplement to revive subjects exhausted from such hard extended activity is also of interest. Campbell[42] draws attention to this need during long expeditions and in mountain accidents and there is sports application. Christensen and Hansen[7] reported that subjects ingesting 200 g of glucose at exhaustion (3·13 MJ) were able to continue work for a further hour. A rise in blood sugar was observed, subjective distress was reduced, but no change in RQ occurred. In an experiment with nine racing cyclists, Brooke and Green,[43] exhaustion of CoH stores was obtained, through work in the manner described above. One of three dietary treatments was then presented, 250 ml GS drink with salts, energy value 1·486 MJ, 250 ml low energy fluid with salts, energy value <20 kJ, and warm, tinned rice pudding with added sucrose approximately isocaloric to the GS supplements. Forty minutes after, exhaustive work restarted at the same load as the first performance: the times to exhaustion a second time are shown in Fig. 6. The differences are statistically significant ($p < \cdot 05$) with 40 min additional work being possible with the GS supplement in comparison with the low energy fluid. No significant differences between the treatments were seen in oxygen uptake or respiratory quotients, but a boost occurred in blood glucose levels with the two high energy supplements. In the recovery context there is one isolated report on the difference between glycogen levels after one exhausting trial when 20% glucose or 20% fructose were infused at 4 g/kg body weight.[28] The glucose infusion elevated muscle glycogen levels in the exhausted muscle to a significantly higher level than the fructose infusion. High CoH supplements to exhausted subjects restore performance capacity, with probably the simpler the sugar, the faster the restoration, the active digestive uptake of glucose being more effective than the passive uptake of fructose. The search to account for these performance differences under the apparent absence of changes in the muscle metabolic mixture has led researchers to hypothesise a central nervous effect.[3] The matter has not been advanced beyond the hypothesis.

In the muscle biopsy studies the close relationships observed between the rate of utilisation of the muscle glycogen and the concomitant values for the respiratory quotients have served to validate the acceptibility of respiratory quotients as indicators of the fuel being combusted in metabolism. The RQ is very susceptible to experimental error, not least by subjects over-breathing; therefore, when biopsy techniques are not available or a more general view of metabolism is required, it is recommended that the RQ and the blood sugar be monitored simultaneously. Sudden high values for RQ can be questioned seriously if the accompanying blood sugar measure remains low. Conversely, RQ measures will describe gradual proportional changes in metabolic fuels at a time when the blood sugar is settling to a lower base line around 60 to 70 mg/100 ml blood.

In our work reported on trained work-habituated racing cyclists, a cessation point at RQ 0·75 to 0·73 was decided upon after one subject early in the pilot work demonstrated his successful tolerance of the increasing distress by finishing the experiment with clinical symptoms of marked hypoglycaemia. In this respect the sportsman's tolerance, developed to resist the distress that is experienced with anaerobic metabolism that results from power demands beyond that needed to elicit $\dot{V}O_2$ max (*see* Table 1), is a source of danger if the tolerance is utilised to resist the feelings of incipient hypoglycaemia. With sports anaerobiosis there is rapid restoration from the threatening disequilibrium of metabolism: cessation of work with hypoglycaemic disequilibrium of CoH metabolism may afford no such immediate relief.

A characteristic observed in the above studies on physical work was the increase in efficiency that occurred with high CoH availability, that is, a reduced requirement for oxygen, and hence energy expenditure, for the same external power demand. The effect was seen when sustaining performance with a glucose syrup drink.[35]

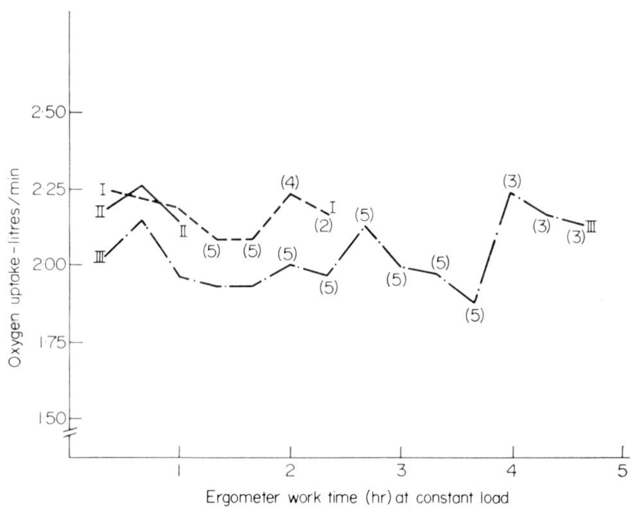

FIG. 7. Oxygen uptake during three work trials (I, II, III) 72 hr apart [6 subjects unless indicated ( )].

Figure 7 shows a similar effect when the muscle glycogen stores have been boosted to high levels by the adaptation of repeated trials and adequate diet. The response is not simply that more energy is liberated per 1·0 mole O_2 when combusting CoH *vs* combusting fat.[9,16] Such a difference would, at such oxygen uptakes, account only for approximately 50 ml of oxygen. The common difference in Fig. 7, for example, is over 150 ml. This phenomenon was also observed by Christensen and Hansen[7] and Benade *et al.*[44] In the latter study, sucrose loads of 100 g or 200 g taken at the third hour of 5 hr shifts by Bantu workers increased RQ in comparison with normal controls and reduced oxygen utilisation by up to 100 ml in approximately 1600 ml O_2/min. In both cases there was a reduction of approximately 6% in the oxygen requirement with high availability of CoH. Goldsmith *et al.*[45] observed differences in efficiency following various isocaloric meals. The increase in $\dot{V}O_2$ against mean pre-meal values was 15% after a high protein meal, 9% after a high fat meal and only 4% after a glucose meal, the carbohydrate meal thus allowing the most efficient basal metabolism to occur. Again, with the nature of the metabolic mixture unable to account directly for the changes in function, particularly in the work performances, hypotheses are directed to the role of the central nervous system.

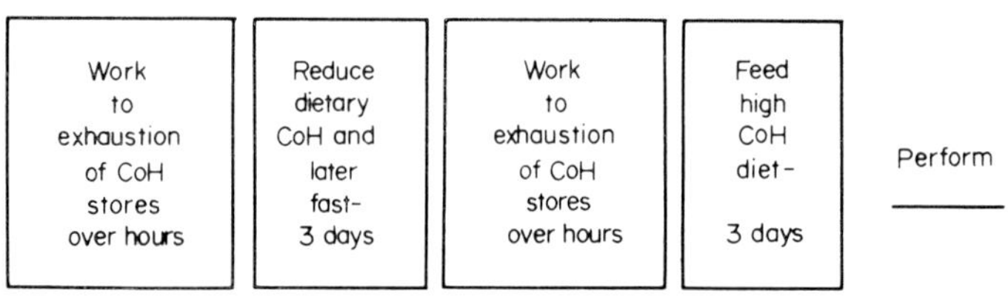

FIG. 8. Scheme to elicit extended performance for hard physical work over hours.

To summarise for the activity of skeletal muscles, in the absence of more obvious limits the muscle glycogen stores appear to limit the performance of hard sustained work over hours. Diets that are high in CoH in the days prior to work are essential to meet the needs of adaptive responses that can be elicited in muscle glycogen resynthesis through prior physical work exhaustion of those stores. With repeated exhaustion there is a marked rebound effect that much facilitates performance: Fig. 8 outlines a programme most likely to achieve this. Why the muscle, at such times and with such work loads, cannot use its other energy substrates, the exogenous supply of free fatty acids,[46] and endogenous supply of muscle triglyceride,[34] is not clear. This substrate is used for muscle energy more as the work intensity is reduced. It does not seem possible to call on fat metabolism alone to maintain power output at loads eliciting 65–75% $\dot{V}O_2$ max when the available CoH stores are exhausted. In both the maintenance of and the recovery from prolonged severe exercise food CoHs are used with positive effect.

CENTRAL NERVOUS STATE

The interaction of the central nervous state, normal performance by human beings and food CoHs is of direct current interest, but there is much less knowledge on these topics. Excluded from consideration in this paper are the clinical problems of obesity, diabetes mellitus, hypoglycaemia and other clinical disturbances of CoH metabolism, although proposals of continua with the clinical state occupying one end are of interest. For example, Danowski[47] considering diabetes mellitus states,

> 'Diabetes mellitus is a spectrum which extends from zero to 100% with clearly non-diabetic individuals at the zero point and clearly diabetic individuals at the 100% point. However, some individuals because of heredity, obesity, pancreatic injury, aging, repeated pregnancy, etc., fall on the 10, 25 or 85% point.'

Clearly, in this statement, there are implications for the performance characteristics of human beings classified as normal, that is, free from identified disease.

The physiological basis for interest in the central nervous system (CNS) and dietary CoHs first should be stated. The primary fuel for the CNS is glucose.[48,49] Measurement of RQ from arterial and mixed venous gas transport in the cerebral circulation results in values such as 0·98. It was thought for many years that glucose was the only CNS fuel. It is clear now this is not so. Normal rate of glucose usage by the human brain is approximately 110 g/day. When available glycogen stores have been depleted by fasting, gluconeogenesis from protein and triglyceride generates only about 67 g/day. The additional nutrient required has been shown[50] to be ketone bodies.

In the brains of fasting patients uptake of acetoacetate and D(−)-3-hydroxybutyrate (D-3-HB) together with the reduced available glucose was sufficient to meet the energy needs of the brain. Zivin and Snarr[51] observe, however, that isolated perfused rat brain could not be maintained on D-3-HB alone; some glucose was necessary. With reduced glucose concentrations in the perfusate there was increased uptake of D-3-HB. At maximum the contribution of fats to CNS fuel was to meet only 14% of the energy expenditure of the rat system: yet up to 60% of this energy requirement can be met by ketone bodies in the human.[50] The difficulties in transferring the results of other animal experiments to make applications to the human are well illustrated by this example. The researchers demonstrate that fat acts as a CNS fuel; the preferred fuel for most of the energy requirement is glucose; it is an essential nutrient for CNS activity.

It is the intention now to consider the effects, upon more delicate skill performance rather than the generation of physical power, of fasting, of depleted CoH stores after physical work and of transient malnutrition from dietary patterns. Where effects are reported, they may often be the result of any of at least four factors, namely:

1. lack of glucose in CNS metabolism,
2. increased CNS metabolism of ketone bodies,
3. increased interoceptive stimulation from ketosis, perceived as distress and therefore commanding part of the attentive space,
4. interaction of all or any parts of 1–3.

To this list may often be added inadequate control of extraneous psychological influences. In most cases no information is available to permit differentiation between these possible aetiological factors.

Partial starvation or fasting has been used to demonstrate deterioration in motor performance. Some of the studies barely come into the category of normal human performance. For instance, Simonson and Brozek[52] reported deterioration of the speed of action of the knee extensor muscles from a mean time of 102 msec in the normal state to a mean time of 130 msec in young men after a 6 month semi-starvation that reduced body weights to approximately 75% of the original weight. Forty-two days of nutritional rehabilitation providing 9·209 to 10·883 MJ/day produced a slight improvement in movement time, with an increased diet of 12·558 to 14·232 MJ/day in another group of subjects showing significant improvement. With undefined specific nutritional disorders and the probability of skeletal muscle protein cannibalisation for gluconeogenesis it is difficult to interpret the results specifically. Klopfer[53] starved subjects for 24 hr and found that perceptual thresholds were elevated. Champion and Field[54] studied subjects fasting 10 hr, 5hr and unfasted. Simple reaction times for the 10-hr fasted group were significantly slower than for the non-fasted group. The difference diminished with repeated assessments as the fasted groups approached the values for the control groups. Two methodological problems are presented by these studies on starvation and extended fasting. First, with awareness of having been starved, subjects' own expectations of performance deteriorations may result in poorer performance. Secondly, with short term assessment methods, subjects may arouse themselves[55] sufficiently to perform normally for the short period required.

Following exhaustion of CoH stores by extended hard physical work as described earlier, subjects have demonstrated emotional responses commonly associated with the hypoglycaemic state. Our subjects, described above, found the sound of a quiet room convector fan intolerably intrusive and had difficulty in focusing vision; Christensen and Hansen[7] noted perceptual disturbances at exhaustion in some subjects. The disturbances were removed in 10–15 min with glucose ingestion. This might be expected if, after exhaustion, values approaching 49 and 46 mg/100 ml for blood glucose (those reported for two subjects by Ahlborg *et al.*[22]) were obtained. Harris[56] reported that when blood glucose levels fall below approximately 75 mg/100 ml, weakness, irritability and fatigue result. Certainly values down to 60 mg/100 ml are commonly observed in extended hard physical work performance and, if study is made, objective evidence of performance decrements in delicate skills may be expected.

Blood glucose levels have been related to emotional responses and performance deteriorations in normal human beings. Psychomotor and affective changes are said to take place when the blood glucose level falls below approximately 70 mg/100 ml. In addition to Harris' work[56] and the emotional changes in marathon runners with low blood glucose,[17] Guetzkow *et al.*[57] observed a correlation of approximately 0·6 between motor reaction time and blood glucose level in the blood glucose range below 65–70 mg/100 ml. Other psychomotor tasks similarly related. In the blood glucose range above this level, test performance and blood glucose were not related.

Murrell[58] did not find a relationship between blood glucose levels raised by ingestion of glucose and rate of production, but this result is difficult to interpret for the post-meal blood glucose levels were initially extremely low in the approximate range 45–55 mg/100 ml. Three subjects were used. Studies in the 1930s had proposed a relationship between productivity or efficiency in workers and blood sugar levels (*e.g.* Haggard and Greenberg[59] and Goldberg[60]). The problem of experimental control is again raised. Novelty in a situation can itself produce an experimental effect in addition to or in the absence of an effect from the treatment variables causing the novelty. One of the classic experiments for this 'Hawthorne' effect was carried out by Roethlisberger and Dickson.[61] Often this problem was controlled inadequately in earlier studies. Commonly the problem is approached by introducing an additional treatment, not expected to have more than novelty effect, and assessing whether the true treatment attribute has a significantly greater effect than the 'control' treatment. However, care still must be taken, for if the 'novelty' response in the short term is likely to be of greater magnitude than the treatment response being searched for and these two do not sum arithmetically, it may mask a treatment effect that is genuine.

The effect on blood glucose levels of ingesting meals has been of much interest, most of it with reference to the clinical blood glucose tolerance test. McDonald *et al.*[62] have commented on the marked variation that occurs in subjects from test to test with replication of the glucose load and time of day. Assessing repeatedly 334 male prisoners, it was typical for peak values for a subject to vary by the mean ±34 mg/100 ml and more than 20% of the population showed variations outside this range. The replicability of the measuring, by Autoanalyser, was very adequate, the standard deviation of duplicates being 1·5 mg/100 ml. The variations were not related in that population to age, race, body weight or a family history of diabetes. There was a low significant correlation (+0·28) between level of fasting blood glucose and degree of individual variability. Such variations lead to the search for performance changes. There is little information documented. An aspect of the glucose load response of particular interest in this context is the undershoot on return to normal values (*see* Fig. 9 from the data of McDonald *et al.*[62]). There has been research upon the effect of feeding on this undershoot. Thornton and Horvath[63] showed, with one mixed meal of 3·139 MJ at breakfast, that 2½ hr later the blood glucose curve was slightly below the fasting level and 5 hr after eating was significantly lower. Providing a second similar meal after 5 hr resulted in a blood glucose level still above fasting $3\frac{1}{2}$ hr after the second meal, at which point it was significantly above the level for one meal alone. Haldi and Wynn[64] reported that high *vs* low CoH breakfasts had no effect on the blood glucose levels $2\frac{1}{2}$ hr later but the CoH load may have been insufficient, being 1·109 MJ and 427 kJ respectively. Mann *et al.*[65] report that oral glucose in comparison to sucrose clears

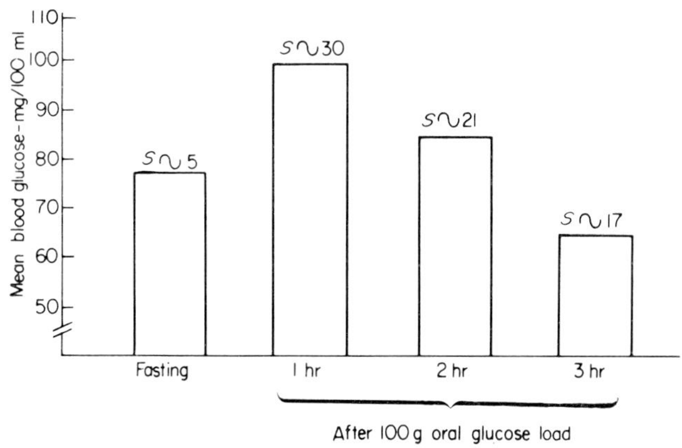

FIG. 9. Blood glucose levels for 334 men, taking 100 g oral glucose load (taken from data of McDonald *et al.*[62]).

the alimentary lipaemia faster and results in a higher blood glucose level and Cook[66] sees a similar result when comparing glucose with fructose loads. There is individuality in the degree of undershoot occurring, as D'Angelo[67] noted: this would be in keeping with Danowski's[47] suggestion of a continuum.

A further source of variation in the blood glucose response to CoH load is the circadian variation reported by Roberts[68] and explored by Jarrett *et al.*[69] Glucose tolerance is lowest in the afternoon and evening, a time when plasma insulin response is less. Jarrett *et al.* review circumstantial evidence to trace the rhythm to the cyclic variation in the activity of the Langerhans' cells. Roberts,[68] in addition, draws attention to the 'twilight biochemical zone' for blood glucose between 50 to 70 mg/100 ml, where hypoglycaemic reactions can be observed. Again it is noted that such levels are observed in normal human performance.

'Stress' from stimulus load may relate to blood sugar levels. Balser and Pacella[70] studied flying personnel with operational fatigue and in 38% found oral glucose tolerance tests with little peak and marked hypoglycaemic undershoot. Intravenous presentation did not show the effects, directing attention to gastric emptying.

Karlan and Cohn[71] reported intravenous load blood glucose tests on 100 soldiers with fatigue. Nine had low blood sugar values. Six of these showed flat curves, the other three rises in the first 30 min and falls in the remaining 90 min. Subjective experiences were of dizziness and nausea; being from intravenous loads, these responses could not be attributed to gastric problems. Frequent meals of complex CoHs and high protein alleviated the conditions. Bloom and Azor[72] report similar symptoms after two days CoH-free diet: the fatigue feelings were alleviated quickly by ingestion of 75 g CoH. Jarosz[73] observed the blood glucose level in patients about to receive lumbar punctures. Five categories of response were observed:

1. non-reactive—small variation,
2. normoglycaemic—slight rise, then fall,
3. hyperglycaemic—rise by 40–52 mg/100 ml,
4. hypoglycaemic—slight rise, then fall to approximately 55 mg/100 ml,
5. paradoxical—fall without initial rise.

This study provides a good indication of the complex sympathetico-hormonal events involved. We just do not know what performance changes occur with this or other life 'stressors'.

It is clear that there is a need to look for subtle changes in attention and the quality of performance in normal human beings in correlation with the range of blood glucose levels commonly occurring. It is equally clear that little sophisticated work is available at present.

Some of the isolated related information can be reviewed briefly. Hutchinson[74] summarises and criticises earlier work which resulted in an inconclusive position. The effects upon reaction times, maximum work rate, efficiency, grip power, etc., of missing breakfast, the studies of Tuttle and his co-workers, are reviewed by the Editor of *Nutrition Reviews.*[75] In the large majority of measures the effect of no breakfast or a very slight nutrient intake was seen in performance deterioration. The difficulty in interpretation is caused by the psychological effect of missing breakfast.

Richards[76] using repeated (five times) short duration tests of visual search, short term memory, coding and error vigilance, could not observe this effect, although there was a tendency for more improvement to occur in performance of three of the tests over a session when the normal breakfast routine was followed, whether this was to take or to omit the meal. However only short duration tests were used. Cass-Beggs and Emery[77] note individual differences in nutrient uptake of workers and suggest that this self-regulation may benefit physiological need and psychological state by alleviating monotony and fatigue. The article did not contain new data on the matter.

Two recent reports of interrelationship between CoH metabolism and error in normal performance are of interest. Proceeding from an initial survey of metabolic work load on foundrymen, Brooke *et al.*[78,79] identified low CoH utilisation by the workers in the early morning, established by dietary survey that slight or no breakfasts were being eaten (mean energy value 1·1 MJ, 700 kJ from CoH) and related this state to recorded accident incidence in the factory over a 16-month period. Significantly more accidents occurred in the morning than in the afternoon, with more in the pre-morning break *vs* post-morning break period. Subsequently, for an 18-week period, 58 men in the hot shops of the factory ingested in the early mornings either 500 ml GS drink with added salts, energy value 2·972 MJ, or 500 ml low energy fluid coloured similarly, energy value <40 kJ. The treatments to subjects were reversed so that each subject acting as his own control experienced a 4-week and a 5-week period on each treatment. Accident incidence for the period was analysed by treatments and time of occurrences. Significantly less accidents occurred under GS ingestion than under control fluid ingestion and the effect was predominantly upon the morning work period. The rate of accidents on the control fluid was similar to that recorded in the earlier survey. By far the highest rate of accidents was recorded in a group of 17 workers who refused to co-operate in the study, but whose records could still be analysed. It appears that there is a causative relationship between inadequate availability of CoH from transient malnutrition and performance error in the population. Thus it is of value to look for evidence of such transient malnutrition and concomitant performance changes in populations whose average carbohydrate and total energy intake is quite adequate over longer periods such as weeks or months.

Durnin[80] has already drawn attention to the marked variation in nutrition occurring in individuals from day to day.

The limited body weight change in this group of workers provided with additional energy intake is of interest. Over the course of the experiment the average increase in body weight was 0·36 kg SD 2·28 kg (non-sign. $p > \cdot 05$). This was in response to approximately 133·7 MJ additional nutrient energy over the 18 weeks. The energy was supplied through glucose syrup, however, and there are a number of reports that animals show less weight gain or adipose tissue deposits on glucose *vs* sucrose in isocaloric amounts; a difference was suggested by Higgins[81] and differences were observed by Feyder[82] with rats and Brook and Noel[83] with baboons. The matter should be clarified with a laboratory study on man.

The other recent concern about CoH intake and performance error has been over driving accidents on motorways. In the correspondence columns of the British Medical Journal, Frais[84] raised the problem of a possible relationship between aggressive driving and blood sugar level, extending the thought to question particularly the competence of the non-stabilised diabetic. Christian[85] then wrote pointing out that a number of lorry drivers crashing for no apparent reason into the centre reservations of the M4 showed very low blood sugar level in many cases and reported that they ate minimal or no breakfast. Subsequently, Leyshon *et al.*[86] commented on the inadequacy of vehicle driving licence application forms in screening out the unstable diabetic. They give details of a case study.

In conjunction with the work done in the foundry these reports raise an important general issue involved[87,88] in achieving optimal well being for normal human beings. In our own laboratories at present work progresses on the relationships between dietary carbohydrate availability, changes in human attention and repeated performances of delicate skills.

REFERENCES

1. Wood, F. (1970). In *Glucose Syrups and Related Carbohydrates*, ed. by G. G. Birch, L. F. Green and C. B. Coulson, Applied Science, London, pp. 93–103.
2. Pettenkofer, M. von and Voit, C. (1866). *Z. Biol.,* **2,** p. 537.
3. Åstrand, P. O. (1967). In *Nutrition and Physical Activity,* ed. by G. Blix, Almqvist & Wiksell, Uppsala.

4. Consolazio, C. F. and Johnson, H. L. (1972). *Am. J. Clin. Nutr.*, **25**, p. 85.
5. Cahill, G. F. and Owen, O. E. (1968). In *Carbohydrate Metabolism and its Disorders*, ed. by F. Dickens, P. J. Randle and W. J. Whelan, Vol. I, p. 497, Academic Press, London.
6. Friedberg, S. J., Harlon, W. R., Trout, D. L. and Estes, H. H. (1960). *J. Clin. Invest.*, **39**, p. 315.
7. Christensen, E. H. and Hansen, O. (1939). *Scand. Arch. Physiol.*, **81**, p. 137.
8. Pappenheimer, J. R. *et al.* (1950). *Fed. Proc.*, **9**, p. 602.
9. Carpenter, T. M. (1964). *Tables, Factors and Formulas for Computing Respiratory Exchange and Biological Transformations of Energy*, 4th Edn, Carnegie Institute, Washington.
10. Consolazio, C. F., Johnson, R. E. and Pecora, L. J. (1963). *Physiological Measurements of Metabolic Functions in Man*, McGraw-Hill, New York.
11. Diem, K. (1962). *Documenta Geigy, Scientific Tables,* 6th Edn, Geigy, Manchester.
12. Mayer, J. and Bullen, B. (1963). *Proc. Int. Congr. Nutr.*, **6**, p. 27.
13. Haldi, J. and Wynn, W. (1946). *Amer. J. Physiol.*, **145**, p. 402.
14. Taylor, A. W., Lappage, R. and Rao, S. (1971). *Med. Sci. Spt.*, **3**, 2, p. 75.
15. Clarke, D., De Jongh, T. W. and Jokl, E. (1943). *Manpower* (*Transvaal*), **1**, p. 30.
16. Krogh, A. and Lindhard, J. (1920). *Biochem. J.*, **14**, p. 290.
17. Levine, S. A., Gordon, B. and Derick, C. L. (1924). *J. Amer. Med. Ass.*, **81**, p. 1778.
18. Saltin, B. and Hermansen, L. (1967). In *Nutrition and Physical Activity*, ed. by G. Blix, Almqvist & Wiksell, Uppsala.
19. Brooke, J. D. and Green, L. F. (1972). *Proc. Nutr. Soc.*, in press.
20. Brooke, J. D. and Firth, M. S. (1973). *Br. J. Spt. Med.*, submitted for publication.
21. Bergström, J. and Hultman, E. (1966). *Scand. J. Clin. Lab. Invest.*, **18**, p. 16.
22. Ahlborg, B., Bergström, J., Ekelund, L. G. and Hultman, E. (1967). *Acta Physiol. Scand.*, **70**, p. 129.
23. Bergström, J. and Hultman, E. (1967). *Scand. J. Clin. Lab. Invest.*, **19**, p. 218.
24. Hultman, E. and Bergström, J. (1967). *Acta Med. Scand.*, **182**, 1, p. 109.
25. Brooke, J. D. (1970). In *Lung Function and Work Capacity*, ed. by J. D. Brooke, The University, Salford.
26. Rowell, L. R., Masoro, E. J. and Spencer, M. J. (1965). *J. Appl. Physiol.*, **20**, 5, p. 1032.
27. Costill, D. L., Kammer, W. F. and Fisher, A. (1970). *Arch. Environ. Health*, **21**, p. 520.
28. Bergström, J. and Hultman, E. (1967). *Acta Med. Scand.*, **182**, p. 93.
29. Karlsson, J. and Saltin, B. (1971). *J. App. Physiol.*, **31**, 2, p. 203.

30. McKechnie, J. K., Reid, J. V. O. and Joubert, S. M. (1970). *Sth Afr. Med. J.*, **44,** p. 728.
31. Adolfsson, S. and Ahren, K. (1971). In *Muscle Metabolism During Exercise*, Plenum, New York.
32. Costill, D. L., Bowers, R., Branam, G. and Sparks, K. (1971). *J. Appl. Physiol.*, **31,** 6, p. 834.
33. Wahren, J., Felig, P., Ahlborg, G. and Jorfeldt, L. (1971). *J. Clin. Invest.*, **50,** 12, p. 2715.
34. Carlson, L. A., Ekelund, L. and Fröberg, S. O. (1971). *Europ. J. Clin. Invest.*, **1,** p. 248.
35. Brooke, J. D., Davies, G. J. and Green, L. F. (1972). *Proc. Nutr. Soc.*, in press.
36. Nefzawi, S. (1963). *The Perfumed Garden*, translated by Sir Richard Burton, Spearman (Panther Ed.), London.
37. Birch, G. G., Green, L. F. and Coulson, C. B. (1970). *Glucose Syrups and Related Carbohydrates*, Applied Science, London.
38. Macdonald, I. (1967). *World Rev. Nutrition Dietetics*, **8,** p. 143.
39. Macdonald, I. (1971). In *Sugar. Chemical, Biological and Nutritional Aspects of Sucrose*, ed. by J. Yudkin, J. Edelman and L. Hough, Butterworth, London.
40. Dill, D. B., Edwards, H. T. and Talbott, J. H. (1933). *J. Physiol.* **77,** p. 4.
41. Fordtron, J. S. and Saltin, B. (1967). *J. Appl. Physiol.*, **23,** 3, p. 331.
42. Campbell, I. A. (1972). *Br. J. Spt. Med.*, **6,** 4, p. 108.
43. Brooke, J. D. and Green, L. F. (1973). *Proc. Nutr. Soc.*, submitted for publication.
44. Benade, A. J. S., Wyndham, C. H., Strydom, N. B. and Rogers, C. G. (1971). *Sth Afr. Med. J.*, **45,** 26, p. 711.
45. Goldsmith, R., Riddell, G. S., Russel, I. F., Sawyer, M. M. and Smith, R. B. (1971). *Proc. Nutr. Soc.*, **30,** 1, p. 4A.
46. Zierler, K. L., Moseri, A., Klassen, G., Rubinowitz, D. and Burgess, J. (1968). *Trans. Assoc. Am. Physns.*, **81,** p. 266.
47. Danowski, T. W. (1963). *Diabetes*, **12,** p. 183.
48. Heald, P. J., McIlwain, H. and Sloane-Stanley, G. H. (1960). In *Handbook of Physiology, Section I, Neurophysiology*, ed. by H. W. Magoun, Vol. 3, Amer. Physiol. Soc., Washington.
49. Sokolov, L. (1960). In *Handbook of Physiology, Section I, Neurophysiology*, ed. by H. W. Magoun, Vol. 3, Amer. Physiol. Soc., Washington.
50. Owen, O. E., Morgan, A. P., Kemp, H. G., Sullivan, J. M., Hernera, M. G. and Cahill, G. F. (1967). *J. Clin. Invest.*, **46,** p. 1589.
51. Zivin, J. A. and Snarr, J. F. (1972). *J. Appl. Physiol.*, **32,** 5, p. 664.
52. Simonson, E. and Brozek, J. (1946). *Fed. Proc.*, **5,** p. 96.
53. Klopfer, F. D. (1952). *Diss. Abstr.*, **12,** p. 382.
54. Champion, R. A. and Field, R. K. (1963). *Austr. J. Psychol.*, **15,** 3, p. 187.
55. Moray, N. (1969). *Attention: Selective Processes in Vision and Hearing*, Hutchinson, London.

56. Harris, S. (1933). *J. Amer. Med. Assoc.,* **101,** p. 1958.
57. Guetzkow, H., Taylor, H. L., Brozek, J. and Keys, A. (1945). *Fed. Proc.,* **4,** p. 28.
58. Murrell, H. (1971). *Occ. Psychol.,* **45,** p. 273.
59. Haggard, H. W. and Greenberg, L. A. (1935). *Diet and Physical Efficiency,* Yale University Press, New Haven.
60. Goldberg, A. P. *et al.* (1934). *Arbeitsphysiol.,* **8,** p. 134.
61. Roethlisberger, F. J. and Dickson, W. J. (1942). *Management and the Worker*, The University Press, Harvard.
62. McDonald, G. W., Fisher, G. F. and Burnham, C. (1965). *Diabetes,* **14,** p. 473.
63. Thornton, R. H. and Horvath, S. M. (1968). *J. Amer. Dietetic Ass.,* **52,** p. 214.
64. Haldi, J. and Wynn, W. (1945). *Fed. Proc.,* **4,** p. 29.
65. Mann, J. I., Truswell, A. S. and Pimstone, B. L. (1971). *Clin. Sci.,* **41,** 2, p. 123.
66. Cook, G. C. (1971). *Am. J. Clin. Nutr.,* **24**(11), p. 1302.
67. D'Angelo, S. (1945). *Amer. J. Physiol.,* **145,** p. 365.
68. Roberts, H. J. (1964). *J. Amer. Geriat. Soc.,* **12,** p. 423.
69. Jarrett, R. J., Baker, I. A., Keen, H. and Oakly, N. W. (1972). *Br. Med. J.,* **1,** 5794, p. 199.
70. Balser, B. H. and Pacella, B. L. (1945). *J. Nerv. Ment. Dis.,* **102,** p. 76.
71. Karlan, S. C. and Cohn, C. (1946). *J. Amer. Med. Assoc.,* **130,** p. 553.
72. Bloom, W. L. and Azor, G. J. (1963). *Arch. Int. Med.,* **112,** p. 333.
73. Jarosz, M. (1970). *Studia Psychol.,* **10,** p. 105.
74. Hutchinson, R. C. (1952). *Nutr. Abstr. Rev.,* **22,** p. 283.
75. Editor (1957). *Nutr. Rev.,* **15,** 7, p. 196.
76. Richards, M. M. C. (1972). *Nutrition,* **26,** 4, p. 219.
77. Cass-Beggs, R. and Emery, F. E. (1965). *Occ. Psychol.,* **39,** p. 247.
78. Brooke, J. D., Toogood, S., Green, L. F. and Bagley, R. (1972). *Proc. Nutr. Soc.,* in press.
79. Brooke, J. D., Toogood, S., Green, L. F. and Bagley, R. (1973). *Proc. Nutr. Soc.,* in press.
80. Durnin, J. V. C. A. (1957). *J. Physiol.,* **136,** 3, p. 34.
81. Higgins, H. L. (1919). *Amer. J. Physiol.,* **41,** p. 258.
82. Feyder, S. (1953). *J. Nutr.,* **9,** p. 457.
83. Brook, M. and Noel, P. (1969). *Nature,* **222,** p. 2562.
84. Frais, J. A. (1972). Letter to the Editor—multiple crashes on motorways, *Br. Med. J.,* 1st April.
85. Christian, M. S. (1972). Letter to the Editor—multiple crashes on motorways, *Br. Med. J.,* 29th April.
86. Leyshon, G. F., Elliott, R. W., Lyons, J. and Francis, H. W. S. (1972). Letter to the Editor—Diabetics and motoring crashes, *Br. Med. J.,* 12th May, p. 405.
87. Editor (1953). *Nutr. Rev.,* **11,** p. 239.
88. Margaria, R., Edwards, H. T. and Dill, D. B. (1933). *Amer. J. Physiol.,* **106,** p. 689.

DISCUSSION

Chairman: Your criterion in the theoretical part of your paper was ability to continue to work. RQ did not change. Is there any measure of efficiency?
Brooke: Yes, I haven't been able to put this in. Looking at the effects of adaptation due to repeated work and the effect of a glucose drink sustaining performance, in both cases the work is more efficient and it is more efficient to the degree that one cannot explain it by the RQ that resulted and therefore a little more energy is available per litre of oxygen. It is a measure of efficiency from oxygen utilisation and the external work required, and it can be a range. It is efficient because of carbohydrate availability.
Questioner: Is it carbohydrate that can be used directly?
Brooke: I think it has to be converted to glycogen. If one feeds glucose and muscle stores of glycogen are high it hasn't much effect, but when the muscle stores are low it is different.
Aminoff: What is the role of liver glycogen as compared to muscle glycogen in the endurance test reported?
Brooke: Muscle glycogen stores are far more important, from the Scandinavian work where direct measures were made.
Aminoff: Which glycogen store is depleted first? Is it the liver store?
Brooke: Liver stores are depleted later when local muscle stores are running down.
Aminoff: So for endurance, liver stores might be quite important?
Brooke: Yes, but when one feeds prior to work one is boosting local stores.
Green: It is to be noted that, in the Scandinavian work, although the muscle glycogen was reduced to a very low level, the blood glucose remained at 'normal' levels. This is quite an interesting point in relation to the question. Maybe the liver plays a part in keeping it normal.
Brooke: I have steered away from making reference to that at all because there is the situation where the glucose levels out at about 80 to 70 and changes continue to be seen in the RQ.
Macdonald: Were the endurance trials randomised and double blind?
Brooke: Yes, in both cases, they were randomised and they were double blind. The experimenters passing out drinks did not know what they were and the subjects would only have been able to tell what they were because carbohydrate has such a distinctive taste. They were given no indication by the experimenters. I was sceptical about the results I have tabled and about the recovery work in particular: they lay in a file for a couple of months before I sorted out what had happened on each of the days, and was very surprised when I saw it starting to come out as strongly as it did.
Greenwood: I think most of us don't take carbohydrate as glucose syrups. I wonder whether Dr Brooke was considering doing similar experiments with more conventional forms of carbohydrate, such as bread.
Brooke: The difficulty here is that one is feeding in quite high energy levels. In the work we were sustaining over hours we were feeding in 375 cals every hour for four hours, which I think would be a lot of bread.

Questioner: In our experiments remarkable results were achieved on a diet including bread.

Parker: In the experiments you described on physical work endurance performance, the comparison between the provision of isocaloric energy feeds, in the form of pure glucose solution and as sucrose sweetened rice pudding, obviously introduced a difference due to the rate of glucose absorption, which would be much greater in the case of pure glucose. Would you care to comment on this? I am presuming that rice pudding would not be digested and absorbed quite as rapidly as glucose fed directly.

Brooke: I think this is the immediate thought, that energy would not be made available as quickly and it was only a 40-minute period and had we left them an hour or an hour and a half the effect might have been equal. The fact that we got energy in so quickly is extremely useful when one turns to sportsmen. In Britain we have 12-hour and 24-hour time trial racing where men see how far they can ride and must not race closer than 10 yards to a competitor and they get a 'knock' and run out of carbohydrate, and some get pulled off by the coaches and some fall in a ditch. This is the sort of situation where to feed energy in quickly and in not too long a time begins to have an effect, would be extremely useful and would extend to other situations where exhaustion occurs.

Parker: Are you implying that there is a psychological effect as well? You mention people being irritable with low glucose levels.

Brooke: I think there is a central nervous effect. You know how difficult it is to identify a psychological effect. Any clinicians here will know there must be some twilight area between the normal state of a person and severe disturbance.

Macdonald: Would the ideal drink consist of fat and carbohydrate, carbohydrate for instant effect and fat for slower?

Brooke: I think it would depend on the intensity of the work. The difficulty with cyclists is that when these stores are exhausted they don't seem to be able to maintain that intensity of work just burning fat. There is body fat available if one drops the load down so they work at 50% of capacity, they can burn body fat with a low RQ, but if you hold the work at 75% of the maximum they can't do this.

Nicol: Can your findings on physical effort be transferred to the field of mental stress with particular reference to airline pilots and company management?

Brooke: This appears in work about factory accidents. It isn't a physical work effect, I think it must be a central nervous one. It appears there is this relationship coming out between accidents and error and low carbohydrate availability for a short period of time. We have a setup and have people working in the lab on mentally demanding tasks and getting them up to maximum capacity performance and are manipulating the carbohydrate availability.

Chairman: This reflects the experiments by Mills on breakfast 25 years ago. Animals and children with no breakfast were below maximum capacity and with a small breakfast they improved. This was the same idea, a mental effect as well as a physical.

16

Carbohydrate Intolerance

H. B. McMichael

Middlesex Hospital, London, England

ABSTRACT

In normal man, the rate of digestion and absorption of carbohydrates is limited by the mucosal cell membrane transport of monosaccharides. Genetically determined defects arise in the hydrolysis of lactose, sucrose and trehalose, and in the transport of glucose and galactose. The osmolarity of ingested food affects its rate of transit through the bowel and therefore may influence total absorption.

All the stages of carbohydrate absorption are impaired in malnourished subjects, and this is particularly a problem in the treatment of such children in the developing countries. The hydrolysis of lactose is particularly impaired. By utilising different modes of digestion and absorption, and perhaps also because of their different subsequent metabolism, there may be an important role for sucrose and fat as calorie sources in these subjects. Benefits may be expected from continuous nasogastric tube feeding. Some features of carbohydrate foods which are desirable from the absorption viewpoint will be discussed.

Intolerance of ingested carbohydrates has two aspects. First, unabsorbed carbohydrate causes diarrhoea, abdominal distension and pain.[1] Secondly, impaired absorption may be nutritionally important. Significant nutritional disturbance rarely results in Western societies, where other energy sources are easily available. However, in less affluent societies carbohydrate intolerance is usually associated with malnutrition,[2] so that problems arise in using this cheap form of nutrition for those whose need is great.

In order to examine the problems constructively, we must first consider the physiology of carbohydrate digestion and absorption, in particular which stage of the process is rate-limiting.

RATE-LIMITING FACTORS IN CARBOHYDRATE DIGESTION AND ABSORPTION

Starch is hydrolysed in the intestinal lumen to maltose, maltotriose and α-limit dextrins by pancreatic amylase. This stage is extremely efficient,[3] but its functions can also be performed by the hydrolytic enzymes localised to the brush-border of the intestinal mucosal cells. Patients who have had the entire pancreatic gland removed are still able to absorb large amounts of carbohydrate.[4] There is no evidence that pancreatic dysfunction ever limits carbohydrate digestion and absorption, although pancreatic enzyme output is impaired in malnourished subjects.[5]

Starch breakdown products and ingested disaccharides are hydrolysed by γ-carbohydrases at the lumen–mucosal cell interface.[6] These enzymes can be readily assayed, using disaccharides as substrates,[7] on pieces of human intestinal mucosa which can be easily obtained by peroral biopsy techniques.[8] There is no correlation between the intestinal mucosal disaccharidase activity and the rate of absorption of the appropriate disaccharide in normal subjects.[3,9] Furthermore, the rates of absorption of sucrose[10] and maltose[11] have been compared directly with those for the component monosaccharides, and equal results obtained. The comparable data on lactose[12] are unfortunately difficult to interpret, since they were done in a racial group with a high incidence of lactase deficiency, and the authors' definition of lactase deficiency was an arbitrary one. The wide standard deviation of their results strongly suggests that lactase-deficient subjects were inadvertently classified as 'normal'. It would appear that the disaccharidases do not limit carbohydrate absorption in the normal subject.

The cell membrane transport of monosaccharides is the crucial phase limiting absorption rates in the normal subject.

There are probably three monosaccharide transport systems, besides simple diffusion (which is very minor and probably of no nutritional importance). The 'glucose–galactose pump' has been extensively studied *in vitro*[13] but relatively little work has been done *in vivo*, particularly in man. Holdsworth and Dawson[14] studied monosaccharide absorption by a steady-state intestinal perfusion system in conscious man and found no inhibition of glucose absorption by galactose. I have recently confirmed this finding in the jejunum of anaesthetised rats,[15] but galactose markedly inhibits glucose absorption in the ileum. Other findings are that uranyl nitrate and phlorizin inhibit glucose and galactose differentially. The results suggest that there are probably two transport systems for glucose, only one of which is shared by galactose. The third system is that apparently used only by fructose.[16] Its existence has been demonstrated *in vivo*[14,17] and *in vitro*.[18]

Optimal carbohydrate absorption in stress situations is likely to be achieved by using all three systems.

SPECIFIC ENZYME AND CARRIER DEFECTS

Congenital, genetically determined defects affect sucrase, lactase,[19] trehalase,[20] and the 'glucose–galactose carrier.'[21] These are all rare and, provided they are diagnosed, are simply treated by avoidance of the appropriate foods.

By contrast, many human adults (in common with most other mature mammals) have a greatly reduced mucosal lactase activity.[22] In this situation, the disaccharidase becomes rate-limiting for absorption and 'intolerance' arises, with varying severity of symptoms.[9] Although ingestion of milk persistently from infancy may delay the regression of lactase, it does not prevent it in the majority of susceptible subjects.[23] Furthermore, prolonged lack of lactose ingestion does not produce lactose intolerance.[24] Racial groups with reduced lactase activity in adulthood include virtually all those in which malnutrition occurs endemically.

The lactase activity in these subjects is, however, reduced rather than absent,[25] even when using an assay technique which measures the brush-border lactase separately from the intracellular β-galactosidases.[26] These subjects are able to absorb some lactose, as evidenced both by direct perfusion studies[11] and elevation of blood sugar after lactose ingestion.[9] Their capacity to absorb lactose is approximately 25% of normal.[9,11]

IMPORTANCE OF DIETARY OSMOLARITY

Few direct studies on dietary osmolarity have been performed. It has been shown that the contents of the bowel are essentially isotonic with respect to body fluids from the upper small intestine to the rectum.[27–29] Adverse effects of hyperosmolar feeds have been observed in the so-called 'dumping syndrome'[30] and during attempts at jejunal feeding.[31] I recently treated a patient who had had a resection of her ileum. During dietary manipulations, her daily number of bowel actions was reduced from 12 to 4 by replacing her carbohydrate source of a glucose-containing mixture by bread and potatoes. Further evidence of the effect of osmolarity and transit rate on absorption is seen in the comparison of the blood sugar rise after lactose and after equivalent amounts of glucose plus galactose. Monosaccharides, with a greater osmotic effect, evidently pass more rapidly over a greater area of intestine, resulting in a higher and earlier blood sugar rise compared with that after lactose.[9] While this may be of no importance in normal subjects, those with a reduced intestinal reserve capacity for absorption (*e.g.* subjects with malnutrition) may absorb less monosaccharide because of the rapid transit. Furthermore, the intralumenal sugar concentration is influenced.

A numerical example may clarify these points. A carbohydrate meal of 100 g glucose would be diluted in the small intestine to a carbohydrate concentration of about 3·3 g/100 ml in approximately 3 litres electrolyte solution (assuming a typical intrajejunal Na^+ concentration of 50 mEq/litre). A comparable meal of maltose would result in only half the volume of fluid, providing less stimulus for peristalsis, and the concentration of carbohydrate would be higher, predictably resulting in a higher rate of absorption per unit segment of gut.[11]

RATE-LIMITING FACTORS IN MALNOURISHED SUBJECTS

The structure of the small intestine is abnormal in malnourished subjects.[32] The rate of glucose absorption is reduced in subjects with damaged small intestine,[33] including those with malnutrition.[2] Malabsorption of ingested carbohydrate is evidently an important factor in the diarrhoea of these subjects,[34] which accords with its dominant dietary osmotic role. Mucosal damage depresses all disaccharidases, but depresses lactase activity more than the other disaccharidases, both in subjects not susceptible to lactase regression[35] and in malnourished children susceptible to lactase regression.[36] This effect on disaccharidases is not surprising, in view of their extremely rapid turnover during the maturation of the intestinal mucosal cell.[37]

James[2] has demonstrated by direct perfusion studies that absorption of lactose is impaired in malnourished children to a greater degree than absorption of glucose, so that lactase activity appears to become rate-limiting. The relevance of this to diarrhoea has been shown by the studies of Prinsloo and colleagues.[38] They demonstrated that faecal weight was greatly increased by administration of lactose, but not by exchange of other disaccharides and glucose. It was observed, however, that the diarrhoea associated with lactose ingestion did not appear to harm the children, at least as determined by the rise in serum albumin level during therapy. This raises important questions as to the role of carbohydrates in malnutrition, and, speculatively, whether stimulation of insulin by carbohydrate ingestion may have disadvantageous effects.

POSSIBLE ADVANTAGES OF FAT AND SUCROSE

The following observations are prompted in part by those of Prinsloo and colleagues,[38] and in part by recent observations on two severely malnourished adults treated by me.

Subject A

This patient had a massive resection of his small intestine, and was slowly dying of malnutrition, in spite of numerous dietary manipulations. We decided to give him energy supplements intravenously, while maintaining his oral ingestion of protein. While receiving 500 g glucose/day intravenously for two weeks his serum albumin dropped from 2·0 to 1·0 g/100 ml, with an equivalent deterioration in the clinical state. This suggested that uptake of amino acids into his skeletal tissues, stimulated by insulin, might be resulting in a relative decrease of protein available for hepatic synthesis.

Subject B

This patient had an oesophageal stricture with severe malnutrition. She also had renal disease, so that we were cautious in our administration of protein supplements. While on intravenous therapy with 300 g glucose and 7 g nitrogen, her albumin dropped from 2·0 to

1·0 g/100 ml. We then gave her the identical mixture through a tube directly into the stomach. Her albumin rose to 3·0 g/100 ml, with appropriate clinical improvement. This appears to demonstrate the importance of site of maximal protein uptake in malnourished subjects.

Two energy foods which do not stimulate insulin secretion (and therefore would not stimulate non-hepatic use of amino acids) are fats and fructose. The latter may cause a lactic acidosis[39] unless given with some glucose,[40] suggesting the use of sucrose. Furthermore, administration of sucrose would enable the fructose carrier to be utilised. Since fat does not require any specific carrier across the lipid cell membrane, its use may be appropriate provided steatorrhoea is not present. Slowing of intestinal transit by use of appropriate carbohydrates (and use of non-osmolar fat) may facilitate fat absorption.

ROLE OF CONTINUOUS TUBE FEEDING

The advantages of continuous feeding throughout 24 hours are obvious in subjects with malabsorption problems, yet such feeding has rarely been used in clinical practice. By utilising the absorptive capacity of the 8 hours of the night, we were able to raise the serum albumin level of subject A (described above) to 3·7 g/100 ml and he was able to leave hospital fit to walk 2 kilometres and to drink with his friends. No complications have been observed during such continuous feeding regimes in 15 subjects. Using a tube of only 1 mm internal diameter, patient discomfort is minimal.

THE IDEAL FOOD FOR MALNOURISHED SUBJECTS

The ideal food should utilise all the available absorptive pathways, should be of low osmolarity, should not stimulate excessive insulin release and should be available in some form appropriate for administration throughout the 24 hours via a fine nasogastric tube.

The ideal carbohydrate from the osmolarity aspect would be maltotriose, since this would not be hydrolysed by pancreatic amylase. But starch is nearly as good after hydrolysis, and 'better' during the short period prior to its hydrolysis. In practice, any maltodextrin or starch mixture, solubilised if necessary, is satisfactory provided it contains little free glucose.

The food should contain sucrose to take advantage of the fructose carrier and to reduce insulin stimulation. Fat should be present for similar reasons. If medium chain triglycerides could be produced cheaply, they might be particularly useful.

In the absence of data I am reluctant to suggest the ratio of these foodstuffs, but I think I ought to attempt this. Since the capacity to absorb glucose is greater than that for fructose, I think a ratio (by weight) of 2 maltodextrin to 1 sucrose may be appropriate (*i.e.* 3 glucose to 1 fructose), and that up to half the maltodextrin could be replaced by lactose. Fat may perhaps provide half as much energy as carbohydrate.

To tabulate as percentage of energy source:

Fat (? some medium chain triglyceride)	33%
Sucrose	22%
Lactose	(up to) 22%
Maltodextrins	(remainder, *e.g.* 23%)

The protein content will be between 15% and 30% of the total weight. The sodium content should not be high, since this increases the osmolarity, and malnourished subjects are often oedematous, with raised total body sodium content.

SUMMARY

In normal man, the rate of digestion and absorption of carbohydrates is limited by the mucosal cell membrane transport of monosaccharides. Genetically determined defects arise in the hydrolysis of lactose, sucrose and trehalose, and in the transport of glucose and galactose. The osmolarity of ingested food affects its rate of transit through the bowel and therefore may influence total absorption.

All the factors concerned with carbohydrate absorption are impaired in malnourished subjects, and this is particularly a problem in the treatment of such children in the developing countries. The hydrolysis of lactose is particularly impaired. By utilising different modes of digestion and absorption, and perhaps also because of their lesser effect in stimulating insulin release, there may be an important role for sucrose and fat as energy sources in these subjects. Benefits may be expected from continuous nasogastric tube feeding. An attempt has been made to suggest optimal sources of food energy.

REFERENCES

1. McMichael, H. B., Webb, J. and Dawson, A. M. (1965). *Lancet,* **I,** p. 717.
2. James, W. P. T. (1968). *Lancet,* **I,** p. 333.
3. McMichael, H. B. (1971). *Proc. Nutr. Soc.,* **30,** p. 248.
4. Gaston, E. A. (1948). *New Engl. J. Med.,* **238,** p. 345.
5. Nutrition Reviews (1969). *Nutr. Rev.,* **27,** p. 100.
6. Johnson, C. F. (1969). *Fed. Proc.,* **28,** p. 26.
7. Dhalqvist, A. (1968). *Anal. Biochem.,* **22,** p. 99.
8. Crosby, W. H. and Kugler, H. W. (1957). *Amer. J. digest. Dis.,* **2,** p. 236.
9. McMichael, H. B. (1972). *Acta Hepatogastroenterologica,* **19,** p. 281.
10. Gray, G. M. and Ingelfinger, F. J. (1966). *J. clin. Invest.,* **45,** p. 388.
11. McMichael, H. B., Webb, J. and Dawson, A. M. (1967). *Clin. Sci.,* **33,** p. 135.
12. Gray, G. M. and Santiago, N. A. (1966). *Gastroenterology,* **51,** p. 489.
13. Crane, R. K. (1968). *Handbook of Physiology,* Section 6, Vol. III, ed. by C. F. Code, Amer. Phys. Soc., p. 1323.
14. Holdsworth, C. D. and Dawson, A. M. (1964). *Clin. Sci.,* **27,** p. 371.
15. McMichael, H. B. (1973). *Gut,* in press.
16. McMichael, H. B. (1971). *Proc. International Symposium on the Clinical and Metabolic Aspects of Laevulose,* Calmic Ltd, England, p. 91.
17. Holdsworth, C. D. and Dawson, A. M. (1965). *Proc. Soc. exptl. biol. Med.,* **118,** p. 42.
18. Gracey, M., Burke, V. and Oshin, A. (1972). *Biochim. biophys. Acta,* **266,** p. 397.
19. Rey, J. and Frezal, J. (1967). *Arch. franc. Ped.,* **24,** p. 65.
20. Bergoz, R. (1971). *Gastroenterology,* **60,** p. 909.
21. Meeuwisse, G. and Melin, K. (1969). *Acta paed. scand. Suppl.,* **188,** p. 3.
22. Simoons, F. J. (1969). *Amer. J. digest. Dis.,* **14,** p. 819.
23. Bolin, T. D. and Davis, A. E. (1970). *Aust. Ann. Med.,* **19,** p. 40.
24. Kogut, M. D., Donnell, G. N. and Shaw, K. N. F. (1967). *J. Paed.,* **71,** p. 75.
25. Asp, N-G., Berg, N. O., Dhalqvist, A., Jussila, J. and Salmi, H. (1971). *Scand. J. Gastroent.,* **6,** p. 755.
26. Asp, N-G. and Dhalqvist, A. (1972). *Anal. Biochem.,* **47,** p. 527.
27. Elias, B., Gibson, G. J., Greenwood, L. F., Hunt, J. N. and Tripp, J. H. (1968). *J. Physiol.,* **194,** p. 317.
28. Fordtran, J. S. and Locklear, T. W. (1966). *Amer. J. digest. Dis.,* **11,** p. 503.

29. Wilson, D. R., Ing, T. S., Metcalfe-Gibson, A. and Wrong, O. M. (1968). *Clin. Sci.,* **34,** p. 211.
30. Sessions, R. T., Reynolds, V. H., Ferguson, J. L. and Scott, H. W. (1962). *Surgery,* **52,** p. 266.
31. Masterton, J. P., Dudley, H. A. and MacRae, S. (1963). *Brit. med. J.,* **II,** p. 909.
32. Stanfield, J. P., Hutt, M. S. R. and Tunicliffe, R. (1965). *Lancet,* **II,** p. 519.
33. Holdsworth, C. D. and Dawson, A. M. (1965). *Gut,* **6,** p. 387.
34. Bowie, M. D., Barbezat, G. O. and Hansen, J. D. L. (1967). *Amer. J. clin. Nutr.,* **20,** p. 89.
35. McMichael, H. B., Webb, J. and Dawson, A. M. (1966). *Brit. med. J.,* **II,** p. 1037.
36. Cook, G. C. and Lee, F. D. (1966). *Lancet,* **II,** p. 1263.
37. James, W. P. T., Alpers, D. H., Gerber, J. F. and Isselbacher, K. J. (1971). *Biochim. biophys. Acta,* **230,** p. 194.
38. Prinsloo, J. G., Wittmann, W., Pretorius, P. J., Kruger, H. and Fellingham, S. A. (1969). *Arch. Dis. Childh.,* **44,** p. 593.
39. Schebjami, H. and Scalettar, R. (1971). *Lancet,* **II,** p. 366.
40. Harries, J. T. (1972). *Parenteral Nutrition,* ed. by A. W. Wilkinson, Churchill Livingstone, Edinburgh, p. 268.

DISCUSSION

Birch: Going back to Bergosz's experiment on mushroom intolerance, if mushrooms contain 1% trehalose you would need 1 kg of mushrooms to receive 10 g of carbohydrate which I venture to suggest is the minimum quantity required to elicit symptoms of intolerance.

McMichael: Yes, there are some doubts about this work but Bergosz did carry out a trehalose tolerence test. Concerning your earlier point about whether trehalase is the carrier, amphibia have high trehalase activity (perhaps associated with high trehalose intake from insect haemolymph, etc.) and they do not transport monosaccharides at a particularly high rate.

Birch: My original query stemmed from Sacktor's work (*Biochim. Biophys. Res. Comm.* 1969, **35,** p. 796) which demonstrated the involvement of trehalase in kidney sugar transport.

Barnett: I would like to contest the relative roles of α-amylase and the amylase activity due to the brush-border maltose, that is, that the salivary and pancreatic α-amylase is not important. Dr McMichael cites the digestion of starch in pancreatectomy as evidence, but even in pancreatectomy (removal of the pancreas) the salivary α-amylase remains, and a high proportion of the starch molecules are partially broken down by the enzyme before the enzyme is inactivated in the stomach because it remains active within the food bolus. Human salivary amylase activity is very variable but the mean activity is about 1 g of maltose equivalents produced from 1% amylose.

McMichael: The pancreatic amylase activity is very much greater than that of saliva, and I suspect its role is trivial especially as it is inactivated by gastric acid.

Barnett: If there are two major glucose carriers, how does Dr McMichael explain the complete loss of glucose absorption in the glucose/galactose malabsorption syndrome?

McMichael: There are two possibilities. Perhaps there is one carrier with two carrier sites. Alternatively, absence of the 'high K_m' glucose carrier may be very common and trouble arises when both mechanisms are absent simultaneously. This would also offer an explanation for 'carbohydrate-induced dyspepsia'.

Parker: Since you advocate minimising insulin stimulation in cases of severe malnutrition, why do you advocate the inclusion of maltotriose in an idealised diet, in addition to sucrose, rather than using all sucrose as the energy source?

McMichael: It is not going to be all one or the other. Sucrose has higher assimilability. I think there is some very definite role for some sucrose, that is all.

Pawan: Is there any difference in the age at which the appearance of acquired lactase deficiency is seen between well-nourished and protein-deficient children in those racial or ethnic groups in which lactase deficiency is prevalent?

McMichael: Although lactase activity is severely depressed by malnutrition, Cook and James have both shown that it recovers fairly well. Presumably it then regresses at the expected age.

Grenby: Why does Dr McMichael advocate medium-chain triglycerides in his 'ideal diet'? This might mean patients would not get their requirements of essential fatty acids.

McMichael: I agree that essential fatty acids must be given and would not suggest complete replacement with medium-chain triglycerides. I suggest medium-chain triglycerides because there are problems of fat absorption in these subjects and a medium-chain triglyceride does not require bile salts or micelle formation. It might therefore be of use.

Stock: Continuing on the role of salivary amylase, it has been suggested that its action in digestion is incidental and its main function is to keep the teeth clean. Is this at all possible?

McMichael: I don't know. But I do wonder if it may be related to taste. Long-chain amylose is unpleasant and tasteless but potatoes are slightly sweet. I wonder if this is partial hydrolysis by salivary amylases to aid taste.

Chairman: I suggest lactase is difficult to produce and, in some races, we do not bother to produce it.

McMichael: Yes, there is evidence that lactase is one of the larger disaccharidases. A very interesting hypothesis is that lactase was retained into adulthood in those racial groups where protein deficiency was likely to inhibit performance and where milk was available.

Macdonald: Would you like to speculate why milk sugar is lactose?

McMichael: One of the things about this is, if you feed children on human breast milk, which contains 7% lactose, they flourish, but if you give them cow's milk without it, they suffer and get constipation.

Chairman: Has lactase deficiency been long known?

McMichael: Since 1889.

Chairman: If you have patients with fever you can save them with lactose.

Grenby: What is the significance of Dr McMichael's measurements of serum albumin? Is it a measure of health or malnutrition?

McMichael: The serum albumin is usually low in severe cases of protein malnutrition and increases as the patient improves. Mild malnutrition may exist with a normal albumin. It is also affected by hepatic and renal disease.

17

Indigestible Constituents of Cereals and Other Foodstuffs

N. FISHER

Flour Milling and Baking Research Association, Chorleywood, Herts., England

ABSTRACT

The chemical composition of the indigestible constituents of foodstuffs will be discussed in relation to the 'crude fibre' values usually reported in the literature. The scope and limitations of crude fibre determinations, especially when applied to materials with very low concentrations of indigestible carbohydrates and lignins, will be outlined, stressing the need for better analytical techniques.

The effect of milling techniques on the fibre content of flours is discussed from an historical as well as from a technological viewpoint.

As bran is the major source of the indigestible material in wheat, the present state of knowledge of the composition of wheat bran will be reviewed.

FIBRE CONTENT, ITS LEGAL BASIS AND ITS DETERMINATION

The so-called fibre content of foodstuffs usually refers to the heterogeneous residue obtained after treatment of the food with hot acid and hot alkali under various sets of conditions that may, or may not, be standardised for that particular material, and may therefore give widely different results. In the UK, a method with a legal status is described in a Statutory Instrument.[1] This publication declares (p. 75) 'For the purposes of the Fertilisers and Feeding Stuffs Act, 1926, "fibre"* means the organic matter calculated as the result of

* Not 'crude fibre', a term of uncertain meaning!

treatment of the feeding stuff according to the method described in para 7:2', where the procedure is described in some detail. In this country, the method appears to be the only one laid down by law for certain specified animal feedstuffs which include beet pulp, decorticated oil cake and the by-products of cereal milling. By the same Act, the fibre content of these feedstuffs must be declared by the seller; the actual analytical figure must not exceed the stated figure by more than 1/8th, nor fall below half of its value. The current Statutory Instrument[2] also refers to fibre as meaning the organic matter contained in the dried, defatted residue obtained by digesting a sample of flour or of bread successively with boiling acid and boiling alkali. The fibre content of brown, or of wheatmeal, bread must contain not less than 0·6% of fibre on a dry weight basis. The method to be used is presumably that recognised by the Feeding Stuffs Act. The legal standing of fibre determinations on foods not specified by these Acts is thus less certain.

REPLICABILITY OF FIBRE DETERMINATION

In principle, the procedure used for determination of fibre dates back many years, but the conditions of the test have been modified at various times to improve its replicability between operators and laboratories—an important requirement for a test carrying legal sanctions. It still involves procedures difficult to control precisely, *e.g.* vigour and temperature of boiling, and conditions of filtration. Nevertheless, in experienced hands and with suitable samples, reasonable agreement can be obtained: in a collaborative study organised by the Analytical Methods Committee of the Society of Public Analysts in 1943[3] involving thirteen experienced analysts in seven laboratories, using a sample of high-extraction flour, the declared means for the seven laboratories ranged from 0·86–0·94% about 0·90%, with a coefficient of variation of 3·0%. A similar level of error of determination between laboratories for a well-cleaned wheat bran of fibre content 11% would introduce a standard error of ±0·3% and an uncertainty of ±0·7% in the final declaration. However, it would be expected that for white flour the coefficient of variation would be much higher; reported values of fibre less than 0·1% are clearly of dubious worth.

DISTRIBUTION OF FIBRE WITHIN CEREAL GRAIN STRUCTURES

Most of the fibre of cereals stems from the relatively indigestible, outermost, protective coats of the grain (Fig. 1[4] and Table 1[5,6]), whereas the endosperm, which is almost, although not entirely, digestible, gives a very low fibre figure (0·1–0·2% in the case of white wheaten flour). Thus the husk of the oat grain, which comprises about 30% of its weight, has a fibre content[5] of about 36% (at 4·6% moisture content) and is almost completely indigestible. It is, indeed, an excellent abrasive, but it is easily removed during the milling

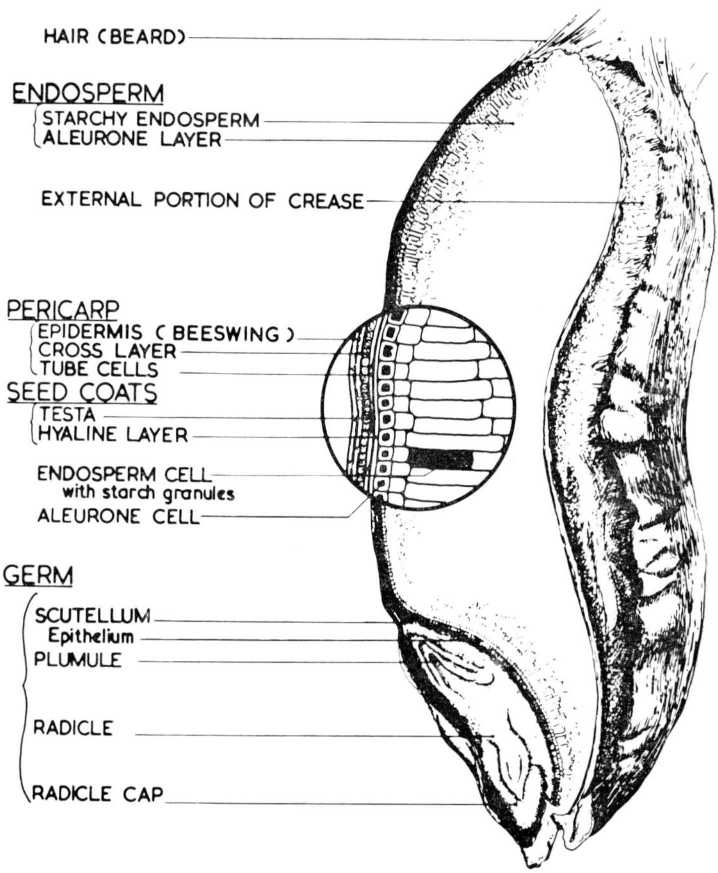

FIG. 1. Longitudinal section of wheat grain through crease and germ.

operation, because it is not attached to the endosperm, as it is in barley.[5] Furthermore, the removal of the oat husk, or hull, by shelling has been a traditional feature of the milling of oatmeal in Britain for many generations. The groat, or inner kernel, of the oat grain, on the other hand, is not a rich source of crude fibre, of which it has only about 1%,[5] most of which is also associated with its thin branny covering, or pericarp. Wheat, after removal of the loose fibrous glumes by the farmer at harvest, has a much lower fibre content, about 2·0%,[7] than either oats or barley.

TABLE 1

Approximate anatomical distribution of the 'crude fibre' of the wheat grain

Tissue	Weight % of grain	Crude fibre content (% of total in grain)
Bran	14	93
Endosperm	83	4
Germ	3	3

In cereal products, the fibre figures are thus roughly proportional, though not equal, to the amount of the outer integuments present. Thus in oat husk the factor is only about one-third, and in wheat about one-seventh because its pericarp is much less resistant than oat husk to the action of the hot acid and alkali of the fibre determination. But undoubtedly a major purpose of the test was, and still is, to place limits upon the excessive and deliberate dilution of feedstuffs with less-digestible, fibrous plant-residues of lower economic value. More recent techniques have involved extraction with detergents,[8,9] or with solvents,[10] and have given results, in the former case, approximating to the actual contents-free weight of the outer layers of the grain.

FIBRE AND THE INDIGESTIBLE MATTER IN FOOD

Irrespective of the precision or accuracy of the determination of fibre, it is legitimate to question whether the result represents the true level of indigestible matter in the food analysed. Determinations of digestibility of such foods show that the true values are often

TABLE 2
Digestibility of bread made from flours of varying extraction rates and fibre contents[11,12]

% Extraction	75	85	90	95	100
% Crude fibre	0·15	0·3	0·8	1·4	2·0
% Digestibility[a]	97·0	93·9	91·5	88·7	86·3
% Indigestible matter	3·0	6·1	8·5	11·3	13·7

[a] Human studies.

considerably higher than those indicated by the crude fibre values (Table 2).

Later work by McCance and Walsham[13] on the digestibility of wholemeal bread gave somewhat higher values of 88–89%.

Clearly, the crude fibre is considerably lower than the indigestible material, and this must be borne in mind when using such values obtained from food composition tables. For wheatmeal fibre values above 0·15%—at which figure the fibre is chiefly due to endosperm cell wall material—an increase of 0·1% in fibre depresses digestibility by about 0·55%,[13] but the factor is likely to vary very widely according to the nature of the fibre and its source.

Another interesting feature of the work of McCance and Walsham[13] on the digestibility of wholemeal bread by human volunteers is their estimate of the percentage of the fibre broken down in its passage through the alimentary canal. The means obtained, 23·4% for Canadian wheat (2·64% N) and 21·6% for English wheat (1·46% N), are not statistically distinguishable (p approx 20%) despite the widely different natures of the two types of wheat in protein content and breadmaking quality.

In more recent work, with more varied diets, Southgate and Durnin[14] found that some 13–15% of the cellulose ingested did not appear in the faeces. Correspondingly, with pentosan (hemicellulose) intakes of about 7 g/day, some 95% failed to appear, whilst for higher intakes (13·5–23 g/day) 72–85% was lost.

THE COMPOSITION OF THE INDIGESTIBLE MATTER IN FOOD

The constituents of the indigestible matter comprise two main classes of compound, the 'unavailable carbohydrates', consisting of cellulose, hemicelluloses, gums and pectins, and the lignins, phenylpropane derivatives originating from aromatic amino acids such as phenylalanine and tyrosine. The method of Southgate[15] for the determination of the amounts of these individual constituents in foodstuffs is a time-consuming task of removal of starch using amylolytic enzymes, and water-soluble sugars using solvent extraction, and successive treatments with acid and ethanol to separate the hemicelluloses and cellulose. The gums and pectins, etc. are separately determined in the hot water-soluble fractions of the defatted, sugar-free sample after removal of any soluble starch. Fraser *et al.*[16] earlier used a

TABLE 3
Pentosan and cellulose contents of various flours

Extraction %	Pentosan %	Cellulose %
80	2·4	0·6
93	3·2	2·8
100	4·0	4·2

combination of amylolytic and proteolytic enzymes and colorimetry and polarimetric methods in their determinations of pentosan and cellulose contents of flours. Table 3, compiled from their (1956) data, shows the pentosan and cellulose contents of flours of 80 %, 93 % and 100 % extraction.

Subsequent results of Fraser and Holmes published in 1959,[17] are compared with those of more recent workers[15,18] in Table 4.

TABLE 4
Comparison of unavailable carbohydrate values in wholewheat flour
(14 % Moisture basis)

	Fraser and Holmes %	Southgate[a] %	Kowalski and Pierkarska % (adjusted to 14 % moisture basis)
Cellulose } Lignins }	4·2	1·2 } 2·8 } 4·0	1·5 } 0·7 } 2·2
Hemicelluloses	6·0	7·6	2·8

[a] Concentrations in residue insoluble in 85 % as methanol: not substantially changed in the original foodstuff.

The discrepancies between the estimates of the different groups of workers are very wide, particularly for the hemicelluloses, and emphasise the need for more convenient methods with greater reliability. A new method for the determination of lignin in forage crops has recently appeared,[19] and is being tested for its applicability to flour and wheat.

THE COMPOSITION OF WHEAT BRAN

Although endosperm cell walls contribute to the cellulose and hemicellulose contents of wheat (the miller does not separate them from the endosperm), the bran is the major source of these materials. Table 5 shows the approximate composition of commercial bran

TABLE 5
Composition of commercial bran

	%		%
Cellulose and lignin	22	Phytin (organic part)	2·0
Hemicellulose	25		
Protein	9·5	Lipid	5·2
Starch	8·5	Sugars	5·0
Ash	5·7	Moisture	14·0

(literature sources[20,21] and FMBRA determinations) which usually contains 10% or more of adherent endosperm. To the best of our knowledge, complete separation of bran and endosperm can be achieved only by manual dissection.

The major hemicellulose in the outer two layers of the bran contains (approx.) arabinose (51%), xylose (39%) and glucuronic acid (9%).[22]

The composition of the total hemicelluloses of bran and germ has been reported by Fraser and Holmes[17] as shown in Table 6.

At this point, it is as well to stress that bran is not simply a source of dietary fibre. The aleurone layer, providing half its total weight, is higher in protein content than endosperm.[23] This protein, however, is not as good in quality as had earlier been thought, its higher lysine content compared with endosperm protein being counterbalanced by lower concentrations of other essential amino acids.

Bran contains 73% of the pyridoxine, 42% of the riboflavin, 33% of the thiamine and 50% of the pantothenic acid of the wheat grain.[5] Although 86% of the nicotinic acid of wheat is found in the bran, about 80% of this is present in unavailable forms as niacytin,[24–26] a complex with polysaccharide and polypeptide moieties, which is converted to trigonelline in the gut. Phenolic compounds,[26–29] and mineral salts,[12,20] occurring in bran may also affect colonic function.

TABLE 6

Composition of the total hemicellulose of bran and germ after hydrolysis

	% Xylose	% Arabinose	% Uronic acid
Bran	64·1	32·7	3·2
Germ	52·1	40·9	7·0

Other less well-known constituents of bran are the *n*-alkyl resorcinols,[28] believed by Wieringa[29] to be responsible for the toxicity and growth-inhibitory effects of his cereal bran extracts upon weanling rats: we have confirmed the latter finding. The presence in bran of phytic acid, which hinders the absorption of calcium and iron, was at first believed to be deleterious in human nutrition,[30] but later findings showed that the body could adapt to the presence of the phytin and restore calcium balance.[31] Recently, however, this problem has again been raised in connection with osteomalacia and rickets in immigrants to Britain consuming chapattis,[32] and there appears to be a need for further investigation of the long-term influence of phytin-rich diets.

THE EFFECTS OF MILLING PROCEDURE ON THE FIBRE CONTENT OF FLOUR

In milling white flour, the major objective is to obtain the maximum yield of endosperm consistent with maintenance of the colour of the product, by minimising the production of bran powder, which cannot easily be separated from powdered endosperm. This aim is facilitated by the rather tough nature of the bran and the friable nature of the endosperm. The cream-white colour of the latter is extremely sensitive to the addition of minute amounts of bran powder—much more so than the fibre content. The addition of 2% bran would greatly affect the flour colour.

White flour was produced even in Roman times by grinding the grain and then sifting, but the yield was low. By the close of the 18th century, the yields of good white flour obtained by current stone milling practice had been greatly improved. Thus in 1795, Samuel Wyatt,[33] in evidence to the Committee of Council, stated that the 'fine household flour makes the white bread in general consumption in London. Seconds, which is sold from 2/- to 3/- per sack under the price of household, goes to mix with household, or to bakers who

TABLE 7

Late 18th century flour milling products: yields of fractions

Flours	%
Fine household	54·6
Seconds	16·3
Thirds	6·8
Fourths	4·0
Offals	**%**
Pollards (total)	16·1
Bran	1·0
Milling loss	1·2
	100·0

sell under price. Thirds is sent coastwise, or *used in London for making brown bread* (our emphasis N.F., J.B.H.). Fourths is .... used for ordinary biscuit mixed with coarse sharps. No part of the pollard is used for the food of man; at the Albion Mills they made out of a given quality of wheat more flour ... than other mills generally did.'

Wyatt supplied the yields of wheat fractions at the Albion Mills (Table 7).

No chemical analyses were available for these flours: the science of chemistry was still in its infancy and analyses for fibre unheard of, but flour of 0·5% fibre, even at a glance, is far from white, and its bread even less so. The small yields of thirds and fourths could not possibly have supplied the bread requirements of the nation, and there would have been little point in separating some 55% of the products as fine white flour unless a reasonable proportion could have been marketed. Later evidence from Lawes and Gilbert[34] of Rothamsted, for flours milled at a small commercial watermill from their own wheats of 1846–48, indicates that their bread flours and presumably those of other mills, would have had a fibre content somewhere between 0·2–0·5%. Thus, a recent fibre determination by FMBRA on a present-day 81% extraction stone-ground flour, only sifted once after grinding, gave a value of 0·5%.

Various improvements in milling practice, *e.g.* the introduction of purifiers and of silk bolting cloths, facilitated further improvements in the extraction of higher amounts of white flours from wheats even before the advent of roller milling in the 1870s, and by the close of the century the bread flours were almost as low in fibre as those of today (0·1–0·2%).

DIETARY FIBRE IN HISTORICAL PERSPECTIVE

It has recently been claimed, by proponents[35–44] of a hypothesis[35–46] linking various so-called 'diseases of civilisation' with deficiency of dietary fibre, that this shortage is due in large measure to some important change in British diet which supposedly occurred around 1880, and that this change allegedly must have reduced the intake of dietary fibre below the level postulated for long-term health. Furthermore, as the roller mill was introduced into Britain at about this time, and had largely replaced the stone mill by the close of the century, it has been suggested that this occurrence was a major factor responsible for this critical drop, around that all-important period, below the safety level of the fibre intake of the national diet.[35] Thus the wide-scale replacement of stones by the steel roller mill was supposed to have reduced the fibre content of flour from a value not far below that of wholemeal,[36] which contains some 14% bran (*see* Table 1) and some 2% fibre, to that of white flour with a fibre figure of 0·1% or even less. This value corresponds to a bran content well below 1%, assuming that endosperm contains no fibre, which is incorrect—indeed, it contains upwards of 3% of unavailable carbohydrate material, chiefly as structural components of its cell walls.

This hypothesis, as it stands, needs correction in at least two important respects: first, the total intake of vegetable fibre has been shown by Robertson[47] not to have fallen over the past 100 years, although the relative contributions of different items of the national diet have changed—increasing consumption of fruit, nuts and vegetables has counter-balanced the declining consumption of cereals and cereal fibre. The second error, already discussed in the previous section, was the supposition that the bread consumed by the general population, prior to roller milling, was not far removed from wholemeal bread.

Some workers[36,48] now appear to recommend an intake of 2 g cereal fibre per head per day as the minimum amount required to maintain health. These workers also consider that cereal fibre is superior to fibre from most other sources, in which case the increased intake of fruit and vegetables (cf. Robertson[47]) would not fully compensate for a fall in cereal fibre intake. This amount of fibre would be provided by about 20 g of clean commercial 'broad bran', or, on average, by about 100 g of wholewheat. The estimate is presumably based on the amounts of bran required by patients with diverticular disease for prolonged remission of their symptoms. Various estimates[47,49–53] of the consumption of flour in the 19th century are shown in Table 8.

TABLE 8
Estimates of flour consumption in the 19th century

Year	Author	Flour (grammes/head/day)	Fibre[a] (grammes/head/day)
1841	Neild	277–345	0·55–1·73
1855	Eliza Acton	270	0·54–1·35
1860	Drummond and Wilbraham	397	0·79–1·98
1861–63	Dr Edward Smith[b] (*a*)	280	0·56–1·40
	Dr Edward Smith (*b*)	560	1·12–2·80
	Dr Edward Smith (*c*)	312–578	0·62–2·89
1880	Greaves and Hollingsworth	348	0·70–1·74
		Mean	0·70–1·98

[a] Calculated for the range 0.2–0.5 g/100 g.
[b] (a) J. Yudkin, (b) J. Robertson, (c) present authors: extremes of range given in final column by the present authors. Values (a), (b) and (c) are all derived from the contemporary estimates of Dr Edward Smith by the authors cited.

Most of the estimates agree remarkably well, and it may be noted that the first, second and fourth estimates were made from surveys, limited though they were, carried out at the time to which they refer.

It is immediately apparent that even if one assumes that average cereal fibre consumption and bran intake are nil today, a decline of 2 g fibre/day would require an intake before 1880 of some 400 g flour of at least 0·5% fibre content. Most estimates put the intake much lower than this, and the extraction rates of the flours suggest that after the 1840s, and probably before, the true fibre levels of much of the bread consumed would have been well below the 0·5% level. Thus, whatever the other merits of the case, the strictures against roller milling lack a firm basis of fact. In this connection, it is pertinent to note that during the last war it was the Medical Research Council[54] which stressed that the fibre content of flour and bread should be kept as low as possible, and recommended an extraction rate for flour of 85%, later reduced to 80% (fibre content 0·3%[55] cf. 3% for wholemeal).

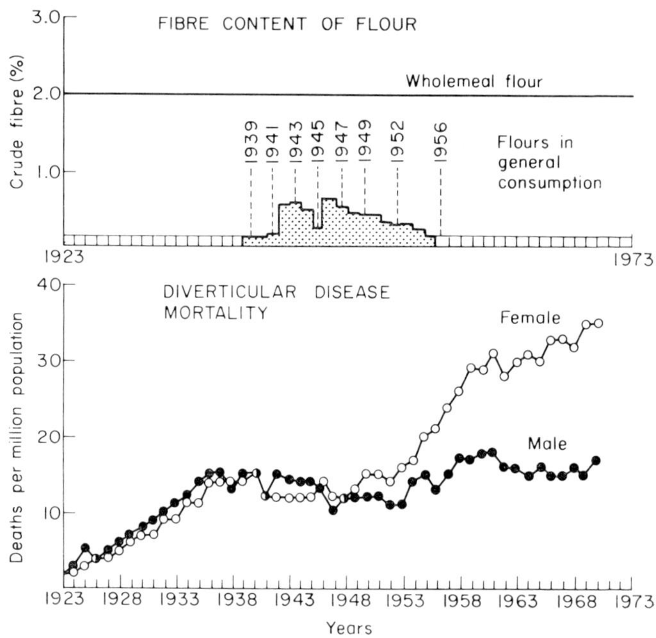

FIG. 2. Top: fibre content of flour. Bottom: diverticular disease mortality.

A further criticism of white flour is based on the supposed association between the fibre content of national flour in the war years and the levelling-off of mortality from diverticular disease. Figure 2, drawn from the data of the Registrar General, extends the earlier graph drawn by Cleave, Campbell, Painter and Burkitt[35,45] and adds a histogram of official data for the fibre content of flour for the years 1939–56.[56]

It is evident that no significant rise in the fibre content of wartime flour occurred until 1942, whereas the levelling-off in diverticular disease mortality started in 1935–36. The highest level attained by the fibre content of flour was 0·6%, less than one-third of that of wholemeal flour. The wide divergence between male and female mortality rates from diverticular disease after 1952–53, when prior to that time these rates were very similar for both sexes, also seems at odds with the present hypothesis of the role of wheat bran fibre as a major factor influencing the shape of the graphs.

PROPERTIES OF FIBRE CONSTITUENTS IN RELATION TO THEIR POSSIBLE PHYSIOLOGICAL EFFECTS

It has been known for many years that the so-called fibrous constituents of the diet influence the bulk, nature, consistency and transit time of the faeces.[45,57–64] The contributions of the individual constituents of dietary fibre (the general term suggested by Southgate and Trowell[65] to cover unavailable carbohydrates and other indigestibles) to these attributes of the faeces are not yet understood, though some of their properties are already known. The hemicelluloses readily take up large quantities of water, swelling considerably in consequence: thus psyllium and ispaghula preparations (*plantago spp.*), used as bulk laxatives for many years, can take up 12–14 times their weight of water. As wheat bran can also absorb water very rapidly, it may be that this property of its hemicellulose constituent is of importance in the physiological effect of bran upon the faecal residues, although as mentioned already, the hemicelluloses are broken down much more than cellulose or lignin in the gut. Not all individuals, however, tolerate bran,[36] and attention has been drawn to adverse effects sometimes occurring with bulking agents.[66] Nor should it be forgotten that high fibre diets lead to increased faecal excretion of nitrogenous compounds and fat.[13] The lignins can bind bile acids and their salts,[63,67] thus aiding their elimination from the body, but little is known about the amounts and properties of the lignin in our customary plant foods—cereals, vegetables, fruits and nuts, etc. Apparently, cholesterol is also absorbed by lignin,[67] and cereal roughage rich in fibre has been found to lower blood cholesterol levels. This property is shared by the pectins, and it is of some interest that Eastwood, in a study on serum triglyceride and cholesterol concentrations in Cistercian monks,[68] found a hypocholesterolaemic effect in a group whose dietary fibre was derived entirely from non-cereal sources.

Cellulose is a much less effective water absorbent than hemicellulose, and the extent of its influence on faecal properties and transit times is uncertain as yet, though wood cellulose preparations have been reported as having an irritant effect in the gut.[69] Methyl cellulose, on the other hand, is well known for its water-binding propensity, and Hodgson[70] has reported beneficial effects with human patients.

Diets rich in fibre are reported to be associated with a lower concentration of anaerobic bacteria in the colon than is found for low residue diets, and it has been suggested that the anaerobes may be involved in the production of some unsaturated steroids which are the precursors of carcinogens,[71,72] though as yet there is little experimental support for this hypothesis.

However the evidence is assessed, it is clear that cereal fibre is not unique in its properties and physiological effects, therapeutic or otherwise. Peas, cabbage, kohlrabi, carrots, radishes and spinach are among the vegetables in which cellulose, hemicellulose and lignin have been identified and quantitatively determined.[15,18]

Crude preparations of apple fibre[73] have been shown to share with bran fibre and wholemeal, as compared with white flour, the property of increasing the length and weight of the gastrointestinal tracts of rats, the effect being greater for apple than for bran fibre. In as yet unpublished trials carried out at FMBRA with weanling Wistar rats, we have confirmed the action of the bran in increasing the wet weight of the colon, caecum and rectum, the effect being correlated with the percentage of bran added to a diet otherwise low in dietary fibre but adequate in other nutrients essential for rapid growth. With increasing levels of bran, the effect persisted even to the point where the bran had caused a diminution of growth rate compared with the control.

The only form of processing covered by the present paper has been the milling of wheat and other cereals. There is, as yet, insufficient information available on the effect of other forms of processing on the content and properties of fibre constituents of foods. Future work will thus require, in addition to improvements in analytical techniques, direct comparisons of fresh versus processed products, as well as improved fractionation techniques, to allow the conduct of strictly controlled animal and human trials with well-defined fractions of such foods.

REFERENCES

1. *The Fertilisers and Feeding Stuffs Regulations* (1968). Statutory Instrument No. 218, HMSO, London.
2. *The Bread and Flour Regulations* (1963). Statutory Instrument No. 1435, HMSO, London.
3. Analytical Methods Committee Report (1943). *Analyst,* **68,** p. 276.
4. McDermott, E. E. (1960). See Ref. 5 and *A Kernel of Wheat*, Copyright 1964, Wheat Flour Institute, 309, West Jackson Boulevard, Chicago, Ill. 60606.
5. Kent, N. L. (1966). *Technology of Cereals with Special Reference to Wheat,* Pergamon Press, Oxford.
6. Elton, G. A. H. and Fisher, N. (1970). *Inf. Bull. Brit. Nutr. Found.,* No. 4, p. 17.
7. Fraser, J. R. and Holmes, D. C. (1956). *J. Sci. Fd. Agric.,* **7,** p. 589.
8. Van Soest, P. J. (1966). *J. Ass. Off. Agric. Chemists,* **49,** p. 546.
9. Moss, H. J. and Stenvent, N. L. (1971). *Austr. J. Agric. Res.,* **22,** p. 547.
10. Zentner, H. (1965). *Analyst,* **90,** p. 303.
11. Macrae, T. F., Hutchinson, J. C. D., Irwin, J. O., Bacon, J. S. D. and McDougall, E. I. (1942). *J. Hyg.,* p. 423; Moran, T. and Pace, J. (1942). *Nature,* **150,** p. 224.
12. Lord Horder, Dodds, Sir C. and Moran T. (1954). *Bread,* Constable, London.
13. McCance, R. A. and Walsham, C. M. (1948). *Brit. J. Nutr.,* **2,** p. 26.
14. Southgate, D. A. T. and Durnin, J. V. G. A. (1970). *Brit. J. Nutr.,* **24,** p. 517.
15. Southgate, D. A. T. (1969). *J. Sci. Fd. Agric.,* **20,** p. 331.
16. Fraser, J. R., Brandon-Bravo, M. and Holmes, D. C. (1956). *J. Sci. Fd. Agric.,* **7,** p. 577.
17. Fraser, J. R. and Holmes, D. C. (1959). *J. Sci. Fd. Agric.,* **10,** p. 506.
18. Kowalski, J. and Piekarska. (1957). *Rocz. P.Z.H.,* **8,** p. 557.
19. Morrison, I. M. (1972). *J. Sci. Fd. Agric.,* **23,** p. 455.
20. Pomeranz, Y. (ed.) (1971). *Wheat Chemistry and Technology,* AACC Monograph Series, Vol. III.
21. Hinton, J. J. C. and (the late) Martin, H. F., personal communication.

22. Adams, G. A. (1955). *Can. J. Chem.,* **33,** p. 56.
23. Stevens, D. J., McDermott, E. E. and Pace, J. (1963). *J. Sci. Fd. Agric.,* **14,** p. 284.
24. Kodicek, E. (1940). *Biochem. J.,* **34,** pp. 712, 724; (1960). *ibid.,* **76,** 27P.
25. Das, M. L. and Guha, B. C. (1960). *J. Biol. Chem.,* **235,** p. 2971.
26. Mason, J. B., Gibson, N. and Kodicek, E. (1971). *Biochem. J.,* **125**(4), 117p.
27. Abrol, Y. P. and Uprety, D. C. (1971). *Curr. Sci.,* **40,** p. 414.
28. Wenkert, E., Loesen, E-M., Mahapatra, S. N., Schenker, F. and Wilson, E. M. (1964). *J. org. Chem.,* **29,** p. 435.
29. Wieringa, G. W. (1967). 'Growth-inhibitory Substance in Rye', Publ. No. 156, Inst. for Storage and Processing of Agricultural Produce, Wageningen.
30. McCance, R. A. and Widdowson, E. M. (1942). *J. Physiol.,* **101,** No. 44, p. 304 quoted in Davidson, S. and Passmore, R. (1969). *Human Nutrition and Dietetics,* 4th Edn, Livingstone, Edinburgh.
31. Walker, A. R. P. (1951). *Lancet,* **ii,** p. 244.
32. Ford, J. A., Colhoun, E. M., McIntosh, W. B. and Dunnigan, M. G. (1972). *Brit. Med. J.,* **3,** p. 446.
33. Bennett, R. and Elton, J. (1900). *History of Corn Milling,* Vol. III, Simpkin, Marshall, p. 290.
34. Lawes, J. B. and Gilbert, J. H. (1857). *Rothamsted Memoirs,* **I,** p. 10; also in *J. Chem. Soc., Lond.* (1858) **10,** 1.
35. Painter, N. S. and Burkitt, D. P. (1971). *Brit. Med. J.,* **2,** p. 450.
36. Painter, N. S., Almeida, A. Z. and Colbourne, K. W. (1972). *Brit. Med. J.,* **2,** p. 137.
37. Burkitt, D. P. (1969). *Lancet,* **ii,** p. 1229.
38. Burkitt, D. P. (1971). *Cancer*, **28,** p. 3.
39. Burkitt, D. P. (1972). *Brit. Med. J.,* **2,** p. 556.
40. Trowell, H. C. (1960). *Non-infective Diseases in Africa,* Edward Arnold, London.
41. Trowell, H. C. (1972). *Heart,* p. 10 (Autumn).
42. Painter, N. S. (1972). *Practitioner,* **208,** p. 669.
43. Painter, N. S. and Truelove, S. C. (1964). *Gut,* **5,** pp. 201, 207.
44. Painter, N. S., Truelove, S. C., Ardran, G. M. and Tuckey, M. (1965). *Gastroenterology*, **49,** p. 169.
45. Cleave, T. L., Campbell, G. D. and Painter, N. S. (1969). *Diabetes, Coronary Thrombosis and the Saccharine Disease,* 2nd Edn, John Wright, Bristol.
46. Burkitt, D. P. (1972). *Inf. Bull. Brit. Nutr. Found.,* No. 7, p. 29, May.
47. Robertson, J. (1972). *Nature,* **238,** p. 290.
48. Painter, N. S. (1972). *Diverticular Disease of the Colon*, Abbot Laboratories Ltd, Queenborough, Kent.
49. Neild, W. (1841). *J. Statistical Soc., Lond.,* **4,** p. 322.
50. Acton, E. (1857). *The English Bread Book*, Longman, London.
51. Drummond, J. C. and Wilbraham, A. (1957). *The Englishman's Food,* 2nd Edn, Revised by D. F. Hollingsworth, Jonathan Cape, London.

52. Barker, T. C., Oddy, D. H. and Yudkin, J. (1970). *The Dietary Surveys of Dr Edward Smith*, 1862–63, Staples Press, London.
53. Greaves, J. P. and Hollingsworth, D. F. (1964). *Proc. Nutr. Soc.,* **23,** p. 136.
54. The Specifications for National Flour (1941). *Nature,* **147,** p. 665.
55. Moran, T. and Drummond, Sir Jack (1945). *Lancet,* **ii,** p. 698.
56. Staff of Research Association of British Flour Millers: National Bread: Data mostly published in *Nature* (1942–44).
57. Fraser, J. R. (1951). *J. Sci. Fd. Agric.,* **2,** p. 193.
58. Fraser, J. R. (1958). *J. Sci. Fd. Agric.,* **9,** p. 125.
59. Bunge, G. (1902). *Physiological and Pathological Chemistry.*
60. Rubner, M., Quoted in *Textbook of Physiology and Biochemistry,* 7th Edn., 1968, Bell, G. H., Davidson, J. N. and Scarborough, H., Livingstone, Edinburgh.
61. McCance, R. A., Prior, K. M. and Widdowson, E. M. (1953). *Brit. J. Nutr.,* **7,** p. 98.
62. Eastwood, M. A., Hamilton, T., Kirkpatrick, J. R. and Mitchell, W. D. (1973). Proc. 250th Mtg. Nutr. Soc. Abstr. comms., 22A.
63. Eastwood, M. A. (1972). 'Vegetable Dietary Fibre, Food-fad or Farrago', Van den Berghs & Jurgens, Nutrition Award Lecture.
64. Burkitt, D. P., Walker, A. R. P. and Painter, N. S. (1972). *Lancet,* **ii,** p. 1408.
65. Southgate, D. A. T. and Trowell, H. C., personal communication.
66. Goodman, L. S. and Gilman, A. (1970). *The Pharmacological Basis of Therapeutics,* 4th Edn, Macmillan, London.
67. Eastwood, M. A. and Hamilton, D. (1968). *Biochem. Biophys. Acta,* **152,** p. 165.
68. Eastwood, M. A. (1969). *Lancet,* **ii,** p. 1222.
69. Moinuddin, J. F. (1970). *Nutr. Revs.,* **28,** p. 109.
70. Hodgson, J. (1972). *Brit. Med. J.,* **3,** p. 729.
71. Aries, V., Crowther, J. S., Drasar, B. S., Hill, M. J. and Williams, R. E. O. (1969). *Gut,* **10,** p. 334.
72. Hill, M. J., Crowther, J. S., Drasar, B. S., Hawksworth, G., Aries, V. and Williams, R. E. O. (1971). *Lancet,* **i,** p. 95.
73. Szczygiel, A. (1962). *Nahrung,* **6,** p. 701.

DISCUSSION

Hollingsworth: Referring to Dr Fisher's statement that Jean Robertson has shown little change in total consumption of fibre in the United Kingdom between 1880 and 1970, her data for 1880 are based on consumption data compiled by myself and Dr Greaves which exclude vegetables other than potatoes, fruits and cereals other than wheat. Therefore, her 1880 total fibre should not be compared with present-day total fibre.

Fisher: I am very well aware of this. Can I also point out that there is another factor which nobody has taken into account which is that food consumption data for later years did not include meals taken outside the home. There has been an increase, I think you will agree, in the number of meals taken outside the home.

Green: The analytical 'fibre' definition is different from that of the physiologists; would Dr Fisher care to comment on the difference?

Fisher: I don't think anybody else has successfully worked out the relationship. Fibre in fact is an artifact: you have chosen an arbitrary set of conditions and what is left you call fibre. What the physiologist wants to know is what materials are present in the colon. I don't want to give the impression in any way that we are decrying the importance of this—it is very interesting and an important field of study—but fibre as such is not a guide in that respect.

Questioner: What the physiologist does is measure what is in the faeces.

Chairman: I think it wasn't analysed.

Fisher: McCance did determine fibre in the faeces.

Questioner: Supposing you want to determine fibre in the faeces, do you do it the way the analyst does it?

Fisher: I think this is entirely arbitrary. The foodstuff manufacturer is obliged by law to use a method. If there is no legally laid down method it is every man for himself.

Southgate: In considering faecal analysis for indigestible carbohydrates, one really should be analysing the faeces for unavailable carbohydrates. If one is concerned with the digestibility of crude fibre, one can analyse food and faeces by the standard procedure although this is not straightforward. Secondly, one must be extremely cautious when comparing faecal analyses with dietary intake because of the high concentrations of micro-organisms in the large intestine which are very active towards all undigested materials.

Pawan: Is there any evidence that adaptation to a high-fibre diet in man produces alteration of gut bacteria population and in this way increases breakdown of 'fibre' to absorbable substances which may be of nutritional significance?

Fisher: We have no data on this. I think I would have to quote Painter and Burkitt. If you compare people of high-fibre diet with people of low-fibre diet—if you take people on a low-fibre diet and put them on a high-fibre diet—then they apparently usually experience a considerable period (3 weeks) of discomfort and so on but after that they are supposed to settle down and they do very well. It is a personal note I am sounding here because, by one of the ironies of fate, I experienced the symptom and was put on a high-residue diet: it wasn't successful, but I can vouch for the discomfort. I don't know if there is any adaptive process possible by which more use could be made of presently unavailable constituents. There is some evidence that the bacterial population of the colon changes according to the residue in the diet, but the only point is that the concentration of anaerobes in the colon increases with low-fibre diets and this is speculated to be one of the possible causes of the production of carcinogens and incidence of bowel cancer in Western countries. This is a frightening thing to put to the public and there is not a great deal of evidence that this does happen.

Pawan: The water absorptive capacity of methyl cellulose is sometimes used in certain products and suggested as a way of helping obese persons to reduce food intake. Recently there has been another product on the market —a gum. I won't say the name, but it is fairly well known. Can you tell me how this compares in water retaining capacity with methyl cellulose?

Fisher: Off hand, I don't know the answer. A number of pharmaceutical firms are producing these gums as laxatives. Other gums that have been produced have been of the modified cellulose type—a lot of them could be broken down and I don't know what the effect would be. I believe Beechams have a representative here and I believe they are one of the firms interested in this field.

Mullen: Are there any potential problems that might arise from ingesting large quantities of wheat bran? I specifically refer to the controversial question you referred to as to whether high levels of phytic acid might cause problems with mineral metabolism.

Fisher: I think, to be fair, Mr Painter says that the patients he has put on bran and who have been following his instructions for several years have had no trouble whatsoever on this diet. But then it isn't just simply adding bran to the diet, always several changes have been made. There have been reports in the literature and it is referred to in the brief note in the BMJ review by Moinuddin in 'Nutrition'. At this conference somebody has told me that there is a consultant surgeon who is asking him for Bagasse waste products which he wants to feed to his patients. It is important how finely Bagasse is ground—it could be extremely harmful. One of the things quoted by Moinuddin as being harmful to the gut was wheat cellulose, and one has therefore to be very careful.

Chairman: Fraser was critical of the use of fibre and mentioned scouring of the intestine. Can you not lose layers of the intestine if you have so much more indigestible material? It has been said in the United States that they don't like the idea of a high-fibre diet.

Fisher: Yes, I have seen evidence in the literature to confirm that last point. Mr Painter says that something like 8% of his patients cannot tolerate bran. I would not draw any distinction between wholemeal and wheat bran on that basis. In Africans with enormous amounts of fibre in their diet it is a rather amazing exercise to look at their figures for transit time, and you find some of the people on very low-fibre diets have just as short a transit time as some of those on extremely high-fibre diets.

Parker: Many years ago we tried to find ways of preparing Bagasse and we were always in trouble with its physical structure and could not overcome it. The possibility of using Bagasse as a source of unassimilable dietary fibre should be regarded cautiously. The fibrils are short, sharp and extremely hard and I can recall that attempts to modify Bagasse as a fodder source for ruminants were completely unsuccessful owing to the results of physical damage to the alimentary tract.

Fisher: Just for the fun of it I should say there was a time when millers thought they had an excellent use for oat husk, which made a very good medium for polishing castings, but the thing died out. I think one should be rather cautious about which fibre one chooses.

Grenby: Having just heard that fibre in apples can increase the weight and length of the gut, is there any advantage in this? Should we aim for a longer and heavier gut.

Fisher: I would like to know the answer myself. I am not a medical man but I have had to look at a lot of medical literature recently. Dr McMichael might comment on this, but one of the first signs of impending diverticular disease is the thickening of the wall of the gut and it is the proliferation of the muscle layers of the gut which creates weaknesses where the blood vessels go through and which allows excessive pressures in the gut. Whether a heavier gut is any advantage to you I just don't know.

McMichael: I feel I must offer some support for Messrs Painter and Burkitt. Paradoxically, the intracolonic pressures are lower if there is a large bulk in the colon. The aspect of cancer is also reasonably based in that delayed transit would give time for carcinogens to be produced, and also allowed to remain in contact for relatively long periods.

Fisher: We will have to disagree on this. Despite the exploration of patients with diverticular disease this could not be demonstrated. The increase in pressure in the gut in these people is induced by the injection of prostaglandins and the justification for this is that it maximises effects which occur physiologically after the ingestion of a meal, but I don't think one could be absolutely dogmatic. There is the evidence of Hodgkin's patients who had methyl cellulose. I am not decrying them, what I am saying is that Painter and Burkitt have gone out of their way not to do critical experiments; they have had many opportunities of carrying out controlled trials, and I understand they are unwilling to do so. Mr Painter says it would be unethical of him, believing as he does that the only treatment for diverticular disease is a high-residue diet, to put patients on a low-residue diet.

Greenwood: I wish to support Dr Fisher's comment to Dr McMichael that not only do we feel strongly about the effects of fibre in the diet, but even more strongly that there is no experimental evidence for a negative correlation between fibre and carcinogenic substances in the gut.

Fisher: There are some very interesting statistics on the incidence of bowel cancer in various countries and in the case of Canada the statistics are divided by regions and if you look at the data for Alberta you will find the incidence is twice as great as in Saskatchewan.

da Rocha Afodu: Mr Burkitt did some experiments on Africans, blacks as well as whites, using different diets and found that the time of passage of the rejected food from ingestion was actually much facilitated by good fibre. This is just evidence.

Fisher: I am sorry, I must contradict that. The experiment he did was to measure transit times. He has done a tremendous amount of work on this and he hasn't proved any production of carcinogens. The work on carcinogens is the work of Fraser, Hill and other people on the relative incidence of anaerobes in the gut.

da Rocha Afodu: I will take up Dr McMichael's saying that it isn't proved that lactase is an inducible enzyme. There are African groups whose main diet is blood and others whose main diet is milk, and I would think these two groups retain their lactase. I am firm in this opinion, and I hope in the future somebody will prove lactase can be induced.

Chairman: May I ask why it should be induced? There are people in Great Britain who are lactase deficient but will drink and tolerate milk.

da Rocha Afodu: These are isolated cases, much fewer than in China and Japan.

McMichael: You are absolutely right. There are certain racial groups in Africa that retain lactase. The Masai are one.

da Rocha Afodu: What I am driving at is that the content of fibre in the diet is a factor in the retention of lactase.

Fisher: I think I acknowledged there hasn't been a dramatic drop in the amount of fibre in the diet. I would also make the point that wheat fibre has always been preferred.

Index